Essentials of Chinese Medicine

Zhanwen Liu
Editor

Liang Liu
Associate Editor

Warner Fan
English Consultant

Shiping Zhang
Associate English Consultant

Editorial Team
Baixiao Zhao
Chunguang Xie
Cunku Chang
Haihong Zhu
Hongyi Hu
Kui Wang
Lanzheng Li
Songping Luo
Yuxiang Zhai
Zhaoxiang Bian

Essentials of Chinese Medicine

Volume 2

Clinical Fundamentals in Chinese Medicine

Springer

Editor

Zhanwen Liu
Dept. Health Preservation & Rehab
Beijing University of Chinese Medicine
11 Beisanhuan East Road
Chaoyang 100029, Beijing
PR China
liuzhanwen4569@sina.com

Associate Editor

Liang Liu
School of Chinese Medicine
Hong Kong Baptist University
Kowloon Tong
Kowloon
Hong Kong/PR China
liuliang@hkbu.edu.hk

ISBN 978-1-4471-6039-7 ISBN 978-1-84882-593-2 (eBook)
DOI 10.1007/978-1-84882-593-2
Springer Dordrecht Heidelberg London New York

British Library Cataloguing in Publication Data
A catalogue record for this book is available from the British Library

Cover design: eStudio Calamar S.L.

Printed on acid-free paper

Springer is part of Springer Science+Business Media (www.springer.com)

Foreword

The Essentials of Chinese Medicine is a text book intended for international students who wish to gain a basic understanding of Chinese Medicine (CM) at the university level. The idea of writing such a text was originated from the Sino-American Consortium for the Advancement of Chinese Medicine (SACACM), which was founded in February 2000. In 1995, the British Hong Kong Administration set up a Preparatory Committee for the Development of Chinese Medicine to look into ways of bringing Chinese medical practice and herbal trade under proper control and regulation. After the reunification of Hong Kong with mainland China in 1997, the Government of the Hong Kong Special Administrative Region continued the efforts to uplift the practice of CM to a fully professional level through legislation.

To help bring up a new generation of professional CM practitioners, the Hong Kong Baptist University (HKBU) obtained approval from the Government's university funding authority to develop a School of Chinese Medicine to prepare students who will meet the future professional requirements through public examinations. In order to establish itself quickly as a rigorous provider of university level CM education, HKBU sought alliance with eight major CM universities in the Chinese Mainland, and one US university which was interested in developing CM education within its medical college. As a result, the Consortium known as SACACM was formed, with ten founding institutions from Beijing, Shanghai, Nanjing, Shandong, Guangzhou, Chengdu, Heilongjiang, Hong Kong, and the United States. (The University of Macau and the Macao University of Science and Technology joined the Consortium 2 years later.)

One of the first projects the Consortium decided to pursue was the writing of a high quality CM text book in English to be endorsed by the member institutions as the foundation for the study of traditional Chinese medicine. The Beijing University of Traditional Chinese Medicine, being one of the oldest and better developed institutions in the field, was nominated to be the coordinating university for the project, with the active assistance of the State Administration of Traditional Chinese Medicine of China (SATCM). The initial funding for the project was provided by the Hong Kong Baptist University and the Ohio University of the USA. An editorial committee was formed to decide on the general coverage and level of the text, and each of the member universities of CM were requested to nominate their senior professors to write the assigned chapters according to their fields of specialty. These authors were to prepare their scripts in both Chinese and English with the help of the Editor. After the English version of the text was checked against the Chinese version for accuracy and consistency, it was sent to an expert who is well versed in both Chinese and Western Medicine and at the same time fluent in both the Chinese and English languages at the mother tongue level. The expert was invited to go over the entire text line by line to make sure that both the language style and the terms used are understood by the international students whose native language is English.

The above steps looked innocent enough, but the execution of the entire process was extremely time consuming and tedious. It has also proven to be a very meaningful, if not "ground-breaking," move which makes the text truly different from publications of similar nature. I am happy that after 9 years of hard work and perseverance this text is finally ready for the press. I do hope that when it comes out, it will prove to be a significant contribution to the education of CM internationally.

Founding Chair, SACACM Daniel C. W. Tse
February 2009

Preface

"Health for all" is still an important task for the World Health Organization (WHO) to accomplish in the twenty-first century The accomplishment of this task requires mutual cooperation and common efforts of various medical sciences, which includes Chinese medicine. WHO has increasingly emphasized the development of traditional medicine and has made great efforts to promote its development. Because traditional medicine is deeply rooted in history and culture, it is part of the traditions of a country and employs healing practices handed down from generation to generation.

Large portions of the population in a number of developing countries still rely mainly on traditional practitioners, including traditional birth attendants, herbalists, and bone-setters, and local medicinal plants to satisfy their primary health care needs. Although modern medicine is now available in many countries, traditional medicine has maintained its popularity because of its historical and cultural impact. People believe in it, and it is still effective against many common diseases, has few side effects, and is economically preferable to modern medicine.

Nowadays, the modern medical model is changing It is gradually shifting from its original medical model of biomedicine into a physiological–psychological–sociological–medical model, which emphasizes that the people the natural environment, ecological conditions and society are all aspects of a united whole. With the transformation into the new medical model, alternative medicine and therapies are developing very rapidly. The study of Chinese Medicine (CM) in the west is both timely and challenging. It is timely because of public demand for traditional medicines to be provided by safe, efficient and competent practitioners. It is challenging because of the greater demand for science-based treatment and evidence-based practice. These perspectives suggest that the integration of orthodox medicine with complementary or alternative medicine is a historical trend in the world medical scene. Therefore, the role of CM in medical treatment and healthcare will certainly become even more important in the world medical scene in the twenty-first century.

CM is an integral part of Chinese culture. Over the centuries, various activities and aspects of the practice of CM have made tremendous contributions to the prosperity of the Chinese nation. Its good reputation resulted from its great vitality is demonstrated by the fact that when compared with other traditional medicine its clinical application has never declined over the past several thousand years.

CM appears to have a bright future in the world There appears to be a growing reliance on it by people everywhere. This seems to be an irresistible historical trend. Working together to develop CM will not only be in line with the developing trend in the world, but also will fundamentally solve existing problems and increase competitive advantages. Collaboration among universities will benefit cultural exchange, the blending of the East and the West, and the global development of CM. However, much work needs to be done in order to meet the health requirements of human beings and to promote the course of internationalization of CM, especially the compilation of textbooks suitable for medical students in western countries in addition to international readers.

With the encouragement of the State Administration of Traditional Chinese Medicine of China, the compilation of this textbook series was initiated by the Sino-American Consortium for the Advancement of Chinese Medicine which was made up of the Ohio University in Athens, Ohio, Beijing University of CM, Chengdu University of TCM, China Academy of Chinese Medical Sciences, Guangzhou University of TCM, Heilongjiang University of TCM, Hong Kong Baptist University, Nanjing University of TCM, Shandong University of TCM, and Shanghai University of TCM, The Beijing University of CM was the lead institution of this project. It gathered experts from the member institutions to compile the series and translate it into English which is now known as *Essentials of Chinese Medicine*. This textbook series contains three volumes: Volume 1 ***Foundations of Chinese Medicine***; Volume 2, ***Clinical Fundamentals in Chinese Medicine***; and Volume 3 ***Essentials of the Clinical Specialties in Chinese Medicine***. These volumes systematically introduce the basic theories, the diagnostic methods, the therapeutic methods based on symptom differentiation, and the knowledge of principles of health preservation and rehabilitation. They explain the basic methods and theories of acupuncture and moxibustion, as well as expounding upon 154 kinds of Chinese herbs; each Chinese medicinal herb is illustrated. The textbooks also introduce 84 Chinese herbal formulas and 11 associated formulas commonly used in clinical practice. Furthermore, it elucidates treatments of commonly and frequently encountered diseases in internal medicine, surgery, gynecology, pediatrics, ophthalmology and otorhinolaryngology.

In the arrangement of contents and compilation, the following features characterize this textbook series:

1. Emphasis on the basic knowledge of CM

Medical students who want to learn CM, especially students in western countries, need to adapt CM to Western medical terms and conditions, but this adaptation can only take place on the solid foundation of the theories of CM. There can be no mastery of CM without a true understanding of the theories and practice of CM. The first volume introduces the terminology and methodology of Chinese medicine in order to improve the critical thinking of medical students and practitioners. It also contains a detailed explanation of the basic theories. The second volume covers the fundamentals of clinical practice. The more solid the foundation is, the easier it will be to have a better understanding and mastery of CM

2. Concise and systematic content

On the basis of developments of CM in education and research in the past, great efforts have been made to highlight the essence of CM through accurate exposition and to introduce them to the world. These textbooks systematically introduce the basic theories, diagnostic methods, acupuncture skills, knowledge of Chinese herbs, knowledge of formulas, as well as clinical application. Mastery of these textbooks will lay a foundation for the further study of CM.

3. Suitability for teaching and self-study

In this textbook series, at the end of most chapters guidance is provided on the aims of study, the objectives of study and exercises for review. The structure combines the features of textbooks and modular handbooks. Therefore, it is highly suitable for self-study by medical students.

4. Reinforcing effects of illustrations

To facilitate the understanding of CM, the textbook series contains many illustrations. There are black and white photographs, line graphs, tables in the text with necessary indexes, color photographs of the tongue, and color photographs of 151 Chinese herbs. These illustrations provide a better appreciation of CM and promote its learning.

5. Case studies

In Volume 3 and Part III of Volume 2 each section contains a successful case study. These case studies enhance the understanding of CM.

6. Standardization

This textbook series is reasonable in structure and distinct in categorization. Most of the technical terms of CM have been standardized in translation with an index glossary. Simultaneously, habitual terms used in countries using English as the mother tongue have been considered in the translation and compilation.

In order to ensure academic standards and an accurate English translation of this textbook series, we invited international experts of the CM profession and the English language to review and revise the English translation.

Professor Zheng Souzeng, the former President of Beijing University of Chinese Medicine, was the Director of the Compilation Board. Dr. Warner Fan of the United States is the English Consultant who has gone through the whole text to ensure the language consistency throughout the text.

International advisors invited include Ryan Thompson from Canada, Ioannis Solos from Greece and Georgia Ross from the United States of America. They and others have given much help in the compilation of this series of books. We are grateful to them for very useful suggestions and revisions.

Note on Conventions Used in the Text

Several conventions of usage have been adopted in the English version of this textbook, and are intended to make the students' task easier.

A number of concepts in traditional Chinese medicine cannot be adequately translated. The terms representing them are therefore presented in transliteration, using the *Pinyin* system. Where the term is already in common usage but in this text are used as technical terms, they are capitalized. Examples include Qi, Yin, Yang, the Five Elements (Metal, Wood, Water, Fire, Earth), the six exogenous pathogenic evil (Wind, Heat or Summer Heat, Cold, Phlegm, Dampness, Fire) and their endogenous counterparts, all the acupoints, the four Levels (Defensive, Qi, Nutritive, and Blood), etc. Where there is no risk of confusion between ordinary and technical usage, they are not capitalized. Examples include the zang and fu organs, the sanjiao, etc.

In the discussion of CM *materia medica*, all materials are referred to as "herbs," even though many are derived from animal or mineral sources. This is the time-honored approach, as comparable medieval European books are often entitled "Herbals." In traditional CM, herbs are seldom prescribed alone. A prescription is referred to here as a "formula."

In addition, the name of each formula is given as one word, in *pinyin* transliteration of the Chinese name. In Chapter 7 of volume 2, which contains the main descriptions of the herbs, each entry is headed by the name of the herb in *pinyin* with its botanical name in brackets. The first line then gives the actual Chinese name in characters and the herb's pharmaceutical name (in Latin). When an herb is mentioned in the text elsewhere, at its first appearance it is followed in brackets by its genus name if it is described in Chapter 7 of volume 2 or by its botanical name, both genus and species, if it is not. It is hoped that doing so will make it easier for the student who chooses to look it up in the Appendix III: Herbs or in Chapter 7 of volume 2. When the herb is mentioned again in the same passage, only the name in *pinyin* is given.

Strictly speaking, the clinical manifestations of an illness include both symptoms and signs. The symptoms are supposed to be what the patient feels and perceives subjectively, whereas the signs are what the physician finds objectively. Take fever, for example. The symptom is the hot sensation, especially in the face and head, that the patient feels, whereas the sign is the higher than normal temperature as measured with a thermometer. In accordance with the recent trend towards simplification, however, in this text the word "symptoms" encompasses both symptoms and signs.

Acknowledgements

International Advisors
Bruce D. Dublin (USA)
Daniel C. W. Tse (HK, PRC)
Daniel K. C. Shao (HK, PRC)
Edward Gotfried (USA)
Georgia Ross (USA)
Ioannis Solas (Greece)
Qichang Zheng (Macau, PRC)
Robert Glidden (USA)
Rosalind Chan (HK, PRC)
Ryan Thompson (Canada)
Shouzeng Zheng (PRC)
Xiaoping Wang (PRC)
Xiaozhuo Chen (USA)
Yanling Fu (PRC)
Yitao Wang (Macau, PRC)
Zaizeng Jiang (PRC)
Zhongzhen Zhao (HK, PRC)

Member-Institutions of The Sino-American Consortium for the Advancement of Chinese Medicine
Beijing University of Chinese Medicine (PRC)
Chengdu University of Traditional Chinese Medicine (PRC)
China Academy of Chinese Medical Sciences (PRC)
Guangzhou University of Traditional Chinese Medicine (PRC)
Heilongjiang University of Traditional Chinese Medicine (PRC)
Hong Kong Baptist University (HK, PRC)
Macau University of Science and Technology (Macau, PRC)
Nanjiang University of Traditional Chinese Medicine (PRC)
Ohio University, Athens (USA)
Shandong University of Traditional Chinese Medicine (PRC)
Shanghai University of Traditional Chinese Medicine (PRC)
University of Macau (Macau, PRC)

Institute for the Advancement of Chinese Medicine (A wholly owned subsidiary of Hong Kong Baptist University)

David W.F. Fong (HK, PRC)
Carry P.C. Yu (HK, PRC)

In grateful acknowledgement to Dr. Daniel C. W. Tse, President Emeritus of Hong Kong Baptist University and Founding Chair of the Sino-American Consortium for the Advancement of Chinese Medicine, who initiated this Textbook writing project in Year 2000 and persevered to keep the project moving until it was completed.

Note on Organization of Volume 2

This volume is composed of three parts.

Part I, in five chapters, introduces the meridians, the acupoints, and the principles of acupuncture and moxibustion.

Part II, in two chapters, introduces the properties and general clinical application of Chinese *materia medica* and provides a detailed description of 154 herbs that are most commonly used in treatment of patients and their illnesses.

Part III, in two chapters, introduces the principles of constructing composition of herbal formulas from herbs and provides a detailed description and analysis of 84 of the most useful formulas, in 17 categories. It also presents a large number of case studies.

We hope that armed with the knowledge gained from Volume 2 the learners and practitioners will be ready to learn about the clinical illnesses presented by patients.

Contents

Contributors

Baixiao Zhao, M.D., Ph.D. School of Acupuncture, Beijing University of Chinese Medicine, Beijing, P.R. China

Chunguang Xie, Ph.D. Chengdu University of Traditional Chinese Medicine, Chengdu, P.R. China

Cunku Chang, M.D. Department of History of Chinese Medicine, Heilongjiang University of Traditional Chinese Medicine, Haerbin, P.R. China

Haihong Zhu, M.B. Department of Traditional Chinese Medicine, Affiliated Hospital of Shandong University of Traditional Chinese Medicine, Jinan, P.R. China

Hongyi Hu, Ph.D. Academic Affair Office, Shanghai University of Traditional Chinese Medicine, Shanghai, P.R. China

Kui Wang, Ph.D. China Academy of Chinese Medical Sciences, Beijing, P.R. China

Lanzheng Li, Ph.D. Guangzhou University of Traditional Chinese Medicine, Guangzhou, P.R. China

Liang Liu, M.D., Ph.D. School of Chinese Medicine, Hong Kong Baptist University, Hong Kong, P.R. China

Shiping Zhang, M.B., Ph.D. School of Chinese Medicine, Hong Kong Baptist University, Hong Kong, P.R. China

Songping Luo, Ph.D. Guangzhou University of Traditional Chinese Medicine, Guangzhou, P.R. China

Warner Fan, M.D. Previous Colonel Doctor, Medical Corp., United States Air Force, U.S.A.

Yuxiang Zhai, Ph.D. Department of Science of Epidemic Febrile Disease, Nanjing University of Traditional Chinese Medicine, Nanjing, P.R. China

Zhanwen Liu, B.S. Department of Health Preservation and Rehabilitation, Beijing University of Chinese Medicine, Beijing, P.R. China

Zhaoxiang Bian, Ph.D. School of Chinese Medicine, Hong Kong Baptist University, Hong Kong, P.R. China

Part I
Meridians, Acupuncture and Moxibustion

Chapter 1
Meridians: General Introduction

Section 1 Introduction

I Basic Concepts

The theory of the meridians (*jingluo*) concerns the system of vessels that sustains the entire human body, providing the means of linking all parts of the body. "Meridians" is the general term, encompassing both *jing* and *luo*. The *jing* are the main meridians (or simply, meridians), which are the pathways linking the upper and lower body, the viscera (interior) and the skin, sinews, bones and other tissues (exterior). The *luo* are the smaller collateral branches of the main meridians; they subdivide into smaller and smaller branches, and these in turn form a network of vessels that reaches every part of the body.

In the interior the meridians are intimately related to the visceral organs. In the exterior they are intimately related to the limbs and joints. Being the conduits between the interior and the exterior of the body they integrate all the organs and tissues into an organic whole. The meridian system provides the pathways for the movement of Qi and blood, for the regulation of Yin–Yang, and for the various organs to influence one another under both physiologic and pathologic conditions. The application of acupuncture and moxibustion also relies upon the meridian system.

The theory of the meridians is an important component of the CM theoretical system.

II Functions of Meridians

The meridian system is central to human physiology and pathology and its theory is indispensable in CM diagnostics, therapeutics and the prevention of disease and health presentation.

Z.W. Liu and L. Liu (eds.), *Essentials of Chinese Medicine: Volume 2*,

1 Physiology

The meridians, main and collateral, form a pervasive network that integrates every part of the human body into an organic whole. They provide the infrastructure that makes possible the circulation of Qi and blood, the actions of Yin–Yang, the nourishment of the organs and tissues and the defense of the body against exogenous disease evils. They are essential for the integration of the many parts of the body and the harmonization of visceral functions and other vital activities.

The Spiritual Pivot states: "Human Qi, blood, essence and spirit are what enable life. The meridians are what enable the movement of Qi and blood, the efficacy of Yin–Yang, the nourishment of the sinews and bones and the facilitation of the joints."

CM also uses the phrase "meridian Qi" to refer to the physiological capacity of the meridians.

2 Pathology

The meridians have an intimate relationship with the onset and development of disease. If meridian-Qi is disturbed, the ability of the meridians to transport Qi and blood is impaired. Then Yin–Yang cannot be regulated and the vital activities of the body cannot be protected. When that happens, exogenous disease evil can succeed in attacking the body and cause illness. After gaining access the disease evils can further follow the pathways of the meridians and transmit from the exterior to the interior or from the interior to the exterior. Conversely, illnesses that arise in the visceral organs can also follow the pathways of the meridians to extend into the exterior and the limbs.

3 Diagnostics

In general, whenever an illness displays changes in any part of the exterior of the body it is possible, by exploiting the knowledge of the pathways of the meridians, to ascertain which visceral organs are diseased and by which meridians the abnormalities are transmitted. For example, flank and inguinal pain mostly reflect disorder of the liver and the liver meridian since the liver meridian winds around the genital organs and distributes to the flanks and ribs.

4 Treatment

In clinical practice the theory of the meridians is widely used to guide the treatment of every type of disease. The meridians are the thoroughfare by which medicines express their actions and instrumental stimulations elicit their responses.

Treatment by acupuncture and moxibustion aims to provide stimulation at designated acupoints along the meridians in order to restore the functions of the meridians and regulate the actions of Yin–Yang, Qi and blood of the body's visceral organs, thereby to achieve the therapeutic goal.

By the same token, in pharmacotherapy the active principles of the herbs are carried to the diseased organs or tissues by means of the meridians. Based on the accumulated observations over many centuries the ancient CM physicians founded the theory of meridian-affinity of herbs, according to which each herb has a special affinity for a certain meridian and visceral organ.

5 *Prevention of Disease and Health Preservation*

In clinical practice the regulation of the meridians is also used to prevent disease. For example, the acupoint Zusanli (ST-36) is an important health-promoting point. Moxibustion at the acupoints Zusanli (ST-36), Zhongwan (CV-12) and Guangyuan (CV-4) has health-promoting and general tonic effects. Moxibustion at the acupoint Dazhui (GV-14) can prevent the common cold. Moxibustion at the acupoints Zusanli (ST-36) and Xuanzhong (GB-39) can prevent stroke.

Section 2 Composition of Meridian System

The composition of the meridian system is summarized in Table 1.1.

I Twelve Main Meridians

The 12 main meridians (or simply meridians) are the principal vessels of the meridian system. On the basis of the regions through which they pass and the Yin or Yang nature of their associated *zang–fu* organs they are classified as three Yang meridians of the hand, three Yin meridians of the foot, three Yin meridians of the hand and three Yin meridians of the foot. The Yin meridians pertain to the *zang* organs and the Yang meridians to the *fu* organs, and each of the 12 is named in accordance with its specific associated visceral organ, as shown in the table.

These 12 main meridians inter-link with one another through their collateral meridians. Functionally they are organized into six sub-systems, each encompassing a *zang* organ and its dyadic *fu* organ (see Volume 1, Part I, Chapter 3, Section 4, Subsection II). For example, the lung and the large intestine form a *zang–fu* dyad. Hence, the Lung Meridian of Hand-Taiyin also pertains to the large intestine, and the Large Intestine Meridian of Hand-Yangming also pertains to the lung.

Table 1.1 Composition of meridian system

Main meridians	Twelve regular meridians	Yin Meridians of Hand	Lung Meridian of Hand-Taiyin
			Pericardium Meridian of Hand-Jueyin
			Heart Meridian of Hand-Shaoyin
		Yang Meridians of Hand	Large Intestine Meridian of Hand-Yangming
			Sanjiao Meridian of Hand-Shaoyang
			Small Intestine Meridian of Hand-Taiyang
		Yang Meridians of Foot	Stomach Meridian of Foot-Yangming
			Gallbladder Meridian of Foot-Shaoyang
			Bladder Meridian of Foot-Taiyang
		Yin Meridians of Foot	Spleen Meridian of Foot-Taiyin
			Liver Meridian of Foot-Jueyin
			Kidney Meridian of Foot-Shaoyin
	Eight irregular meridians	Du Meridian (Governor Vessel)	
		Ren Meridian (Conception Vessel)	
		Chong Meridian	
		Dai Meridian	
		Yinwei Meridian	
		Yangwei Meridian	
		Yinqiao Meridian	
		Yangqiao Meridian	
	Twelve divergent meridians		
	Twelve muscle meridians		
	Twelve cutaneous meridians		
Collateral meridians	Fifteen collaterals		
	Minute collateral		
	Superficial collaterals		

The functional meridian systems are interconnected, so that together they form an endless closed circuit that reaches every part of the human body. In this way, Qi and blood flow through them and reach every part of the body in a cyclical circulation.

The flow pattern formed by the meridian system begins in the lung and ends in the liver and progresses from the interior to the exterior and from the upper body to the lower. The three Yin meridians of the hand start from the chest and course down the medial aspect of the upper limb to fingertips. The three Yang meridians of the hand start at the fingertips and course up the lateral aspect of the upper limb to the head and face. The three Yang meridians of the foot start from the head and face and course through the trunk and lower limb to the toetips. The three Yin meridians of the foot start from the foot and course up the medial aspect of the lower limb through the abdomen to the chest.

The distribution of the 12 meridians follows three rules. (1) The Yin meridians course along the medial aspects of the limbs and in the chest and abdomen. The Yang meridians course along the lateral aspects of the limbs. (2) All the hand meridians course along the upper limbs; and all the foot meridians along the lower limbs. (3) Among the Yang meridians, the courses of the Yangming meridians are anterior, those of the Taiyang meridians are posterior, and those of the Shaoyang meridians are intermediate. Among the Yin meridians, the courses of the Taiyin meridians are anterior, those of the Shaoyin meridians are posterior, and those of the Jueyin meridians are intermediate. The only exception is at 8 *cun* above the medial malleolus, where the Foot Taiyin and the Foot Jueyin reverse their relative positions – the Foot Taiyin in the intermediate and the Foot Jueyin in the anterior position. (For *cun* as a unit of measurement see Volume 2, Part I, Chapter 2, Section 4.)

For Qi and blood circulation the order of the 12 main meridians is as follows:

From Lung Meridian of Hand-Taiyin
To Large Intestine Meridian of Hand-Yangming
To Stomach Meridian of Foot-Yangming
To Spleen Meridian of Foot-Taiyin
To Heart Meridian of Hand-Shaoyin
To Small Intestine Meridian of Hand-Taiyang
To Bladder Meridian of Foot-Taiyang
To Kidney Meridian of Foot-Shaoyin
To Pericardium Meridian of Hand-Jueyin
To Sanjiao Meridian of Hand-Shaoyang
To Gallbladder Meridian of Foot-Shaoyang
To Liver Meridian of Foot-Jueyin, and back
To Lung Meridian of Hand-Taiyin

II Eight Irregular Meridians

There are eight main meridians that differ in important respects from the 12 regular meridians. They are the Du, Ren, Chong, Dai, Yinwei, Yangwei, Yinqiao and Yangqiao Meridians. Note that the 1989 Geneva Convention on Acupoint Nomenture names the Du Meridian the Governor Vessel and the Ren Meridian the Conception Vessel.

Unlike the 12 regular meridians, these irregular meridians are not associated with the *zang–fu* organs and do not link the exterior and the interior of the body. Their paths also differ from those of the regular meridians. Of these eight only the Du and the Ren Meridians have associated acupoints.

The irregular meridians have two main functions. (1) They augment the interrelationship between the 12 regular meridians. (2) They regulate quantitatively the Qi and blood in the regular meridians, such as storage and drainage.

III Fifteen Collaterals

Each of the 12 regular main meridians has a major collateral meridian. The Du and the Ren Meridians also have a major collateral meridian each. In addition, the spleen has a major collateral meridian. Thus, all together there are fifteen such major collateral meridians. They are respectively named for the meridians or organ from which they arise.

The main function of these 15 collateral meridians is to strengthen the association of the Yin and Yang meridians and that between meridians in the exterior and in the interior. For example, the Ren Collateral connects the Qi of all the meridians in the abdomen. The Du Collateral connects the Qi of all the meridians in the back. The Spleen Collateral connects the Qi of all meridians on the sides of the chest.

Of the collateral meridians of the body some course through the superficies of the body. These are also known as the Superficial (or Floating) Collaterals. Also, the collateral meridians themselves give rise to many smaller branches, and these in turn to many yet smaller branches, and so on. The smallest branches, known as the "minute collaterals," are too numerous to count. The branches form a network that pervades the entire body and serves as the pathway whereby Qi and blood reach every part of the body to provide nourishment.

IV Twelve Divergent Meridians

The 12 divergent meridians are branches that derive from the 12 regular meridians. They emerge from and join the regular meridians and serve to link them to the deeper parts of the body.

These divergent meridians arise from the regular meridians mostly in the regions around the elbows and knees and course to the thoracic and abdominal cavities, where they join their respective *zang–fu* organs. Thence they continue to course to the head and neck region, where they emerge to the exterior of the body. There the Yang divergent meridians rejoin those Yang meridians from which they arise, and the Yin divergent meridians join the respective Yang meridians that link the exterior and the interior.

In this way the divergent meridians augment the interconnection between the *zang–fu* organs, enhance the intimate relationship between the regular meridians and all parts of the body, and broaden the scope of acupuncture and moxibustion therapy.

V Twelve Muscle Meridians

The 12 muscle meridians are the conduits which distribute the Qi of the 12 regular meridians to the muscles, tendons and joints, and which are the external connecting regions of the 12 regular meridians. Each of these muscle meridians corresponds to the superficial region controlled by the regular meridian that gives rise to it. Each begins at the finger or toe tips and runs on to the head and trunk. Instead of entering the *zang–fu* organs they travel along the body's surface and connect with the joints and bones.

The main functions of the muscle meridians are to regulate the bones and joints to ensure smooth flexion and extension and fluid motion of the body.

VI The 12 Cutaneous Regions

The 12 cutaneous regions refer to the body's surface areas on which the functions of the respective 12 regular meridians are reflected and the Qi of the collateral meridians is distributed. The mapping of these cutaneous regions reflects the courses of the 12 regular meridians.

Since the cutaneous regions are the most superficial part of the body tissues, they serve as the protective barrier for the human body.

Guidance for Study

I Aim of Study

This chapter introduces the basic concepts, organization and functions of the main and collateral meridians. This basic knowledge is essential for understanding acupuncture and moxibustion.

II Objectives of Study

After completing this chapter the learners will

1. Know the basic meaning of the meridians and collaterals
2. Know the components of the meridian system
3. Be familiar with the concept of the distribution of the 12 meridians in the superficial part of the body and the order of flow of Qi in the 12 regular meridians
4. Be familiar with the functions of the main and collateral meridians

III Exercises for Review

1. What are the main meridians and their collaterals?
2. What are the components of the system of the meridians and the collaterals?

3. State the order of flow of Qi in the 12 regular meridians.
4. What is the main functions of the 12 regular meridians?
5. Describe how the 12 regular meridians are reflected in the superficial parts of the body.

Chapter 2
Overview of Acupoints

Section 1 Classification and Nomenclature of Acupoints

The acupoints are the specific sites where Qi of the *zang–fu* organs and meridians flows to the body's surface. They are also the sites where acupuncture or moxibustion treatment is applied. The main acupoints are on the meridians, while the meridians pertain to the *zang–fu* viscera. The relationship between the acupoints, the meridians and the *zang–fu* organs is intimate and inseparable.

I Classification of Acupoints

There are numerous acupoints distributed over the human body. In general they fall into the following three categories.

1 Acupoints of the 14 Meridians

Also known as the "regular acupoints," acupoints of the 14 meridians are distributed along the 12 regular and the Du and Ren meridians. These acupoints all have specific locations, defined names and associated meridians, and may all be used to treat disorders of the related meridians and collaterals.

The acupoints of the 14 meridians number 361 in total. They are the most commonly used acupoints in clinical practice.

2 Extra-Meridian Acupoints

These are acupoints not associated with any of the 12 regular meridians or Du or Ren meridians; hence they are named the "extra-meridian acupoints." They also have specific locations and defined names.

Z.W. Liu and L. Liu (eds.), *Essentials of Chinese Medicine: Volume 2*,

These extra-meridian acupoints are effectively used in the treatment of certain diseases.

3 *Ashi Acupoints*

These do not have names or defined locations, but emerge as acupoints that may be used for the application of acupuncture or moxibustion to suppress pain or other pathological responses reflected in these acupoints. For this reason they are also known as "pain-suppressing acupoints," "reflexive acupoints" or "unfixed acupoints."

II Nomenclature of Acupoints

Traditionally, acupoints of the 14 meridians are named by analogy. Because the flow of Qi and blood is similar to the flow of water, the prominences and depressions of the bones and tendons are compared to hills and valleys. The characteristic shape of each local site is also exploited by comparison to animals, plants or utensils. In addition, some acupoints are named for architectural features or for astronomical or meteorological phenomena. Others are named using anatomical terms or therapeutic properties.

In English literature, all acupoints are assigned an alphanumeric code. For the acupoints on the 14 meridians the alphabetical part is a two-letter designation of the meridian (e.g. LI for Large Intestine Meridian, HT for Heart Meridian), and the numeric part is the order of the acupoint on that meridian. For the extra-meridian acupoints not on the meridians, the alphabetical part refers to their location (e.g. EX for being extra-meridian, UE for Upper Extremity, HN for Head/Neck). The specific acupoints are described in Volume 2, Part I, Chapter 3 and Appendix II.

The following lists give examples. For each acupoint the name is given in *pinyin* followed in brackets by its alphanumeric designation and a translation of the Chinese name.

Section 2 Acupoints in Therapeutics

The acupoints are not merely where visceral and meridian Qi flows to the body surface. They are also sites where evil Qi can lodge when the physiological functions are disturbed, and they are sites where stimulation by acupuncture or moxibustion can unblock the meridians, regulate Qi and blood, promote the dynamic balance of Yin–Yang and harmonize the *zang–fu* organs. Appropriate application of acupuncture at acupoints may therefore be useful for supporting the genuine and repelling the evil Qi. While all the acupoints share some properties, each also has its specific properties.

In general, the acupoints have three types of therapeutic properties.

I Local Treatment

Each acupoint may be used to treat disturbances of the tissue and organs at its site or the area around it. This is a therapeutic property shared by all acupoints.

For example, in the area around the eye the acupoints Jingming (BL-1), Chengqi (ST-1) and Sibai (ST-2) may all be used to treat eye diseases. In the epigastric region the acupoints Zhongwan (CV-12), Jianli (CV-11) and Liangmen (ST-21) are used for disorders of the stomach. In the area around the ear the acupoints Tinggong ((SI-19), Ermen (SJ-21), Tinghui (GB-2) and Yifeng (SJ-17) may be used to treat ear disorders.

II Remote Treatment

This is the basic property employed in acupuncture and moxibustion therapy.

All the acupoints of the 14 meridians, especially those of the 12 regular meridians on the limbs distal to the elbows and knees, may be used to treat disorders of distant *zang–fu* organs, functional systems and sense organs associated with the meridian of the acupoints selected. In general, all the acupoints of any particular meridian may be used to treat disorders of this meridian. All the acupoints of the exteriorly–interiorly related meridians may be used complementarily to treat disorders of those meridians. Some acupoints may even be effective for the systemic treatment of the entire body.

For example, the acupoint Hegu (LI-4) may be used to treat not only disorders in the hands and wrists but also those of the head and face, as well as fever due to exogenous pathogens. The acupoint Zusanli (ST-36) may be used to treat not only disorders of the lower limbs but also those of the entire digestive system; it may even be used to strengthen the body's resistance to disease, thereby preventing disease and prolonging lifespan.

III Special and Specific Therapeutic Properties

Accumulated clinical experience shows that stimulation of certain acupoints can elicit different beneficial responses under different conditions. For example, in certain patients with diarrhea puncturing the acupoint Tianshu (ST-25) relieves the diarrhea; but in other patients with constipation puncturing Tianshu may induce defecation. In certain patients with tachycardia puncturing the acupoint Neiguan (PC-6) may lower the heart rate; and in other patients with bradycardia puncturing Neiguan may raise the heart rate.

In addition to these special properties, acupoints also have properties that are relatively specific. For example, puncturing the acupoint Dazhui (GV-14) has an antipyretic effect and puncturing the acupoint Zhiyin (BL-67) helps correct malposition of the fetus.

Section 3 Acupoints with Specific Properties

Some of the acupoints of all 14 meridians have specific properties; they are called "specific acupoints." Because each of them has a unique therapeutic property these specific acupoints are given special names on the basis of their therapeutic functions.

I Shu Acupoints

The "five Shu" is the general term for a set of five acupoints – Jing (Well), Ying (Spring), Shu (Stream), Jing (River) and He (Sea) – for each of the 12 regular meridians. They are located in order from the distal ends of the extremities to the elbow or knee. Since each of the 12 regular meridians contains these five acupoints, in all there are 60 such acupoints.

The ancient CM physicians conceptualized the flow of meridian-Qi of these Shu acupoints by analogy to the flow of water in nature, from small trickles on the surface to larger and deeper streams and rivers finally to the sea. They used this analogy to explain the varying depth and volume of meridian-Qi as it courses by these acupoints along each meridian and hence the different properties of these acupoints.

The Jing (Well) acupoints are located in the tips of the fingers or toes. At Jing meridian-Qi is still very small in volume, like the water of a spring that has just emerged from the ground. The Ying (Spring) acupoints are anterior to the metacarpophalangeal or metatarsophalangeal joints. At Ying meridian-Qi is larger in volume, like a stream that has just formed. The Shu (Stream) acupoints are posterior to the metacarpophalangeal or metatarsophalangeal joints. At Shu meridian-Qi is full, like a gushing stream. The Jing (River) acupoints are located above the wrist or ankle. At Jing meridian-Qi is more full, like a river forming from the confluence of many streams. Finally, the He (Sea) acupoints are located around the elbow or knee. At He meridian-Qi is abundant, like the sea that forms from several rivers. Upon leaving the He acupoints, meridian-Qi flows into the *zang–fu* organs.

In general, treatment at the Jing (Well) acupoint is indicated for mental disorders and restlessness or agitation. Treatment at the Ying (Spring) acupoint is indicated in Heat illnesses. Treatment at the Shu (Stream) acupoints is indicated for heaviness in the body and pain in the joints. Treatment at the Jing (River) acupoint is indicated for labored breathing with coughing or pharyngolaryngeal disorders. Treatment at the He (Sea) acupoint is indicated for diseases of any of the *fu* organs, such as the gastrointestinal tract.

II Yuan (Source) and Luo (Connecting) Acupoints

The Yuan acupoints are where genuine Qi of the *zang–fu* organs transit and tarry. Each of the 12 regular meridians has a Yuan acupoint, located in a limb. These are together known as the "twelve Yuan." The Yuan acupoints are important in the treatment of illnesses of the meridians and the *zang–fu* organs.

The Yuan acupoints of the six Yin meridians are not distinct but overlap with the Shu (Stream) acupoints. The Yuan acupoints of the six Yang meridians, on the other hand, are distinct, and are located posterior to the Shu (Stream) acupoints.

Each of the major collateral meridians has a Luo (Connecting) acupoint, located at the place where the collateral meridian branches off the main meridian. Since there are all together 15 major collateral meridians the Luo acupoints are together known as the "fifteen Luo." (For the 15 major collateral meridians, see Volume 1, Part I, Chapter 1, Section 2, Subsection III.)

The Luo acupoints are used in acupuncture or moxibustion treatment of disorders of the meridians that are in exterior–interior relationship and in the regions around them.

III Back-Shu and Front-Mu Acupoints

The Back-Shu acupoints are the sites in the back of the body to which the visceral organs' Qi flows. Each of the *zang–fu* organs has a Back-Shu acupoint, so there are 12 in all. They are given names according to these organs. The Back-Shu acupoints all belong to Yang. They are located along the two sides of the spinal column along the Bladder Meridian of Foot-Taiyang. In general, their vertical order follows that of the visceral organs and they are mostly located near their respective organs. The Back-Shu acupoints are important sites where Yin-type illnesses are treated by a Yang-type approach.

The Front-Mu acupoints are the sties in the chest or abdomen to which the visceral organs' Qi flows. Again, each of the *zang–fu* organs has a Front-Mu acupoint, so there are 12 in all. The Front-Mu acupoints all belong to Yin. They are located on the chest or abdomen. Among them six belong to the Ren and Du Meridians, two to the liver meridian, two to the gallbladder meridian, one to the lung meridian and one to the stomach meridian. The Front-Mu acupoints are important sites where Yang-type illnesses are treated by a Yin-type approach.

When a *zang–fu* organ is diseased, its corresponding Back-Shu or Front-Mu acupoint often manifests abnormalities, such as tenderness on pressure. Hence, these acupoints are important in the diagnosis and treatment of diseases of their corresponding *zang–fu* organs.

IV Influential Acupoints

The Eight Influential Points are the eight points where the vital essence and energy of the *zang* organs, *fu* organs, Qi, blood, tendons, vessels, bones and marrow join together. These points are distributed on the trunk and limbs.

V Xi (Cleft) Points

The Xi (Cleft) acupoints are the sites of gathering for meridian-Qi of various meridians. There are all together 16 Xi (Cleft) acupoints – one for each of the 12 regular meridians, and one for each of four of the irregular meridians (Yinwei, Yangwei, Yinqiao and Yangqiao). They are distributed on the four limbs distal to the elbow or knee joints, with a few exceptions.

Each Xi acupoint may be used to treat acute disorders in the areas governed by its meridian or in its related *zang–fu* organ.

VI Lower-He (Sea) Acupoints

The Lower-He (Sea) acupoints are the six sites where meridian-Qi of the three Foot Yang Meridians and the three Hand Yang Meridians flow and gather in the three Foot Yang Meridians. These six acupoints are located around the knee joints. They are important in the treatment of diseases of the *fu* organs.

VII Confluence Acupoints

Each Confluence acupoint is the site where meridian-Qi of an irregular meridian joins Qi of a regular meridian. Thus there are eight Confluence acupoints, and they are distributed around the wrist and ankle joints.

Section 4 Techniques of Locating Acupoints

In the clinical application of acupuncture and moxibustion the therapeutic results depend upon accurate location of the acupoints. In order to locate the positions of the acupoints the physician must master the techniques of locating them.

I Finger Measures

This defines the basic unit of measurement, the *cun*. (Literally, the word *cun* means "inch," but the Chinese inch differs in length from the English inch.) The length and width of the patient's fingers are taken as the standard. The following measures are the most commonly used in clinical practice. Note that the *cun* as defined here and in the next subsection is not a fixed measure of length, but varies with the patient's body size.

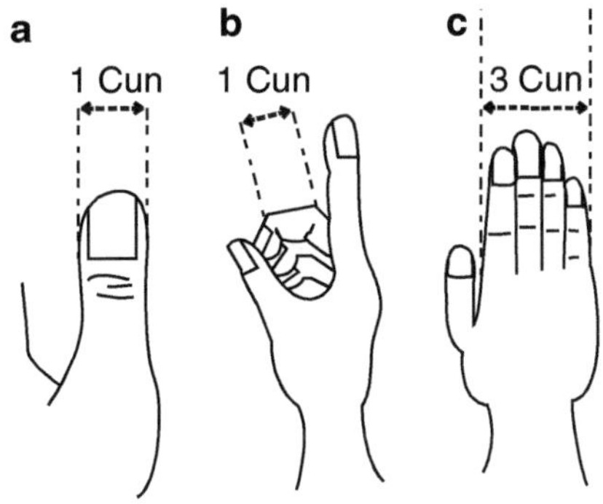

Fig. 2.1 (**a**) Thumb measure (**b**) Middle finger measure and (**c**) four fingers measure

Middle Finger Measure: Ask the patient to flex the middle finger. The distance between the two ends of the interphalangeal creases is taken as 1 *cun* (see Fig. 2.1b). This is used to measure the vertical distances for locating on the limbs the acupoints.

Thumb Measure: The width of the interphangeal joint of the patient's thumb is taken as 1 *cun* (see Fig. 2.1a).

Four Fingers Measure: Ask the patient to straighten the hand with the fingers close together naturally, as indicated in Fig. 2.1c. The width spanning all four fingers at the level of the dorsal skin crease of the proximal interphalangeal joint of the middle finger is taken as 3-*cun*.

II Comparative Measures

Also known as the "bone-measuring technique" this uses the lengths of bone segments between various joints as measures for locating acupoints. These measures are applicable on any patient – of either sex and of any age or body size. This has become the basic technique for locating acupoints. For details see Figs. 2.2 and 2.3 and Table 2.1.

III Anatomical Landmarks

The normal anatomical landmarks on the body surface provide another technique for locating acupoints. These landmarks fall into two categories.

Fixed landmarks are those that do not change with body movement, such as the five sense organs, nails, nipples, umbilicus, and prominences and depressions of the bones. Acupoints that are adjacent to or on such landmarks may be located directly. Examples include Yintang (EX-HN-3), midway between the two eyebrows,

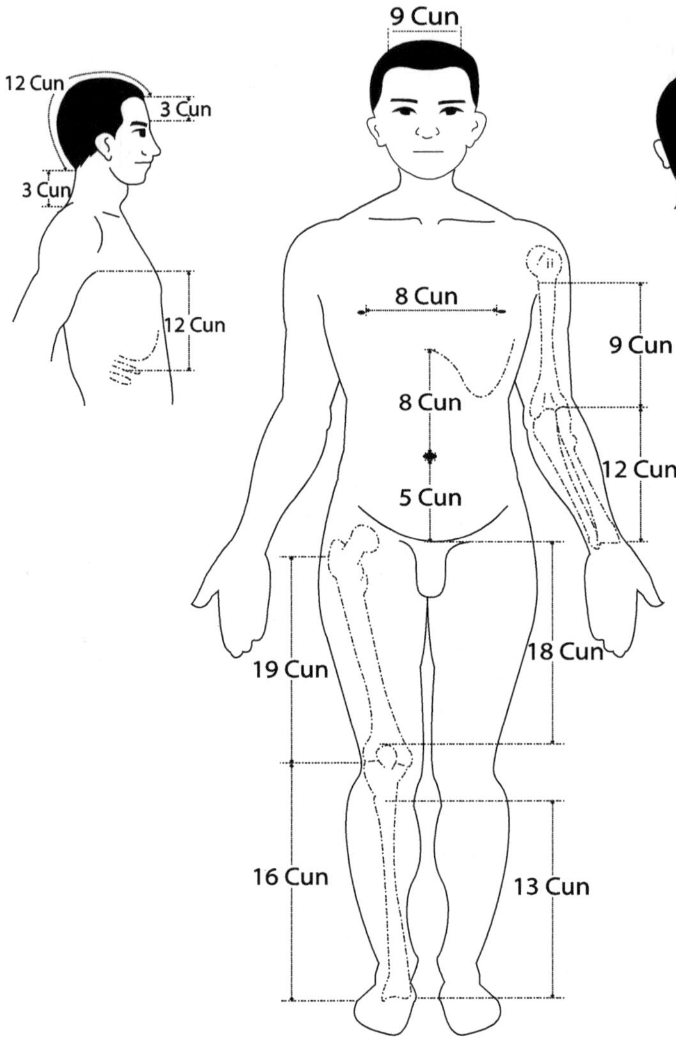

Fig. 2.2 Comparative measures – anterior

Tanzhong (CV-17), midway between the two nipples, Tianshu (ST-25), lateral to the umbilicus, and Yanglingquan (GB-34), anterior and inferior to the small head of the fibula.

Moving landmarks are spaces, depressions, wrinkles and other features that are revealed with voluntary motion of the joints, muscles and skin. For example, when the mouth is opened a depression is formed immediately anterior to the tragus of the ear; this is the location of Tinggong (SJ-19). When the hand is curled, the transverse palmar crease appears and Houxi (SI-3) may be located.

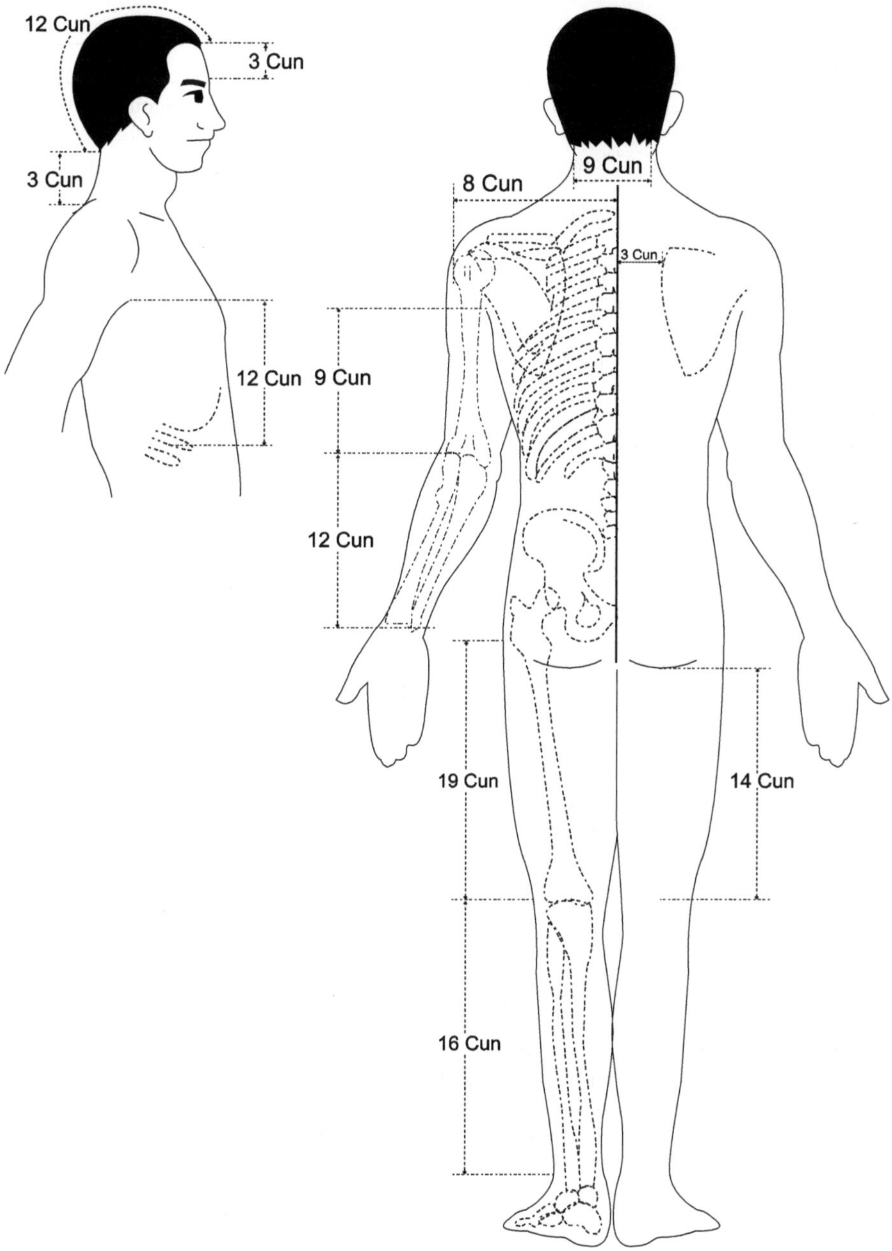

Fig. 2.3 Comparative measures – posterior

Table 2.1 Standards for comparative measures

Body Part	Description	Measure	Explanation
Head	From anterior hairline to posterior Hairline	12 *cun*	Used to measure longitudinal distance of acupoints on head
	From glabella (Yintang) to anterior hairline	3 *cun*	
	From Dazhui (GV-14) to posterior hairline	3 *cun*	
	From glabella to Dazhui (GV-14)	18 *cun*	
	Between the two corners of forehead	9 *cun*	Used to measure transverse distance of acupoints on head
	Between the two mastoid processes	9 *cun*	
Chest and Abdomen	From Tiantu (CV-22) to sternocostal angle	9 *cun*	Used to measure longitudinal distance of acupoints on Ren Meridian and other acupoints on abdomen
	From sternocostal angle to center of umbilicus	8 *cun*	
	From center of umbilicus to upper border of symphysis pubis	5 *cun*	
	Between the two nipples	8 *cun*	Used to measure transverse measurement of acupoints on abdomen
Lateral chest	From end of axillary fold to tip of 11th rib	12 *cun*	Used to measure longitudinal distance of acupoints in subcostal region
Back	From medial border of scapula to posterior midline	3 *cun*	Used to measure transverse distance of acupoints on back
	From acromion process of scapula to posterior midline	8 *cun*	
Upper limbs	From end of axillary fold to transverse cubital crease	9 *cun*	Used to measure longitudinal distance of acupoints on arm
	From transverse cubital crease to transverse wrist crease	12 *cun*	
Lower limbs	From level of border of symphysis pubis to medial epicondyle of femur	18 *cun*	Used to measure longitudinal distance of acupoints of Yin Meridians of foot
	From lower border of medial condyle of tibia to tip of medial malleolus	13 *cun*	
	From prominence of greater trochanter to middle of patella	19 *cun*	1. Used for Yang Meridians of Foot 2. Distance from gluteal fold to center of patella is taken as 14 *cun* 3. Anterior level of center of patella is same level as Dubi (ST-35), and posterior level is same level as Weizhong (BL-40)
	From center of patella to tip of lateral malleolus	16 *cun*	
	From tip of lateral malleolus to inferior surface of heel	3 *cun*	

IV Simple Location

These are simple and direct techniques of acupoint location employed in clinical practice. For example, when the fist is clenched, Laogong (PC-8) is just under the tip of the middle finger. Fengshi (GB-31) is at the tip of the middle finger when standing at attention (Fig. 2.4).

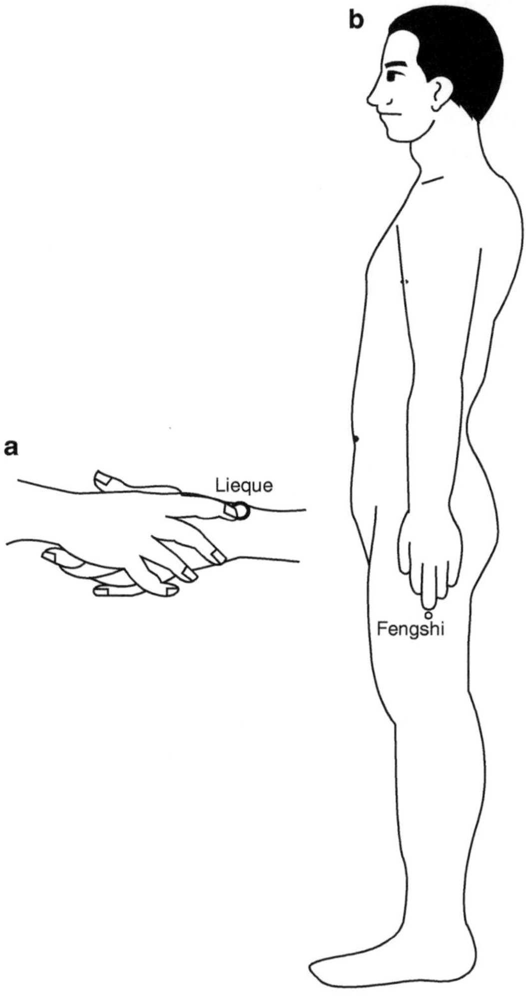

Fig. 2.4 Simple location

Guidance for Study

I Aim of Study

This chapter presents the classification and the nomenclature of the acupoints. It provides an overview of their role in therapeutics and describes the techniques used in locating them.

II Objectives of Study

After completing this chapter the learners will

1. Know the classification and naming of acupoints;
2. Know the therapeutic properties of acupoints;
3. Be familiar with the meaning of acupoints;
4. Know the techniques of locating acupoints.

III Exercises for Review

1. What is an acupoint?
2. What are the categories of acupoints?
3. Describe the main types of therapeutic properties of acupoints?
4. What are the "specific acupoints?" How many groups of "specific acupoints" are there? Describe them briefly.
5. What are the Five Shu acupoints? Discuss their meaning and distribution features.
6. What are the Yuan (Source) acupoints? Where are they located? Describe their properties.
7. What are the Luo (Connecting) acupoints? Describe their distribution and function.
8. What are the eight Confluent Points?
9. Describe the main techniques for locating acupoints.
10. Illustrate how to locate acupoints by the technique of anatomical landmarks. Provide examples.

Chapter 3
Descriptions of Specific Acupoints

This chapter describes the specific acupoints of the 12 regular meridians, the Ren and Du Meridians, and some other acupoints commonly used in treatment with acupuncture or moxibustion.

Section 1 Lung Meridian of Hand-Taiyin

I Pathway

The Lung Meridian of Hand-Taiyin (the Lung Meridian, for short) originates in the middle-jiao. It moves down and connects with the large intestine, then winds back up along the upper orifice of the stomach, passing through the diaphragm and entering the lung. It leaves the lung where the lung communicates with the throat and follows a transverse course to the axilla. Thence it descends along the antero-lateral upper arm, passing in front of the Heart and the Pericardium Meridians, to reach the antecubital fossa. From the antecubital fossa it continues down the antero-lateral forearm, past the thenar eminence, and ends at the lateral side of the tip of the thumb (see Fig. 3.1).

A branch emerges from this meridian at Lieque (LU-7), above the wrist. This branch courses laterally and wraps around the wrist and runs directly to the lateral side of the tip of the index finger, where it links with the Large Intestine Meridian.

II Main Applications

The acupoints of the Lung Meridian are used mainly in the treatment of disorders of the throat, the chest and the lung.

Z.W. Liu and L. Liu (eds.), *Essentials of Chinese Medicine: Volume 2*,

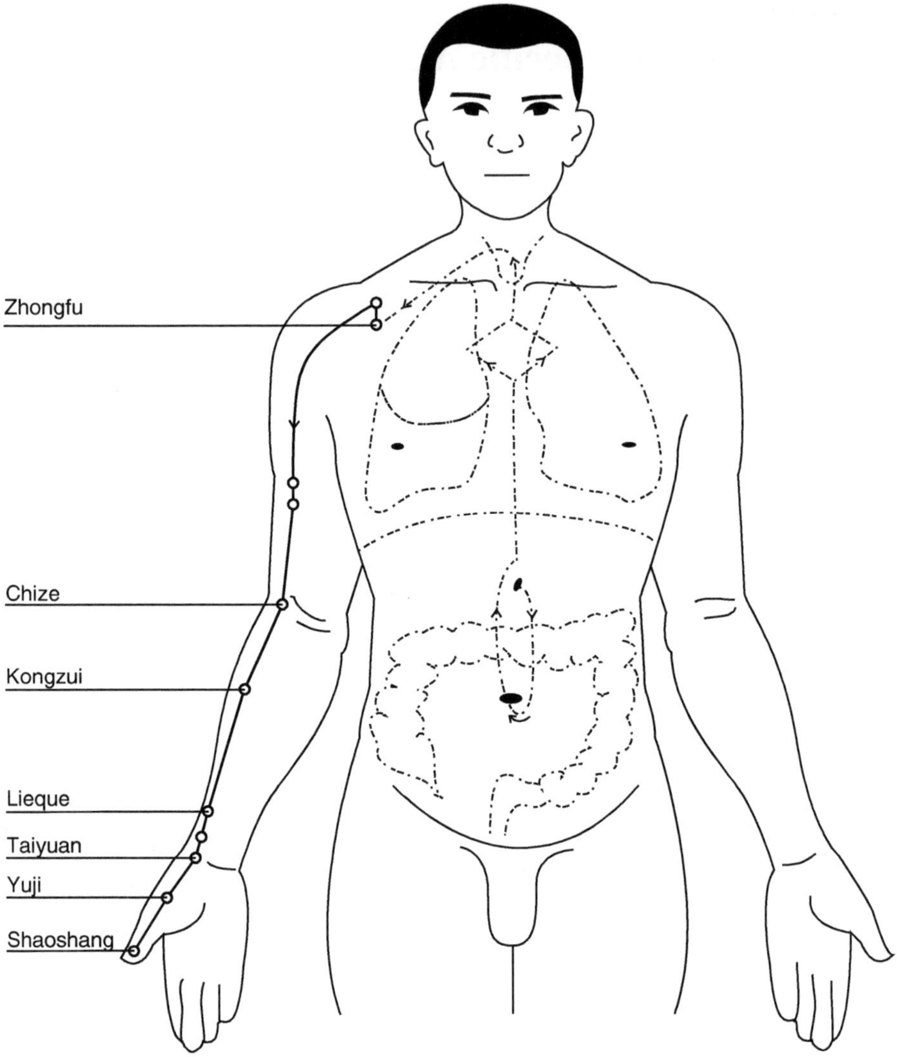

Fig. 3.1 Lung Meridian of Hand-Taiyin

III Commonly Used Acupoints

There are 11 acupoints in all – see Table 3.1. The more useful ones are individually described.

Zhongfu (LU-1)

This is the Front-Mu acupoint of the Lung Meridian. It is also the crossing point of the Lung and the Spleen Meridians.

Table 3.1 Acupoints of the Lung Meridian of Hand-Taiyin

Name	Location	Applications
LU-1	Described separately	
LU-2 Yunmen	Anterior shoulder, in depression of infraclavicular fossa superior to coracoid process of scapula – 6 *cun* from anterior midline	Cough, labored breathing, chest pain
Acupoints on chest: for diseases of lung and chest		
LU-3 Tianfu	Medial side of upper arm, lateral border of biceps muscle, 3 *cun* below anterior end of axillary fold	Labored breathing, nosebleed
LU-4 Xiabai	Medial side of upper arm, on lateral border of biceps, 4 *cun* below anterior end of axillary fold or 5 *cun* above antecubital crease	Cough, labored breathing
LU-5		
LU-6	Described separately	
LU-7		
LU-8 Jingqu Jing (River)	Antero-lateral aspect of forearm, 1 *cun* proximal to wrist crease, in depression between styloid process of radius and radial artery	Cough, labored breathing, sore throat
LU-9		
LU-10	Described separately	
LU-11		
Acupoints on arm: for diseases of throat, chest and lung		

Location: In the superior lateral part of the shoulder, 1 *cun* below Yunmen (LU-2) at the level of the first intercostal space and 6 *cun* from the anterior midline.

Applications: Cough, labored breathing; pain in the chest, shoulder and back; abdominal distention.

Techniques and Notes: Insert the needle obliquely and laterally or subcutaneously for 0.5–0.8 *cun*. Moxibustion may be applied. (For the definitions of "obliquely" and "subcutaneously" (see Volume 2, Part I, Chapter 4, Section 1, Subsection III, Sub-subsection 2).

Chize (LU-5)

This is the He (Sea) acupoint of the Lung Meridian.

Location: In the antecubital crease in the depression lateral to the biceps tendon.

Applications: Sore throat; cough, labored breathing, chest fullness; acute abdominal pain with vomiting or diarrhea; infantile convulsion; and spasmodic pain of the elbow and arm.

Techniques and Notes: Insert the needle perpendicularly 0.8–1.2 *cun*, or prick the point to cause slight bleeding. Moxibustion may be applied.

Kongzui (LU-6)

This is the Xi (Cleft) acupoint of the Lung Meridian.

Location: On the antero-lateral aspect of the forearm and on the line connecting Chize (LU-5) and Taiyuan (LU-9), at 7 *cun* above the transverse crease of the wrist.

Applications: Acute hemoptysis, epistaxis, bleeding hemorrhoids; sore throat; cough, labored breathing; arm pain with loss of elbow extension.

Techniques and Notes: Insert the needle perpendicularly 0.5–1.2 *cun*. Moxibustion may be applied.

Lieque (LU-7)

This is the Luo (Connecting) acupoint of the Lung Meridian. It is also the Confluence acupoint of the Ren Meridian and the Lung Meridian.

Location: On the antero-lateral aspect of the forearm, proximal to the styloid process of the radius at 1.5 *cun* above the wrist crease, between the tendons of the brachioradialis and the long thumb abductor muscles.

Applications: Headache caused by exogenous disease evils; cough, nasal congestion; sore throat, toothache; penile pain, hematuria, spermatorrhea; wry eyes and mouth; and weakness in the wrists.

Techniques and Notes: Insert the needle upward and obliquely 0.5–0.8 *cun*. Moxibustion may be applied.

Taiyuan (LU-9)

This is the Shu (Stream) acupoint and the Yuan (Source) acupoint of the Lung Meridian. It is also the Influential acupoint of the vessels.

Location: At the lateral end of the palmar surface of the transverse crease of the wrist, where the radial pulse is palpable.

Applications: Cough, labored breathing; sore throat; chest pain; pulse-less syndrome; headache; hemiplegia; and wrist pain.

Techniques and Notes: Insert the needle perpendicularly 0.3–0.5 *cun*. Be very careful not to puncture the radial artery. Moxibustion may be applied.

Yuji (LU-10)

This is the Ying (Spring) acupoint of the Lung Meridian.

Location: In the depression proximal to the first metacarpophalangeal joint, on the radial side of the midpoint of the first metacarpal bone, and at the demarcation of the lighter and darker skin.

Applications: Sore throat; cough, labored breathing; aphonia; fever.

Techniques and Notes: Insert the needle perpendicularly 0.5–1 *cun*. Moxibustion may be applied.

Shaoshang (LU-11)

This is the Jing (Well) acupoint of the Lung Meridian.

Location: On the antero-lateral aspect of the distal segment of the thumb, 0.1 *cun* from the corner of the nail.

Applications: Cough, sore throat; epistaxis; high fever; unconsciousness; violent mental disorders.

Techniques and Notes: Insert the needle 0.1 *cun* or prick the point to cause slight bleeding. Moxibustion may be applied.

Section 2 Large Intestine Meridian of Hand-Yangming

I Pathway

The Large Intestine Meridian starts at the tip of the index finger (Shangyang, LI-1), runs upward along the lateral side of the index finger and passes through the space between the first and second metacarpal bones (Hegu, LI-4). It enters the depression between the tendons of the long and short thumb extensor muscles. Thence it follows the antero-lateral forearm, reaches the lateral elbow and continues upward along the lateral upper arm until it comes to the end of the shoulder (Jianyu, LI-15). It then courses along the anterior border of the acromion, where it branches. One branch goes up to the 7th cervical vertebra (confluence of the three Yang meridians of the hand and of the foot) (Dazhui, GV-14). The other branch proceeds to the supraclavicular fossa (Quepen, ST12) to connect with the lung, its corresponding *zang* organ. From the lung it continues past the diaphragm and enters the large intestine (see Fig. 3.2).

From the supraclavicular fossa a branch runs to the neck, passes through the cheek, enters the gums of the lower teeth, and curves around the upper lip and crosses path at the philtrum with its mirror-image meridian. From the philtrum the branch of the left Large Intestine Meridian of Hand-Yangming goes to the right side of the nose and the branch of the right Large Intestine Meridian of Hand-Yangming goes to the left of the nose. At the side of the nose the Large Intestine Meridian links with the Stomach Meridian of Foot-Yangming.

II Main Applications

The acupoints of the Large Intestine Meridian are mainly used to treat diseases of the head, the face, and the sense organs; diseases of the digestive system; and diseases of the reproductive system. They are also used in febrile diseases and diseases in the regions along the course of this meridian.

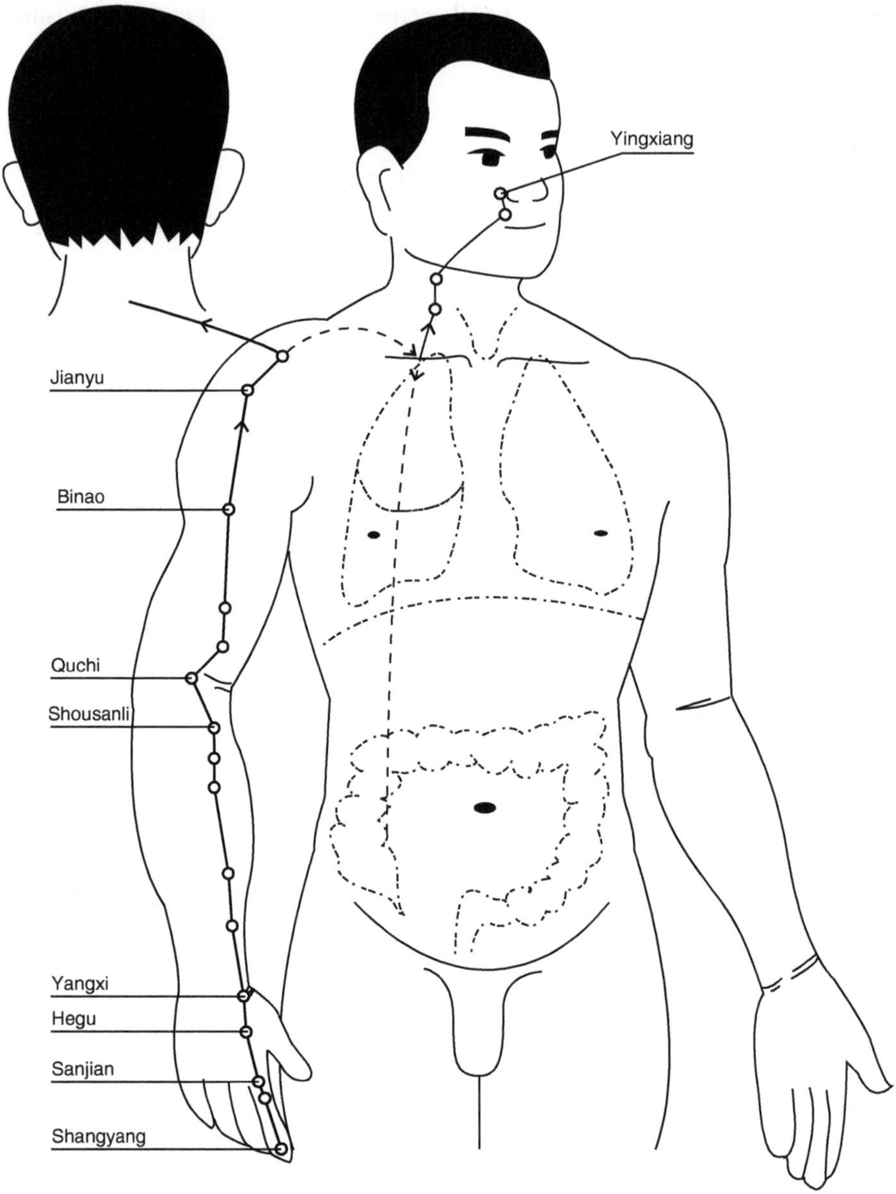

Fig. 3.2 Large Intestine Meridian of Hand-Yangming

III Commonly Used Acupoints

There are 20 acupoints in all – see Table 3.2. The more useful ones are individually described.

Shangyang (LI-1)

This is the Jing (Well) acupoint of the Large Intestine Meridian.

Location: On the lateral side of the distal segment of the index finger, 0.1 *cun* from the corner of the nail.

Applications: Sore throat; toothache; tinnitus and deafness; stroke with loss of consciousness; febrile diseases without sweating; and numbness of the fingers.

Techniques and Notes: Insert the needle perpendicularly 0.1 *cun*, or prick the point to cause slight bleeding. Moxibustion may be applied.

Sanjian (LI-3)

This is the Shu (Stream) acupoint of the Large Intestine Meridian.

Location: Just proximal to the second metacarpophalangeal joint, in the lateral depression formed with the hand in a loose fist.

Applications: Sore throat; toothache; pain in the eye; fever; abdominal distention with borborygmus; and inflammation on the dorsum of the hand and fingers.

Techniques and Notes: Insert the needle perpendicularly 0.3–0.5 *cun*. Moxibustion may be applied.

Hegu (LI-4)

This is the Yuan (Source) acupoint of the Large Intestine Meridian.

Location: On the dorsum of the hand, just lateral to the midpoint of the second metacarpal bone.

Applications: Headache; toothache; sore throat; inflammation of the eye; diseases of the nose; deafness; facial palsy or facial spasm; Heat diseases without sweating, or profuse and persistent sweating; fever with cold-intolerance; menstrual cramps, amenorrhea; stalled labor; stomach pain, abdominal pain, constipation; hemiplegia; infantile convulsions; urticaria; and mumps.

Techniques and Notes: Insert the needle perpendicularly 0.5–1 *cun*. Moxibustion may be applied. Acupuncture at Hegu is **contraindicated for pregnant women**.

Table 3.2 Acupoints of Large Intestine Meridian of Hand-Yangming

Name	Location	Applications
LI-1	Described separately	
LI-2 Erjian Ying (Spring) acupoint	In depression on radial side of index finger, distal to second metacarpophalangeal joint when a loose fist is made	Blurred vision; epistaxis; toothache; dry mouth, sore throat; febrile diseases
LI-3		
LI-4	Described separately	
LI-5		
LI-6 Pianli Luo (Connecting) acupoint	With elbow slightly flexed, on radial side of dorsal surface of forearm, and on line connecting LI-5 and LI-11, 3 *cun* above wrist crease	Eye redness; tinnitus; epistaxis; sore throat; pain in hand and arm; edema
LI-7 Wenliu Xi (Cleft) acupoint	With elbow flexed, on radial side of dorsal surface of forearm and on line connecting LI-5 and LI-11, 5 *cun* above wrist crease	Headache; facial swelling; sore throat; shoulder and arm pain; borborygmus, abdominal pain
LI-8 Xialian	On radial side of dorsal surface of forearm and on line connecting LI-5 and LI-11, 4 *cun* below antecubital crease	Headache; vertigo; eye pain; elbow, arm pain; abdominal pain and distention
LI-9 Shanglian	On radial side of dorsal surface of forearm and on line connecting LI-5 and LI-11, 3 *cun* below antecubital crease	Headache; hemiplegia; pain or numbness of hand, arm, shoulder; borborygmus, abdominal pain
LI-10	Described separately	
LI-11		
Acupoints on hand and elbow: for febrile diseases and diseases of head, face, ear, nose mouth and teeth		
LI-12 Zhouliao	With elbow flexed, on lateral side of upper arm, 1 *cun* above LI-11, on border of humerus	Pain, contracture and numbness of elbow and arm
LI-13 Shouwuli	On lateral side of upper arm and on line connecting LI-11 and LI-15, 3 *cun* above LI-11	Pain, contracture of elbow and arm; scrofula
LI-14	Described separately	
LI-15		
LI-16 Jugu	On shoulder, in depression between lateral end of clavicle and scapular spine	Pain, paresis of shoulder and arm; scrofula
Acupoints on upper arm and shoulder: mainly for diseases of local area		
LI-17 Tianding	On lateral side of neck, on posterior border of sternocleidomastoid muscle beside laryngeal protuberance, at midpoint of line connecting LI-18 and Quepen	Sudden loss of voice, sore throat; scrofula; goiter
LI-18 Futu	On lateral side of neck, beside laryngeal protuberance, between sternal head and clavicular head of sternocleidomastoid muscle	Sore throat, sudden loss of voice; goiter
LI-19 Heliao	On upper lip, directly below lateral border of nostril, at level of GV-26	Nasal congestion; epistaxis; wry mouth; lockjaw
LI-20	Described separately	
Acupoints on neck and face: for diseases of throat and nose		

Yangxi (LI-5)

This is the Jing (River) acupoint of the Large Intestine Meridian.

Location: At the radial end of the dorsal wrist crease, in the depression between the tendons of the short and the long extensor muscles of the thumb when the thumb is extended.

Applications: Headache; toothache; sore throat; weakness in the wrist; and tinnitus or deafness.

Techniques and Notes: Insert the needle perpendicularly 0.3–0.8 *cun*. Moxibustion may be applied.

Shousanli (LI-10)

Location: On the radial side of the dorsal surface of the forearm, on the line connecting Yangxi (LI-5) and Quchi (LI-11) at 2 *cun* below the antecubital crease.

Applications: Toothache; abdominal distention and pain, diarrhea; paralysis of the upper limbs.

Techniques and Notes: Insert the needle perpendicularly 0.5–0.8 *cun*. Moxibustion may be applied.

Quchi (LI-11)

This is the He (Sea) acupoint of the Large Intestine Meridian.

Location: With the elbow flexed, at the lateral end of the antecubital crease, at the midpoint of the line connecting Chize (LU-5) and the lateral epicondyle of the humerus.

Applications: Heat diseases; sore throat; hemiplegia; urticaria; abdominal pain, vomiting, diarrhea; painful inflammation and weakness of the arm; high blood pressure; headache; inflammation of the eye; toothache; and violent mental problems.

Techniques and Notes: Insert the needle perpendicularly 0.8–1.5 *cun*. Moxibustion may be applied.

Binao (LI-14)

Location: On the lateral side of the upper arm, at the insertion of the deltoid muscle on the line connecting Quchi (LI-11) and Jianyu (LI-15), 7 *cun* above Quchi.

Applications: Pain in the shoulder or the arm; diseases of the eye; scrofula; and spasticity of the neck.

Techniques and Notes: Insert the needle perpendicularly or obliquely 0.8–1.5 *cun*. Moxibustion may be applied.

Jianyu (LI-15)

This is the crossing point of the Large Intestine and the Yangqiao Meridians.

Location: On the shoulder, above the deltoid muscle, in the depression inferior to the acromion when the arm is abducted or raised level to the front.

Applications: Pain causing inability to raise the arm; paralysis with numbness of the arm; and urticaria due to Wind or Heat.

Techniques and Notes: Insert the needle perpendicularly or obliquely downward 0.8–1.5 *cun*. Moxibustion may be applied.

Yingxiang (LI-20)

This is the crossing point of the Stomach and the Large Intestine Meridians.

Location: In the naso-labial groove, by the midpoint of the lateral border of the ala nasi.

Applications: Nasal congestion; epistaxis; wry mouth; and lockjaw.

Techniques and Notes: Insert the needle perpendicularly or obliquely upward 0.3–0.5 *cun*. Moxibustion is not advisable.

Section 3 Stomach Meridian of Foot-Yangming

I Pathway

The Stomach Meridian is quite complex. It starts from the side of the ala nasi (Yingxiang, LI-20), ascends to the bridge of the nose where it meets the Bladder Meridian (Jingming BL-1), then turns downward along the side of the nose (ST-1) and enters the upper gum. Reemerging to the surface it curves around the lips and descends to meet the Ren Meridian in the groove between the lower lip and the chin (Chengjiang, Ren-24). Thence it runs posterior-laterally across the lower portion of the cheek at Daying (ST-5). Winding along the angle of the mandible (Jiache ST-6), it ascends in front of the ear, traverses Shangguan (GB-3), and follows the anterior hairline up to the forehead (see Fig. 3.3).

From Daying (ST-5) a facial branch emerges and runs down to Renying (ST-9), and continues along the throat and enters the body in the supraclavicular fossa. It

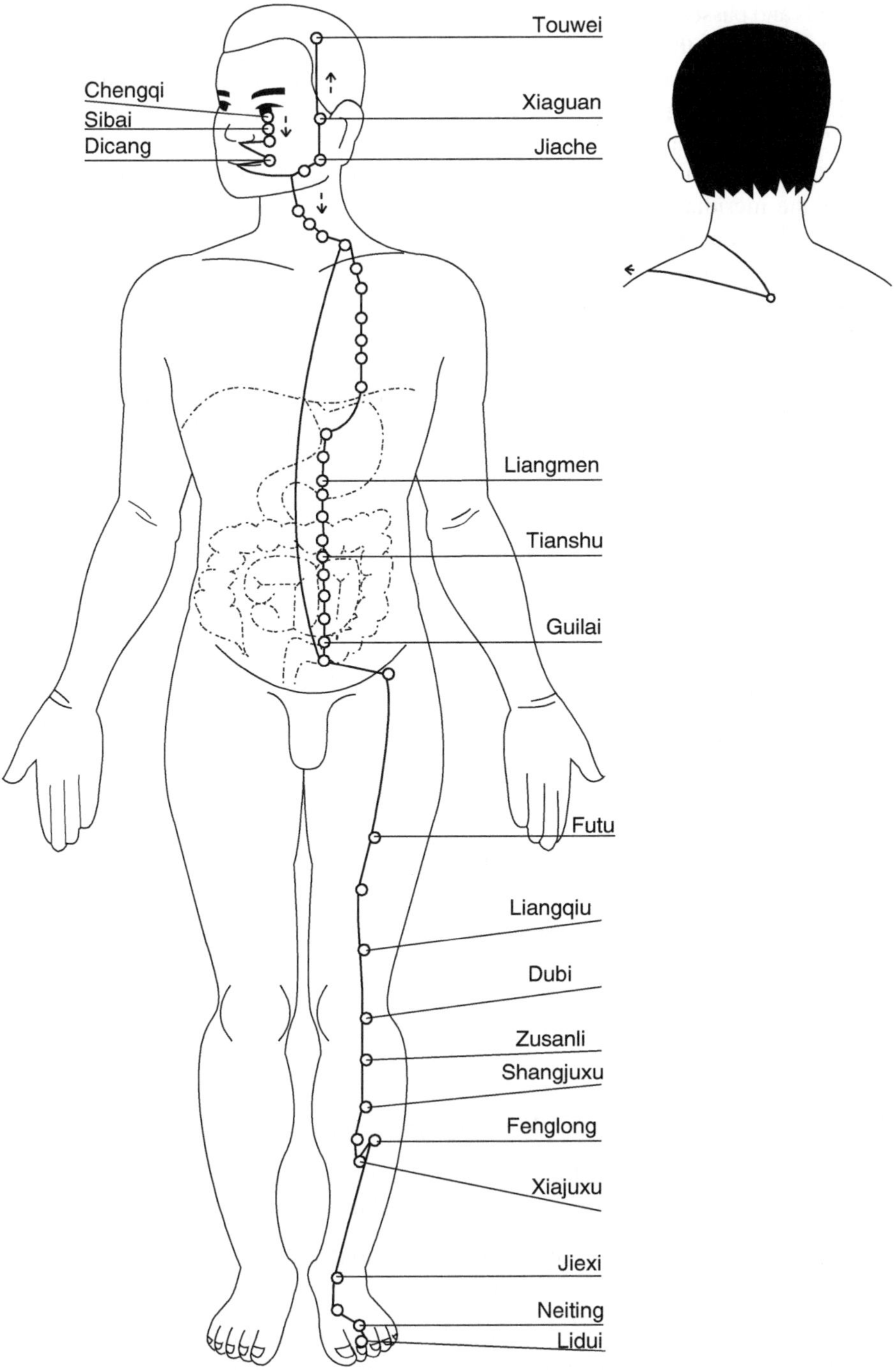

Fig. 3.3 Stomach Meridian of Foot-Yangming

descends and passes through the diaphragm, enters the stomach, its pertaining organ, and connects with the spleen.

From the supraclavicular fossa the straight portion of the meridian runs downward, passing through the nipple, continues by the umbilicus, and enters Qichong (ST-30) on the lateral side of the lower abdomen.

At the lower orifice of the stomach a branch descends inside the abdomen and rejoins the meridian at Qichong (ST-30). The reunited meridian runs downward, traverses Biguan (ST-31), through Futu (ST-32) over the femur, and reaches the knee. From the knee it continues downward along the anterior border of the lateral aspect of the tibia, passes through the dorsum of the foot, and reaches the lateral side of the tip of the second toe.

Near the upper end of the tibia a branch arises at Zusanli (ST-36), 3 *cun* below the knee. It courses downward and enters the lateral side of the middle toe.

A branch at the dorsum of the foot arises at Chongyang (ST-42) and terminates at the medial side of the tip of the great toe, where it links with the Spleen Meridian.

II Main Applications

The acupoints of the Stomach Meridian are mainly used in the acupuncture treatment of diseases of the digestive system, disorders of the head, the face and the sense organs, febrile illnesses, and mental illnesses.

III Commonly Used Acupoints

There are 45 acupoints in all – see Table 3.3. The more useful ones are individually described.

Chengqi (ST-1)

This is the crossing point of the Stomach, the Yangqiao and the Ren Meridians.

Location: With the patient looking directly forward, on the vertical line through the pupil and between the infra-orbital ridge and the eyeball.

Applications: Inflammation of the eye, night blindness, excessive tearing, twitching of the eyelids, and wry mouth and eye.

Techniques and Notes: Push the eyeball upward with the left thumb and insert the needle perpendicularly and slowly 0.3–0.7 *cun* just over the infra-orbital ridge. Do not angle the needle about or twist it. Moxibustion is contraindicated.

Table 3.3 Acupoints of Stomach Meridian of Foot-Yangming

Name	Location	Applications
ST-1	Described separately	
ST-2		
ST-3 Juliao	On face, at intersection of vertical line through pupil and horizontal line just below ala nasi	Wry mouth, eye; twitching of eyelids; epistaxis; toothache; cheek, lip pain
ST-4	Described separately	
ST-5 Daying	Anterior to mandibular angle, just in front of attachment of masseter muscle, where facial artery is palpable	Lockjaw; wry mouth; swelling of the cheek; toothache
ST-6		
ST-7	Described separately	
ST-8		
Acupoints on head and face: for diseases of head, face, eyes, nose, mouth and teeth		
ST-9 Renying	Level with tip of Adam's apple, on path of common carotid artery, at anterior border of sternocleidomastoid muscle	Sore throat; asthma, chest fullness, hypertension
ST-10 Shuitu	On neck, at anterior border of sternocleidomastoid muscle and midpoint of line joining Renying and Qishe	Sore throat; asthma
ST-11 Qishe	On neck, at upper border of medial end of clavicle, between sternal head and clavicular head of sternocleidomastoid muscle	Sore throat; asthma
ST-12 Quepen	At center of supraclavicular fossa, 4 *cun* lateral to anterior midline	Cough, asthma; sore throat; pain in local area
ST-13 Qihu	On chest, below midpoint of lower border of clavicle, 4 *cun* lateral to anterior midline	Asthma, cough, chest congestion
ST-14 Kufang	On chest, in first intercostal space, 4 *cun* lateral to anterior midline	Fullness, pain in chest; cough
ST-15 Wuyi	On chest, in second intercostal space, 4 *cun* lateral to anterior midline	Cough, asthma, fullness and pain in chest and ribs; mastitis
ST-16 Yongchuang	On chest, in third intercostal space, 4 *cun* lateral to anterior midline	Cough, asthma, fullness and pain in chest and ribs; mastitis
ST-17 Ruzhong	On chest, in fourth intercostal space, at center of nipple, 4 *cun* lateral to anterior midline	Serves only as landmark. Not used in acupuncture or moxibustion
ST-18 Rugen	On chest, in fifth intercostal space, directly below nipple, 4 *cun* lateral to anterior midline	Deficient lactation; mastitis, pain in chest
Acupoints on neck and chest: for diseases of throat, chest and lung		
ST-19 Burong	On upper abdomen, 6 *cun* above center of umbilicus and 2 *cun* lateral to anterior midline	Abdominal distention, vomiting, gastric pain, anorexia
ST-20 Chengman	On upper abdomen, 5 *cun* above center of umbilicus and 2 *cun* lateral to anterior midline	Abdominal distention, vomiting, gastric pain, anorexia
ST-21	Described separately	
ST-22 Guanmen	On upper abdomen, 3 *cun* above center of umbilicus and 2 *cun* lateral to anterior midline	Abdominal distention and pain, borborygmus, diarrhea, anorexia, edema
ST-23 Taiyi	On upper abdomen, 2 *cun* above center of umbilicus and 2 *cun* lateral to anterior midline	Gastric pain, indigestion; irritability, mania

(continued)

Table 3.3 (continued)

Name	Location	Applications
ST-24 Huarumen	On upper abdomen, 1 *cun* above center of umbilicus and 2 *cun* lateral to anterior midline	Gastric pain, abdominal distention, vomiting, diarrhea; mania
ST-25	Described separately	
Acupoints on upper abdomen: for diseases of stomach, intestines; mental disorders		
ST-26 Wailing	On lower abdomen, 1 *cun* below center of umbilicus and 2 *cun* lateral to anterior midline	Abdominal pain, diarrhea
ST-27 Daju	On lower abdomen, 2 *cun* below center of umbilicus and 2 *cun* lateral to anterior midline	Lower abdominal distention; dysuria; hernia; spermatorrhea
ST-28 Shuidao	On lower abdomen, 3 *cun* below center of umbilicus and 2 *cun* lateral to anterior midline	Lower abdominal distention; dysuria; hernia
ST-29	Described separately	
ST-30 Qichong	Slightly above inguinal groove, 5 *cun* below center of umbilicus and 2 *cun* lateral to anterior midline	Swelling and pain of external genitalia, hernia; irregular menstruation
Acupoints on lower abdomen: for diseases of external genitalia (male and female)		
ST-31 Biguan	On anterior aspect of thigh and on line connecting anterior superior iliac spine and superior lateral corner of patella, at level of perineum when thigh is flexed, in depression lateral to sartorius muscle	Weakness in legs; hemiplegia; infantile paralysis; aches and pain in waist and legs
ST-32	Described separately	
ST-33 Yinshi	On anterior aspect of thigh and on line connecting anterior superior iliac spine and superior lateral corner of patella, 3 *cun* above this corner	Numbness, weakness, aches and pain of leg and knee; impaired knee flexion
ST-34	Described separately	
ST-35		
Acupoints on thigh and knee: for diseases of local area		
ST-36	Described separately	
ST-37		
ST-38 Tiaokou	On leg, 8 *cun* below Dubi (ST-35), and one middle finger-breadth lateral to anterior crest of tibia	Frozen shoulder; cold pain of the lower extremities; gastric, abdominal pain
ST-39	Described separately	
ST-40		
Acupoints on leg: for mental problems and diseases of stomach and intestine		
ST-41	Described separately	
ST-42 Chongyang Yuan (Source) acupoint	At highest point of dorsum of foot, between tendons of long extensor of hallux and long extensor of toes, where dorsal artery is palpable	Gastric pain, abdominal distention; facial swelling, toothache; psychosis
ST-43 Xiangu Shu (Stream) acupoint	On dorsum of foot, in depression distal to commissure of second and third metatarsal bones	Facial or general edema; swelling, pain of dorsum of foot; redness of eye
ST-44	Described separately	
ST-45		
Acupoints on foot: for diseases of head, face, eyes, nose, mouth, teeth, stomach, intestine; mental disorders		

Sibai (ST-2)

Location: On the face, with the patient looking directly forward, in the depression of the infra-orbital foramen vertically below the pupil.

Applications: Inflammation of the eye, corneal opacity, twitching of the eyelids; wry mouth and eye; and pain in the face.

Techniques and Notes: Insert the needle perpendicularly or obliquely 0.3–0.5 *cun*. Moxibustion is not advisable.

Dicang (ST-4)

This is the crossing point of the Large Intestine, the Stomach and the Yangqiao Meridians.

Location: On the face, lateral to the corner of the mouth, vertically below the pupil.

Applications: Wry mouth; excessive salivation; twitching of the corner of the mouth; and twitching of the eyelids.

Techniques and Notes: With the needle aimed toward Jiache (ST-6) insert the needle subcutaneously 0.5–1.5 *cun*. Moxibustion may be applied.

Jiache (ST-6)

Location: Approximately one width of the middle finger superior and anterior to the mandibular angle at the prominence formed when the masseter muscle contracts (by clenching the teeth).

Applications: Wry mouth; toothache; cheek swelling; and trismus.

Techniques and Notes: Insert the needle perpendicularly 0.3–0.5 *cun*, or subcutaneously with the needle aimed toward Dicang (ST-4) 0.5–1.5 *cun*. Moxibustion may be applied.

Xiaguan (ST-7)

This is the crossing point of the Stomach and the Gallbladder Meridians.

Location: On the face, anterior to the ear, in the depression between the zygomatic arch and the mandibular notch.

Applications: Deafness, tinnitus; wry mouth and eye; trismus; and toothache.

Techniques and Notes: Insert the needle perpendicularly 0.5–1 *cun*. Moxibustion may be applied.

Touwei (ST-8)

This is the crossing point of the Stomach, the Gallbladder and the Yangwei Meridians.

Location: On the side of the head, 0.5 *cun* inside the anterior hairline at the corner of the forehead, and 4.5 *cun* from the midline of the head.

Applications: Dizziness; headache; blurred vision; twitching of the eyelids; and excessive tearing.

Techniques and Notes: Insert the needle 0.5–1 *cun* subcutaneously with the needle aimed posteriorly. Moxibustion is not advisable.

Liangmen (ST-21)

Location: On the upper abdomen, 4 *cun* above the center of the umbilicus and 2 *cun* from the anterior midline.

Applications: Gastric pain, vomiting, anorexia, abdominal distention, and diarrhea.

Techniques and Notes: Insert the needle perpendicularly 0.5–1 *cun*. Moxibustion may be applied.

Tianshu (ST-25)

This is also the Front-Mu acupoint of the Large Intestine Meridian.

Location: On the middle abdomen, 2 *cun* laterally from the center of the umbilicus.

Applications: Abdominal distention, borborygmus, peri-umbilical pain; constipation, diarrhea, dysentery; irregular menstruation, amenorrhea, and dysmenorrhea.

Techniques and Notes: Insert the needle perpendicularly 0.8–1.2 *cun*. Moxibustion may be applied.

Guilai (ST-29)

Location: On the lower abdomen, 4 *cun* below the center of the umbilicus and 2 *cun* from the anterior midline.

Applications: Abdominal pain; amenorrhea, dysmenorrhea, irregular menstruation, vaginal discharge; prolapse of the uterus; impotence, spermatorrhea; and hernia.

Techniques and Notes: Insert the needle perpendicularly 0.8–1.2 *cun*. Moxibustion may be applied.

Futu (ST-32)

ST-32 and LI-18 are both named Futu. Their names in Chinese are quite different.

Location: On the anterior thigh, on the line connecting the anterior superior iliac spine and the superior lateral corner of the patella, 6 *cun* from this corner.

Applications: Pain in the lumbar and iliac regions; coldness in the knee; paralysis or paresis of the lower extremities; and beriberi.

Techniques and Notes: Insert the needle perpendicularly 1–2 *cun*. Moxibustion may be applied.

Liangqiu (ST-34)

This is the Xi (Cleft) acupoint of the Stomach Meridian.

Location: With the knee flexed, on the anterior thigh, on the line connecting the anterior superior iliac spine and the superior lateral corner of the patella, 2 *cun* above this corner.

Applications: Pain and numbness in the knee; acute stomachache, heartburn; mastitis; and numbness and paresis of the lower extremities.

Techniques and Notes: Insert the needle perpendicularly 1–1.5 *cun*. Moxibustion may be applied.

Dubi (ST-35)

Location: With the knee flexed, just below the patella in the depression lateral to the patellar ligament.

Applications: Pain, swelling and impairment of the knee joint; and beriberi.

Techniques and Notes: Insert the needle toward the back and angled slightly medially, 0.8–1.5 *cun*. Moxibustion may be applied.

Zusanli (ST-36)

This is the He (Sea) acupoint of the Stomach Meridian.

Location: On the antero-lateral leg, 3 *cun* below Dubi (ST-35), one middle finger breadth lateral to the anterior crest of the tibia.

Applications: Gastric pain, vomiting, abdominal distention, diarrhea, constipation, dysentery; emaciation due to general deficiency; palpitations of the heart; shortness of breath; dizziness, insomnia; paralysis from a stroke; edema; numbness and pain of the lower extremities; mastitis; mental problems.

Techniques and Notes: Insert the needle perpendicularly 1–2 *cun*. Moxibustion may be applied.

Shangjuxu (ST-37)

This is also the Lower He (Sea) Point of the Large Intestine Meridian.

Location: On the antero-lateral leg, 6 *cun* below Dubi (ST-35), one middle finger breadth lateral to the anterior crest of the tibia.

Applications: Borborygmus, abdominal pain, diarrhea, constipation, intestinal ulcer; and muscular atrophy, numbness, pain and flaccidity of the lower extremities.

Techniques and Notes: Insert the needle perpendicularly 1–1.5 *cun*. Moxibustion may be applied.

Xiajuxu (ST-39)

This is also the Lower He (Sea) acupoint of the Small Intestine Meridian.

Location: On the antero-lateral lower leg, 9 *cun* below Dubi (ST-35), one middle finger breadth lateral to the anterior crest of the tibia.

Applications: Lower abdominal pain, diarrhea with bloody and purulent stools; pain in the back with radiation to the testis; and numbness and paralysis of the lower extremities.

Techniques and Notes: Insert the needle perpendicularly 1–1.5 *cun*. Moxibustion may be applied.

Fenglong (ST-40)

This is the Luo (Connecting) acupoint of the Stomach Meridian.

Location: On the antero-lateral leg, 8 *cun* above the tip of the lateral malleolus, lateral to Tiaokou (ST-38) and two middle finger breadths lateral to the anterior crest of tibia.

Applications: Cough with much sputum; asthma; constipation; paresis of the lower limbs; headache; dizziness; psychosis; epilepsy; and edema.

Techniques and Notes: Insert the needle perpendicularly 1–1.5 *cun*. Moxibustion may be applied.

Jiexi (ST-41)

This is the Jing (River) acupoint of the Stomach Meridian.

Location: At the midpoint of the transverse crease of the ankle joint, in the depression between the tendons of the long extensor of the hallux and the long extensor of the toes.

Applications: Headache, dizziness; abdominal distention, constipation; epilepsy; ankle pain; and paresis of the lower extremities.

Techniques and Notes: Insert the needle perpendicularly 0.5–1 *cun*. Moxibustion may be applied.

Neiting (ST-44)

This is the Ying (Spring) acupoint of the Stomach Meridian.

Location: On the dorsum of the foot, at the margin of the darker and lighter skin proximal to the web between the second and third toes.

Applications: Toothache; sore throat; wry mouth; epistaxis; abdominal distention, constipation, gastric pain; febrile diseases; and swelling and pain of the dorsum of the foot.

Techniques and Notes: Insert the needle perpendicularly 0.3–0.5 *cun*. Moxibustion may be applied.

Lidui (ST-45)

This is the Jing (Well) acupoint of the Stomach Meridian.

Location: On the lateral aspect of the distal segment of the second toe, 0.1 *cun* posterior to the corner of the toenail.

Applications: Epistaxis; toothache; sore throat; febrile diseases; dream-disturbed sleep; and psychosis.

Techniques and Notes: Insert the needle subcutaneously 0.1 *cun*. Moxibustion may be applied.

Section 4 Spleen Meridian of Foot-Taiyin

I Pathway

The Spleen Meridian of Foot-Taiyin starts at the tip of the hallux. It runs along the medial aspect of the hallux along the border between the darker and lighter skin, ascends to the front of the medial malleolus, and continues up the medial aspect of the leg. It then follows the posterior edge of the tibia and passes in front of the Liver Meridian. Continuing along the antero-medial knee and thigh it enters the abdomen, in which it reaches the spleen and connects with the stomach. Thence it ascends through the diaphragm and along the esophagus to reach the root of the tongue where it spreads over its under surface (see Fig. 3.4).

A branch arises at the stomach and goes upward through the diaphragm. It flows into the heart to link with the Heart Meridian.

II Main Applications

The acupoints of the Spleen Meridian are used mainly in the treatment of disorders of the throat, the chest and the lung.

III Commonly Used Acupoints

There are 21 acupoints in all – see Table 3.4. The more useful ones are individually described.

Yinbai (SP-1)

This is the Jing (Well) Acupoint of the Spleen Meridian.

Location: On the medial side of the distal segment of the hallux, 0.1 *cun* posterior to the corner of the nail.

Applications: Metrorrhagia or excessive menses; hematochezia; hematuria; abdominal distention; dream-disturbed sleep; psychosis; and convulsion.

Techniques and Notes: Insert the needle subcutaneously 0.1 *cun*. Moxibustion may be applied.

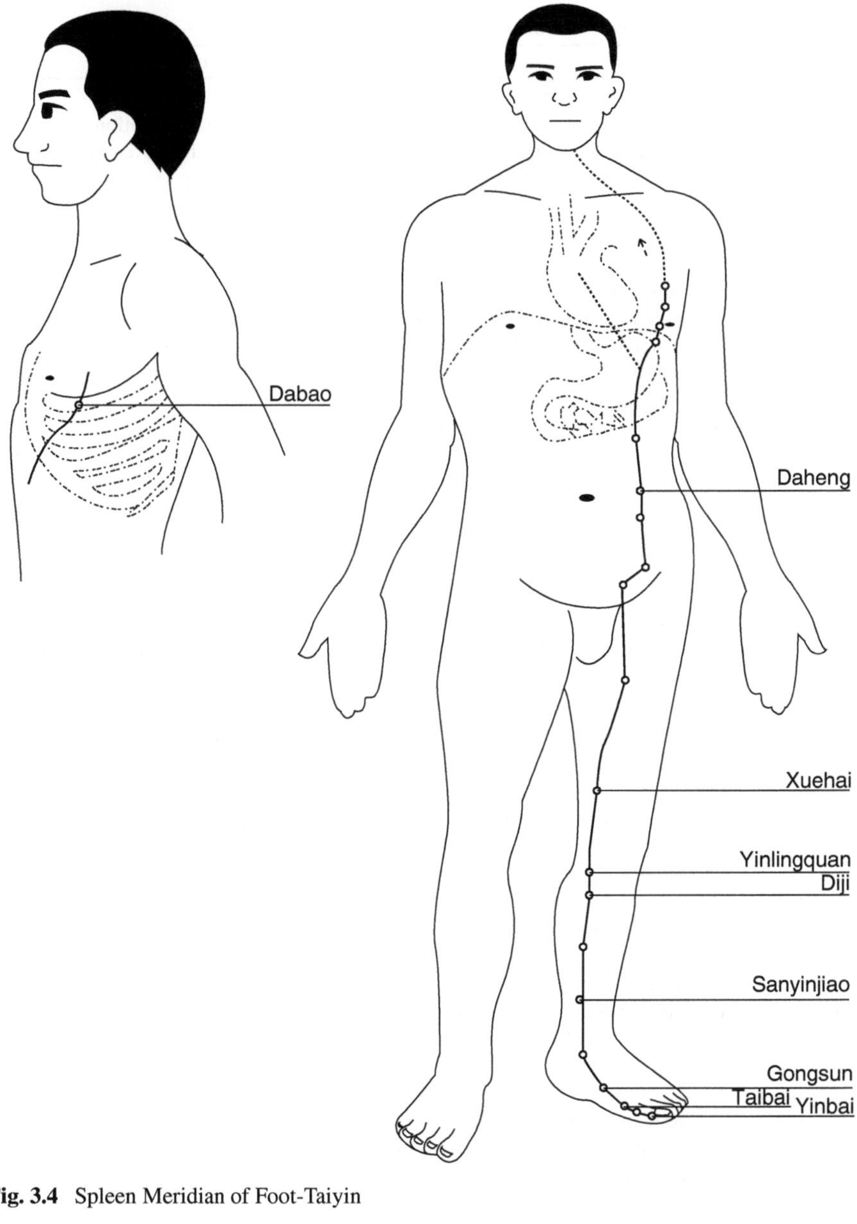

Fig. 3.4 Spleen Meridian of Foot-Taiyin

Taibai (SP-3)

This is the Shu (Stream) and the Source acupoint of the Spleen Meridian.

Location: On the medial aspects of the foot, proximal and inferior to the head of the first metatarsal bone, at the border of the lighter and darker skin.

Table 3.4 Acupoints of Spleen Meridian

Name	Location	Applications
P-1	Described separately	
SP-2 Dadu Ying (Spring) acupoint	On medial side of foot, distal-inferior to first metatarsophalangeal joint, in depression at junction of lighter and darker skin	Abdominal distention, gastric Pain; high fever without sweating
SP-3	Described separately	
SP-4		
SP-5 Shangqiu Jing (River) acupoint	In depression distal-inferior to medial malleolus, midway between tuberosity of navicular bone and tip of medial malleolus	Abdominal distention, diarrhea, constipation, borborygmus; cough; jaundice; pain in foot and ankle; hemorrhoid
SP-6	Described separately	
SP-7 Lougu	Posterior to medial border of tibia, 3 *cun* above SP-6, on line joining tip of medial malleolus and SP-9	Abdominal distention, borborygmus; cold leg and knee; numbness and paresis of knee and leg
SP-8		
SP-9	Described separately	
SP-10		
SP-11 Jimen	On line drawn from SP-10 to SP-12, 6 *cun* above SP-10	Difficult urination, enuresis; inguinal pain and swelling
PSP-12 Chongmen	At lateral end of inguinal groove, 3.5 *cun* lateral to midpoint of upper border of symphysis pubis, lateral to external iliac artery	Orchitis; abdominal pain; hernia; metrorrhagia; vaginitis; hemorrhoid
SP-13 Fushe	On lower abdomen, 4 *cun* below center of umbilicus, 0.7 *cun* above Chongmen (SP-12) and 4 *cun* lateral to anterior midline	Abdominal pain, hernia, appendicitis
SP-14 Fujie	On lower abdomen, 1.3 *cun* below Daheng (SP 15) and 4 *cun* lateral to anterior midline	Peri-umbilical pain; hernia; diarrhea, constipation
SP-15	Described separately	
SP-16 Fuai	On upper abdomen, 3 *cun* above center of umbilicus and 4 *cun* lateral to anterior midline	Abdominal pain, indigestion, constipation, dysentery
SP-17 Shidou	On lateral side of chest and in fifth intercostal space, 6 *cun* lateral to anterior midline	Fullness and pain in chest and subcostal region
SP-18 Tianxi	On lateral side of chest and in fourth intercostal space, 6 *cun* lateral to anterior midline	Chest pain, cough; mastitis, insufficient lactation
SP-19 Xiongxiang	On lateral side of chest and in third intercostal space, 6 *cun* lateral to anterior midline	Fullness and pain in chest and subcostal region
SP-20 Zhourong	On lateral side of chest and in second intercostal space, 6 *cun* lateral to anterior midline	Fullness in chest and subcostal region, cough
SP-21 Dabao Collateral meridian of spleen	On lateral side of chest and on mid-axillary line, in sixth intercostals space	Pain in chest and subcostal region; asthma; total body pain; weakness of all limbs

Applications: Abdominal distention and pain, gastric pain, diarrhea; heaviness in the body; and hemorrhoids.

Techniques and Notes: Insert the needle perpendicularly or obliquely 0.5–0.8 *cun*. Moxibustion may be applied.

Gongsun (SP-4)

This is the Luo (Connecting) acupoint of the Spleen Meridian and is also the Confluence acupoint between the Spleen and the Chong Meridians.

Location: On the medial aspect of the foot, in the depression distal and inferior to the base of the first metatarsal bone, at the border of the lighter and darker skin.

Applications: Gastric pain, vomiting, abdominal pain, diarrhea, hematochezia; chest pain, pressure in the chest, distention in the flank; and irregular menstruation.

Techniques and Notes: Insert the needle perpendicularly 0.5–1 *cun*. Moxibustion may be applied.

Sanyinjiao (SP-6)

Location: On the posterior border of the medial aspect of the tibia, 3 *cun* directly above the tip of the medial malleolus.

Applications: Irregular menstruation, amenorrhea, metrorrhagia, dysmenorrhea; vaginitis with white or red discharge; dystocia (difficult labor or childbirth), postpartum hemorrhage, excessive lochia; spermatorrhea, premature ejaculation, impotence; enuresis, dysuria; edema; borborygmus, diarrhea, abdominal distention; beriberi; myalgia (muscle pain); skin disorders; insomnia; headache; and dizziness.

Techniques and Notes: Insert the needle perpendicularly 1–1.5 *cun*. Moxibustion may be applied. Acupuncture at this acupoint is **contraindicated for pregnant woman**.

Diji (SP-8)

This is the Xi (Cleft) acupoint of the Spleen Meridian.

Location: On the posterior border of the medial aspect of the tibia, on the line connecting Yinlingquan (SP-9) and the tip of the medial malleolus, at 3 *cun* below Yilingquan (SP-9).

Applications: Abdominal pain, diarrhea; edema, reduced ability to urinate; irregular menstruation, dysmenorrhea; and spermatorrhea or impotence.

Techniques and Notes: Insert the needle perpendicularly 1–2 *cun*. Moxibustion may be applied.

Yinlingquan (SP-9)

This is the He (Sea) acupoint of the Spleen Meridian.

Location: On the medial aspect of the leg, in the depression posterior and inferior to the medial condyle of the tibia.

Applications: Abdominal distention, diarrhea; jaundice; dysuria, edema; and knee pain or paralysis of the lower limbs.

Techniques and Notes: Insert the needle perpendicularly 1–2 *cun*. Moxibustion may be applied

Xuehai (SP-10)

Location: With the knee flexed, on the medial side of the thigh, 2 *cun* above the superior medial corner of the patella, on the prominence of the medial head of the quadriceps muscle. Alternately, with the knee flexed cup your right palm to his left knee so that the four fingers are directly above the knee pointing at the hip and the thumb resting at an angle of 45° to the index finger. The Xuehai acupoint is at the tip of your thumb.

Applications: Irregular menstruation, amenorrhea, dysmenorrhea, metrorrhagia; and urticaria, eczema, and erysipelas.

Techniques and Notes: Insert the needle 1–1.5 *cun* perpendicularly or obliquely upward. Moxibustion may be applied.

Daheng (SP-15)

This is the crossing point of the Spleen and the Yinwei Meridians.

Location: On the abdomen, at 4 *cun* lateral to the center of the umbilicus.

Applications: Diarrhea, constipation, and abdominal pain.

Techniques and Notes: Insert the needle perpendicularly 1–1.5 *cun*. Moxibustion may be applied.

Section 5 Heart Meridian of Hand-Shaoyin

I Pathway

The Heart Meridian of Hand-Shaoyin originates in the heart. As it emerges it spreads over the "heart system" (the collaterals connecting the heart with the other *zang–fu* organs). From the "heart system" it follows three paths. The meridian itself is very short. It passes through the diaphragm to connect with the small intestine (see Fig. 3.5).

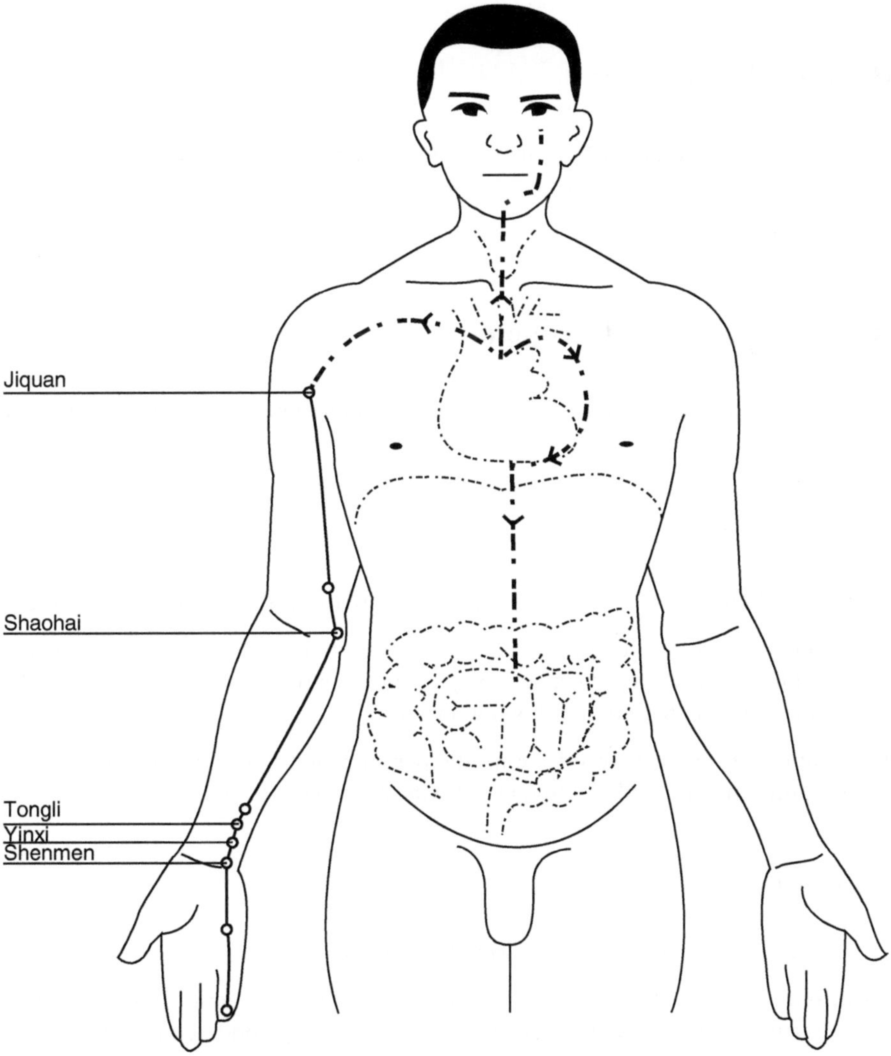

Fig. 3.5 Heart Meridian of Hand-Shaoyin

An ascending branch emerges from the "heart system" and runs along the esophagus to connect with the "eye system" (the collaterals connecting the eyes with the brain).

A straight branch emerges from the "heart system," courses to the lung and continues to the axilla, where it emerges on the surface. It then courses along the posterior-medial arm, behind the Lung and the Pericardium Meridians, past the antecubital fossa and through the region of the pisiform bone (the wrist bone at the medial end of the proximal row of wrist bones), and enters the palm. From the palm it courses along the medial aspect of the little finger to its tip, where it links with the Small Intestine Meridian.

II Main Applications

The acupoints of the Heart Meridian are used mainly in the treatment of illnesses of the heart and chest, mental diseases and diseases of the regions along the path of this meridian.

III Commonly Used Acupoints

There are 9 acupoints in all – see Table 3.5. The more useful ones are individually described.

Jiquan (HT-1)

Location: At the apex of the axillary fossa, where the axillary artery is palpable.

Indications: Pain or palpitations of the heart; chest tightness or shortness of breath; paresis of the upper extremities; hemiplegia due to a stroke; fullness and pain in the chest and flank; and pain in the shoulder and arm.

Techniques and Notes: Insert the needle perpendicularly or obliquely 0.5–1 *cun*. **Do not puncture the axillary artery**. Moxibustion may be applied.

Shaohai (HT-3)

This is the He (Sea) acupoint of the Heart Meridian.

Location: With the elbow flexed, at the midpoint of the line connecting the medial end of the transverse antecubital crease and the medial epicondyle of the humerus.

Table 3.5 Acupoints of Heart Meridian

Name	Location	Indications
HT-1	Described separately	
HT-2 Qingling	On medial side of arm and on line connecting Jiquan (HT-1) and Shaohai (HT-3), 3 *cun* above antecubital crease, in groove medial to biceps muscle	Yellow eyes; flank pain; pain in arm and shoulder
HT-3	Described separately	
HT-4 Lingdao Jing (River) acupoint	On palmer aspect of forearm, on radial side of tendon of flexor carpi ulnaris muscle, 1.5 *cun* proximal to transverse crease of wrist	Cardiac pain, pain in the elbow and arm; hysteria
HT-5		
HT-6	Described separately	
HT-7		
HT-8 Shaofu Ying (Spring) acupoint	Between fourth and fifth metacarpal bones, at part of palm touched by tip of little finger when making fist	Palpitation, chest pain; genital itch; dysuria, enuresis; hotness in palm; easily frightened
HT-9 Shaochong Jing (Well) acupoint	On radial side of distal segment of little finger, 0.1 *cun* posterior to corner of nail	Febrile diseases; stroke with coma; palpitations, cardiac pain; psychosis

Indications: Cardiac pain, numbness of the arm; hand tremors; forgetfulness; pain in the axilla and flank; impaired movement of the elbow joint; and scrofula.

Techniques and Notes: Insert the needle perpendicularly 0.5–1 *cun*. Moxibustion may be applied.

Tongli (HT-5)

This is the Luo (Connecting) acupoint of the Heart Meridian.

Location: On the palmar aspect of the forearm, on the radial side of the tendon of the muscle flexor carpi ulnaris, 1 *cun* proximal to the transverse crease of the wrist.

Indications: Sudden loss of the voice; stiffness of the tongue with difficulty to talk; palpitations with panic; and pain in the wrist and forearm.

Techniques and Notes: Insert the needle perpendicularly 0.3–0.5 *cun*. Moxibustion may be applied.

Yinxi (HT-6)

This is the Xi (Cleft) acupoint of the Heart Meridian.

Location: On the palmar aspect of the forearm, on the radial side of the tendon of the muscle flexor carpi ulnaris, 0.5 *cun* proximal to the transverse crease of the wrist.

Indications: Night sweats; cardiac pain; panic, palpitations; hemoptysis, epistaxis; and sudden loss of voice.

Techniques and Notes: Insert the needle perpendicularly 0.3–0.5 *cun*. Moxibustion may be applied.

Shenmen (HT-7)

This is the Shu (Stream) as well as the Yuan (Source) acupoint of the Heart Meridian.

Location: At the ulnar end of the transverse crease of the wrist, in the depression on the radial side of the tendon of the muscle flexor carpi ulnaris.

Indications: Insomnia and forgetfulness; palpitations due to fright or panic; cardiac pain; restlessness; psychosis; epilepsy; depression with easy crying; and hysteria.

Techniques and Notes: Insert the needle perpendicularly 0.3–0.5 *cun*. Moxibustion may be applied.

Section 6 Small Intestine Meridian of Hand-Taiyang

I Pathway

The Small Intestine Meridian of Hand-Taiyin starts from the medial side of the tip of the fifth finger and courses along the medial-dorsal hand to the wrist. Passing the styloid process of the ulna, it courses along the posterior-lateral forearm, goes between the olecranon of the ulna and the medial epicondyle of the humerus, and continues along the posterior-lateral upper arm to the shoulder joint. Circling around the scapular region it meets Dazhui (GV-14) on the superior aspect of the shoulder. It turns downward to the supraclavicular fossa, where it enters the body and connects with the heart. It then descends along the esophagus, passes through the diaphragm, crosses the stomach and finally enters the small intestine (see Fig. 3.6).

In the supraclavicular fossa a branch ascends along the neck past the cheek to the outer canthus of the eye. It then turns toward the ear and enters it near the tragus. At the lower cheek a branch courses through the infra-orbital region, passes the lateral side of the nose and reaches the inner canthus. There it links with the Bladder Meridian of Foot-Taiyang.

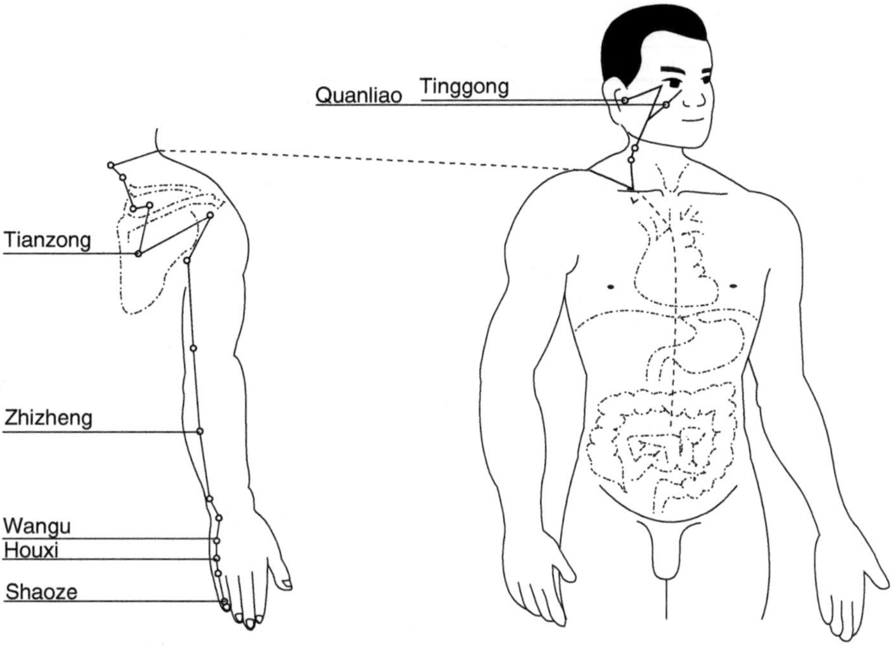

Fig. 3.6 Small Intestine Meridian of Hand-Taiyang

II Main Applications

The acupoints of the Small Intestine Meridian are used mainly in the treatment of diseases of the head, nape, ear, eye and throat, back, shoulder, and the regions along its path. They can also be used to treat febrile and mental diseases.

III Commonly Used Acupoints

There are 19 acupoints in all – see Table 3.6. The more useful ones are individually described.

Shaoze (SI-1)

This is the Jing (Well) acupoint of the Small Intestine Meridian.

Table 3.6 Acupoints of Small Intestine Meridian

Name	Location	Applications
SI-1	Described separately	
SI-2 Qiangu Ying (Spring) acupoint	On ulnar side of hand, distal to fifth metacarpophalangeal joint, at junction of darker and lighter skin	Numbness of fingers; febrile diseases; headache; sore throat
SI-3	Described separately	
SI-4		
SI-5 Yanggu Jing (River) acupoint	At ulnar end of transverse crease on dorsal aspect of wrist, in depression between styloid process of ulna and cuneiform bone of wrist	Headache, dizziness; neck and submandibular swelling; lateral arm pain; hand and wrist pain; febrile diseases; psychosis; epilepsy
SI-6 Yanglao Xi (Cleft) acupoint	On ulnar side of dorsal aspect of forearm, in depression proximal to and on radial side of head of ulna	Blurred vision; pain in the shoulder and arm; acute back pain
SI-7	Described separately	
SI-8 Xiaohai He (Sea) acupoint	On medial side of elbow, in depression between olecranon and medial epicondyle of humerus	Pain or paresis in elbow and arm; psychosis, epilepsy, depression; headache, dizziness; tinnitus, deafness
SI-9 Jianzhen	Posterior-inferior to shoulder joint, 1 *cun* above posterior end of axillary fold with arm adducted	Pain in scapular region; pain and numbness of hand and arm; inability to raise arm
SI-10 Naoshu	On shoulder, above posterior end of axillary fold, in depression inferior to scapular spine	Swelling of shoulder; inability to raise arm from pain in shoulder; scrofula
SI-11	Described separately	
SI-12 Bingfeng	On scapula, at center of supraspinous fossa, directly above Tianzong (SI-11), in depression formed when arm is raised	Inability to raise arm from pain in shoulder; numbness and pain of arm
SI-13 Quyuan	On scapula, at medial end of supraspinous fossa, at midpoint of line connecting Naoshu (SI 10) and spinous process of second thoracic vertebra	Pain and stiffness in scapular region
SI-14 Jianwaishu	On back, 3 *cun* lateral to lower border of spinous process of first thoracic vertebra	Aching of shoulder and back, pain and rigidity of neck
SI-15 Jianzhongshu	On back, 2 *cun* lateral to lower border of spinous process of seventh cervical vertebra	Cough, labored breathing; pain in shoulder and back
SI-16 Tianchuang	On lateral aspect of neck, posterior to sternocleidomastoid muscle and Futu (LI-18), on level of laryngeal protuberance	Tinnitus, deafness; sore throat; stiffness and pain in neck
SI-17 Tianrong	On lateral side of neck, posterior to mandibular angle, in depression on anterior border of sternocleidomastoid muscle	Tinnitus, deafness; sore throat; stiffness and pain in neck
SI-18	Described separately	
SI-19		

Location: On the ulnar side of the little finger, 0.1 *cun* posterior to the corner of the nail.

Applications: Headache; corneal opacity; sore throat; mastitis; insufficient lactation; febrile diseases; and stroke or loss of consciousness.

Techniques and Notes: Insert the needle subcutaneously 0.1 *cun*, or prick the acupoint to cause slight bleeding. Moxibustion may be applied.

Houxi (SI-3)

This is the Shu (Stream) acupoint of the Small Intestine Meridian and also the Confluence acupoint between the Small Intestine Meridian and the Du Meridian.

Location: On the ulnar side of the hand, proximal to the fifth metacarpophalangeal joint, at the end of the transverse crease and the border between the darker and lighter skin, with the hand in a loose fist.

Applications: Headache, stiff neck; lumbosacral pain; spasmodic pain of the finger, elbow and arm; redness of the eye; deafness; psychosis; epilepsy; depression; and night sweats.

Techniques and Notes: Insert the needle perpendicularly 0.5–1 *cun*. Moxibustion may be applied.

Wangu (SI-4)

This is the Yuan (Source) acupoint of the Small Intestine Meridian.

Location: On the ulnar side of the dorsum of the hand, in the depression between the fifth metacarpal and the hamate bones, at the junction of the darker and lighter skin. (The hamate is the carpal bone in the distal row at the ulnar end.)

Applications: Stiffness and pain of the nape and head; tinnitus; corneal opacity; diabetes; jaundice; spasm in the fingers, pain in the wrist, and weakness of the hand.

Techniques and Notes: Insert the needle perpendicularly 0.3–0.5 *cun*. Moxibustion may be applied.

Zhizheng (SI-7)

This is the Luo (Connecting) acupoint of the Small Intestine Meridian.

Location: On the medial-dorsal forearm, on the line joining Yanggu (SI-5) and Xiaohai (SI-8), 5 *cun* proximal to the dorsal transverse crease of the wrist.

Applications: Headache; stiff neck; febrile diseases; dizziness; and aches in the elbow and arm.

Techniques and Notes: Insert the needle perpendicularly 0.3–0.8 *cun*. Moxibustion may be applied.

Tianzong (SI-11)

Location: On the scapula, at the center of the infraspinous fossa, at the level with the fourth thoracic vertebra.

Applications: Pain in the scapular region; pain in the lateral-posterior aspect of the elbow and arm; labored breathing; and mastitis.

Techniques and Notes: Insert the needle perpendicularly or obliquely 0.5–1 *cun*. Moxibustion may be applied.

Quanliao (SI-18)

This is the crossing point of the Sanjiao and the Small Intestine Meridians.

Location: On the face, directly below the outer canthus, in the depression below the zygomatic bone.

Applications: Wry eye and mouth; twitching of the eyelids; toothache; cheek swelling; and facial pain.

Techniques and Notes: Insert the needle perpendicularly 0.3–0.5 *cun* or obliquely 0.5–1 *cun*. Moxibustion may be applied.

Tinggong (SI-19)

This is the crossing point of the Sanjiao, the Gallbladder and the Small Intestine Meridians.

Location: On the face, anterior to the tragus and posterior to the condylar process of the mandible, in the depression formed when the mouth opens.

Applications: Tinnitus, deafness, drainage from the ear; toothache; and impairment of mandibular joint.

Techniques and Notes: Insert the needle perpendicularly 1–1.5 *cun* with the mouth open. Moxibustion may be applied.

Section 7 Bladder Meridian of Foot-Taiyang

I Pathway

The Bladder Meridian of Foot-Taiyang starts from the inner canthus of the eye. It ascends to the forehead, then joins the Du Meridian at the vertex. At the vertex a branch runs to the temple. The main meridian enters and communicates with the brain from the vertex. It then emerges, descends along the posterior neck and bifurcates. Both arms descend between the scapula and the vertebral column (see Fig. 3.7).

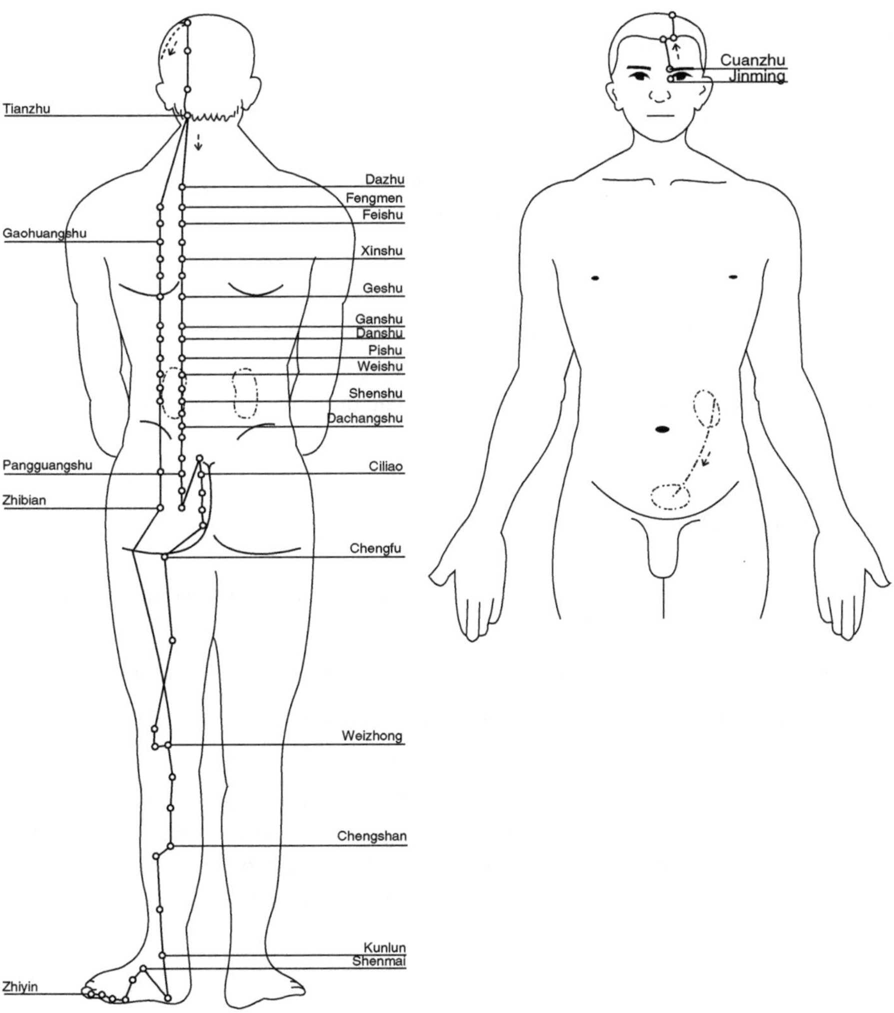

Fig. 3.7 Bladder Meridian of Foot-Taiyang

The more medial arm reaches the lumbar region, where it enters the body through the paravertebral muscle. It connects with the kidney, then continues to the urinary bladder. Before it enters the body in the lumbar region it gives off a branch, which descends through the gluteal region to the popliteal fossa.

The more lateral arm descends along the medial border of the scapula through the gluteal region and reaches the popliteal fossa, where it joins the branch from the other arm. From the popliteal fossa the re-joined meridian continues to descend, through the gastrocnemius muscle, to the posterior aspect of the external malleolus. It continues along the tuberosity of the fifth metatarsal bone and reaches the lateral tip of the fifth toe, where it links with the Kidney Meridian of Foot-Shaoyin.

II Main Applications

The acupoints of the Bladder Meridian are used mainly in the treatment of diseases of the head, nape, eyes, lumbar region and the lower extremities, and mental diseases. The Back-Shu acupoints of this meridian are used in the treatment of diseases of their respective *zang–fu* organs and tissues.

III Commonly Used Acupoints

There are 67 acupoints in all – see Table 3.7. The more useful ones are individually described.

Jingming (BL-1)

This is the crossing point of the Small Intestine, the Bladder, the Stomach, the Yinqiao and the Yangqiao Meridians.

Location: On the face, in the depression slightly above the inner canthus of the eye.

Applications: Inflammation of the eye; corneal opacity; excessive tearing induced by wind; blurry vision, night blindness; and acute low back pain.

Techniques and Notes: With the eye closed push the eyeball gently to the side. Puncture perpendicularly and slowly 0.3–0.5 *cun* along the orbital wall. **Do not twist, lift or thrust the needle more than minimally necessary**. After withdrawal of the needle press the puncture site for 1–2 min to avoid bleeding. **Moxibustion is forbidden**.

Table 3.7 Acupoints of the Bladder Meridian

Name	Location	Applications
BL-1	Described separately	
BL-2		
BL-3 Meichong	On head, directly above BL-2, 0.5 *cun* within hairline, between GV-24 (Shenting) and BL-4	Headache; dizziness; epilepsy; nasal congestion
BL-4 Qucha	On head, 0.5 *cun* within hairline, 1.5 *cun* lateral to GV-24, at junction of medial third and lateral two-thirds of distance from GV-24 to ST-8	Frontal headache; blurred vision; eye pain; nasal congestion
BL-5 Wuchu	1 *cun* directly above anterior hairline, 1.5 *cun* from midline	Headache; dizziness; blurred vision
BL-6 Cheng-guang	2.5 *cun* above anterior hairline, 1.5 *cun* from midline	Headache; eye diseases; nose diseases
BL-7 Tongtian	4 *cun* above anterior hairline, 1.5 *cun* from midline	Headache; dizziness, nose diseases
BL-8 Luoque	5.5 *cun* above anterior hairline, 1.5 *cun* from midline	Dizziness; tinnitus; psychosis; blurred vision
BL-9 Yuzhen	On occiput, 2.5 *cun* superior to posterior hairline, 1.3 *cun* from midline, in depression at upper border of occipital protuberance	Headache; eye pain; nose diseases
BL-10		
BL-11		
BL-12	Described separately	
BL-13		
BL-14 Jueyinshu Back-Shu acupoint of Pericardium	On back, 1.5 *cun* from midline, at level of lower border of spinous process of fourth thoracic vertebra	Cardiac pain; palpitations of heart; chest tightness; cough; vomiting
BL-15	Described separately	
BL-16 Dushu	On back, 1.5 *cun* from midline, at level of lower border of spinous process of sixth thoracic vertebra	Cardiac pain; abdominal pain and distention; borborygmus; hiccup
BL-17		
BL-18		
BL-19	Described separately	
BL-20		
BL-21		
BL-22 Sanjiaoshu Back-Shu acupoint of Sanjiao	On back, 1.5 *cun* from midline, at level of lower border of spinous process of first lumbar vertebra	Edema; dysuria; epigastric pain; abdominal distention, vomiting, borborygmus

(continued)

Table 3.7 (continued)

Name	Location	Applications
BL-23	Described separately	
BL-24 Qihaishu	On back, 1.5 *cun* from midline, at level of lower border of spinous process of third lumbar vertebra	Low back pain; dysmenorrhea; borborygmus; hemorrhoids
BL-25	Described separately	
BL-26 Quanyuan-shu	On back, 1.5 *cun* from midline, at level of lower border of spinous process of fifth lumbar vertebra	Low back pain; abdominal distention; diarrhea; enuresis
BL-27 Xi-Aochang-shu Back-Shu acupoint of Small Intestine	On sacrum, 1.5 *cun* from middle sacral crest, level with first sacral foramen	Spermatorrhea; enuresis; white vaginal discharge; abdominal pain; diarrhea; pain in low back and leg
BL-28	Described separately	
BL-29 Zhonglushu	On sacrum, 1.5 *cun* from middle sacral crest, level with third posterior sacral foramen	Low back stiffness and pain; diabetes; dysentery
BL-30 Baihuanshu	On sacrum, 1.5 *cun* from middle sacral crest, level with fourth sacral foramen	Low back and leg pain; white vaginal discharge; irregular menstruation; spermatorrhea
BL-31 Shangliao	On sacrum, at first sacral foramen	Low back pain; irregular menstruation; vaginal discharge; dysuria and defecation; spermatorrhea; impotence
BL-32	Described separately	
BL-33 Zhongliao	On sacrum, at third sacral foramen	Irregular menstruation; vaginal discharge; low back pain; dysuria; constipation
BL-34 Xialiao	On sacrum, at fourth sacral foramen	Low back pain; dysuria; constipation or diarrhea
BL-35 Huiyang	On sacrum, 0.5 *cun* lateral to tip of coccyx	Impotence; spermatorrhea; vaginal discharge; diarrhea; hemorrhoids
BL-36	Described separately	
BL-37 Yinmen	On posterior thigh, 6 *cun* below BL-36 on line connecting BL-36 and BL-40	Low back pain and stiffness; numbness or paresis of lower extremities
BL-38 Fuxi	On lateral end of popliteal crease, 1 *cun* above BL-39, medial to tendon of femoral biceps muscle	Pain, numbness, spasm around popliteal fossa
BL-39 Weiyang Lower He (Sea) acupoint for Sanjiao	On lateral end of popliteal crease, medial to tendon of femoral biceps muscle	Abdominal distention; dysuria; low back pain and stiffness; pain and spasm of lower extremities
BL-40	Described separately	

(continued)

Table 3.7 (continued)

Name	Location	Applications
BL-41 Fufen	On back, 3 *cun* from midline, at level of lower border of spinous process of second thoracic vertebra	Stiffness and pain in neck, shoulder, and back; numbness of elbow and arm
BL-42 Pohu	On back, 3 *cun* from midline, at level of lower border of spinous process of third thoracic vertebra	Cough, labored breathing; pulmonary tuberculosis; shoulder and back pain
BL-43	Described separately	
BL-44 Shentang	On back, 3 *cun* from midline, at level of lower border of spinous process of fifth thoracic vertebra	Cough, labored breathing, chest tightness; back pain
BL-45 Yixi	On back, 3 *cun* from midline, at level of lower border of spinous process of sixth thoracic vertebra	Cough, labored breathing; pain in shoulder and back
BL-46 Geguan	On back, 3 *cun* from midline, at level of lower border of spinous process of seventh thoracic vertebra	Vomiting, eructation; dysphagia; back pain and stiffness
BL-47 Hunmen	On back, 3 *cun* from midline, at level of lower border of spinous process of ninth thoracic vertebra	Chest and subcostal pain; back pain; vomiting
BL-48 Yanggang	On back, 3 *cun* from midline, at level of lower border of spinous process of tenth thoracic vertebra	Borborygmus, diarrhea, abdominal pain; jaundice; diabetes
BL-49 Yishe	On back, 3 *cun* from midline, at level of lower border of spinous process of 11th thoracic vertebra	Abdominal distention, borborygmus, vomiting dysphagia
BL-50 Weichang	On back, 3 *cun* from midline, at level of lower border of spinous process of 12th thoracic vertebra	Epigastric pain; abdominal distention; back pain
BL-51 Huangmen	On lower back, 3 *cun* from midline, at level of lower border of spinous process of first lumbar vertebra	Abdominal pain; constipation; abdominal mass
BL-52 Zhishi	On lower back, 3 *cun* from midline, at level of lower border of spinous process of second lumbar vertebra	Spermatorrhea; impotence; pain in external genitals; dysuria; edema; pain and stiffness in back and flank
BL-53 Baohuang	On buttock, 3 *cun* from middle sacral crest, level with second sacral foramen	Borborygmus, abdominal distention; low back pain; dysuria
BL-54	Described separately	
BL-55 Heyang	On posterior leg, 2 *cun* below BL-40, on line connecting BL-40 and BL-57	Low back and leg pain; aches and pain or paresis of lower extremities
BL-56 Chengjin	On posterior leg, 5 *cun* below BL-40, on line connecting BL-40 and BL-57, at center of belly of gastrocnemius muscle	Spasm of gastrocnemius; hemorrhoids; acute low back pain
BL-57	Described separately	
BL-58 Feiyang Luo (Connecting) acupoint	On posterior leg, 7 *cun* directly above BL-60, about 1 *cun* inferior and lateral to BL-57	Headache; dizziness; nasal congestion; epistaxis; back pain, leg weakness; hemorrhoids

(continued)

Table 3.7 (continued)

Name	Location	Applications
BL-59 Fuyang Xi (Cleft) acupoint of Yangqiao	3 *cun* directly above BL-60, on lateral aspect of gastrocnemius	Heaviness in head, headache; pain in low back and leg; paresis of lower extremities; redness and swelling of lateral malleolus
BL-60	Described separately	
BL-61 Pucan	On lateral foot, posterior and inferior to lateral malleolus, directly below BL-60, in depression lateral to calcaneum at border of darker and lighter skin	Paresis of lower extremities; heel pain; epilepsy; knee swelling
BL-62	Described separately	
BL-63 Jinmen Xi (Cleft) acupoint	On lateral foot, directly below anterior border of lateral malleolus, in depression behind cuboid bone	Epilepsy; infantile convulsions; low back pain; paresis and pain of lower extremities
BL-64 Jinggu Yuan (Source) acupoint	On lateral foot, below tuberosity of fifth metatarsal bone, at border of darker and lighter skin	Headache; stiff neck; pain in low back and leg; epilepsy; corneal opacity
BL-65 Shugu Shu (Stream) acupoint	On lateral foot, posterior and lateral to head of fifth metatarsal bone, at border of lighter and darker skin	Headache, stiff neck; psychosis; dizziness; low back pain; pain in posterior lower extremities
BL-66 Tonggu Ying (Spring) acupoint	On lateral foot, in depression anterior and lateral to fifth metatarsophalangeal joint, at border of lighter and darker skin	Headache, stiff neck; dizziness; epistaxis; psychosis
BL-67	Described separately	

Cuanzhu (BL-2)

Location: On the face, in the depression on the medial end of the eyebrow, or in the supra-orbital notch.

Applications: Frontal headache; supra-orbital pain; inflammation of the eye; twitching of the eyelids; drooping of the eyelid; low back pain; and hiccup.

Techniques and Notes: Insert the needle subcutaneously 0.5–0.8 *cun*. **Moxibustion is not advisable**.

Tianzhu (BL-10)

Location: On the nape of the neck, about 1.3 *cun* lateral to the midpoint of the posterior hairline, in the depression on the lateral border of the trapezius muscle.

Applications: Headache; stiff neck; shoulder and back pain; dizziness; inflammation of the eye; nasal congestion; and sore throat.

Techniques and Notes: Insert the needle perpendicularly or obliquely 0.5–0.8 *cun*. **Do not puncture deeply, or with the tip of the needle angled upward or inward**. Moxibustion may be applied.

Dazhu (BL-11)

This is the one of the eight Influential acupoints (that of bones) and also the crossing point of the Small Intestine and the Bladder Meridians.

Location: On the back, 1.5 *cun* from the posterior midline, at the level of the lower border of the spinous process of the first thoracic vertebra.

Applications: Cough; fever; spasm of the neck; headache; and shoulder and back pain.

Techniques and Notes: Insert the needle obliquely 0.5–0.8 *cun*. Moxibustion may be applied.

Fengmen (BL-12)

This is the crossing point of the Bladder and the Du Meridians.

Location: On the back, 1.5 *cun* from the posterior midline, at the level of the lower border of the spinous process of the second thoracic vertebra.

Applications: Diseases of exogenous Wind; cough; headache; fever; dizziness; stiff; chest and back pain.

Techniques and Notes: Insert the needle obliquely 0.5–0.8 *cun*. Moxibustion may be applied.

Feishu (BL-13)

This is also the Back-Shu acupoint of the lung.

Location: On the back, 1.5 *cun* from the posterior midline, at the level of the lower border of the spinous process of the third thoracic vertebra.

Applications: Cough, labored breathing, hemoptysis; recurrent fever; night sweats; nasal congestion; and certain skin problems.

Techniques and Notes: Insert the needle obliquely 0.5–0.8 *cun*. Moxibustion may be applied.

Xinshu (BL-15)

This is also the Back-Shu acupoint of the heart.

Location: On the back, 1.5 *cun* from the posterior midline, at the level of the lower border of the spinous process of the fifth thoracic vertebra.

Applications: Heart pain; palpitations of the heart; chest tightness, shortness of breath; insomnia; forgetfulness; epilepsy, depression; night sweat; nocturnal spermatorrhea; cough; and hematemesis.

Techniques and Notes: Insert the needle obliquely 0.5–0.8 *cun*. Moxibustion may be applied.

Geshu (BL-17)

This is one of the eight Influential acupoint (that of blood).

Location: On the back, 1.5 *cun* from the posterior midline, at the level of the lower border of the spinous process of the 17th thoracic vertebra.

Applications: Stomachache, vomiting, hiccup, eructation; hematochezia; hematemesis; cough, labored breathing; and night sweat.

Techniques and Notes: Insert the needle obliquely 0.5–0.8 *cun*. Moxibustion may be applied.

Ganshu (BL-18)

This is the Back-Shu acupoint of the liver.

Location: On the back, 1.5 *cun* from the posterior midline, at the level of the lower border of the spinous process of the ninth thoracic vertebra.

Applications: Jaundice; flank and subcostal pain; hematemesis; eye diseases; backache; night blindness; psychosis, epilepsy, and depression.

Techniques and Notes: Insert the needle obliquely 0.5–0.8 *cun*. Moxibustion may be applied.

Danshu (BL-19)

This is the Back-Shu acupoint of the gallbladder.

Location: On the back, 1.5 *cun* from the posterior midline, at the level of the lower border of the spinous process of the tenth thoracic vertebra.

Applications: Jaundice; flank and subcostal pain; a bitter taste; vomiting; cholecystitis (inflammation of the gallbladder) and cholelithiasis (gallstones).

Techniques and Notes: Insert the needle obliquely 0.5–0.8 *cun*. Moxibustion may be applied.

Pishu (BL-20)

This is the Back-Shu acupoint of the spleen.

Location: On the back, 1.5 *cun* from the posterior midline, at the level of the lower border of the spinous process of the 11th thoracic vertebra.

Applications: Abdominal distention; jaundice; vomiting, diarrhea, dysentery, hematochezia; edema; and back pain.

Techniques and Notes: Insert the needle obliquely 0.5–0.8 *cun*. Moxibustion may be applied.

Weishu (BL-21)

This is the Back-Shu acupoint of the stomach.

Location: On the back, 1.5 *cun* from the posterior midline, at the level of the lower border of the spinous process of the 12th thoracic vertebra.

Applications: Stomachache, vomiting, abdominal distention, borborygmus, impaired digestion; chest and epigastric pain.

Techniques and Notes: Insert the needle obliquely 0.5–0.8 *cun*. Moxibustion may be applied.

Shenshu (BL-23)

This is the Back-Shu acupoint of the kidney.

Location: On the back, 1.5 *cun* from the posterior midline, at the level of the lower border of the spinous process of the second lumbar vertebra.

Applications: Enuresis; dysuria; edema; spermatorrhea; impotence; irregular menstruation; white vaginal discharge; low back pain; bone diseases, hemiplegia due to stroke; tinnitus, deafness; cough and labored breathing.

Techniques and Notes: Insert the needle perpendicularly 0.5–1 *cun*. Moxibustion may be applied.

Dachangshu (BL-25)

This is the Back-Shu acupoint of the large intestine.

Location: On the back, 1.5 *cun* from the posterior midline, at the level of the lower border of the spinous process of the fourth lumbar vertebra.

Applications: Abdominal distention; diarrhea or constipation; bleeding hemorrhoid; low back pain; and urticaria.

Techniques and Notes: Insert the needle perpendicularly 0.8–1.2 *cun*. Moxibustion may be applied.

Pangguangshu (BL-28)

This is the Back-Shu acupoint of the bladder.

Location: On the sacrum, 1.5 *cun* from the medial sacral crest, level with the second sacral foramen.

Applications: Difficulty with urination; enuresis; diarrhea or constipation; low back pain or stiffness; and leg pain.

Techniques and Notes: Insert the needle perpendicularly or obliquely 0.8–1.2 *cun*. Moxibustion may be applied.

Ciliao (BL-32)

Location: On the sacrum, at the second sacral foramen.

Applications: Irregular menstruation, dysmenorrhea, red vaginal discharge; dysuria; enuresis; spermatorrhea; impotence; low back pain; and numbness and paresis of the lower extremities.

Techniques and Notes: Insert the needle perpendicularly 1–1.5 *cun*. Moxibustion may be applied.

Chengfu (BL-36)

Location: On the posterior aspect of the thigh, at the midpoint of the gluteal fold.

Applications: Pain in the low back and gluteal region; hemorrhoids; paresis of the lower extremities.

Techniques and Notes: Insert the needle perpendicularly 1–2 *cun*. Moxibustion may be applied.

Weizhong (BL-40)

This is the He (Sea) acupoint of the Bladder Meridian.

Location: At the midpoint of the popliteal transverse crease, between the tendons of the femoral biceps and semitendinosus muscles.

Applications: Low back and flank pain; paresis of the lower extremities; hemiplegia; spasticity of the muscles of the popliteal fossa; abdominal pain; vomiting or diarrhea; enuresis; dysuria; erysipelas; rashes and generalized itch.

Techniques and Notes: Insert the needle perpendicularly 1–1.5 *cun*, or prick the popliteal vein with a three-edged needle to cause slight bleeding. Moxibustion may be applied.

Gaohuang (BL-43)

Location: On the back, 3 *cun* from the posterior midline, at the level of the lower border of the spinous process of the fourth thoracic vertebra.

Applications: Cough, labored breathing; pulmonary tuberculosis; anorexia; loose feces; emaciation and lassitude; forgetfulness; spermatorrhea; night sweat; and shoulder and scapular pain.

Techniques and Notes: Insert the needle obliquely 0.5–0.8 *cun*. Moxibustion may be applied.

Zhibian (BL-54)

Location: On the buttock, 3 *cun* from the medial sacral crest, at the level of the fourth sacral foramen.

Applications: Lumbosacral pain; paresis of the lower extremities; dysuria; constipation or hemorrhoids.

Techniques and Notes: Insert the needle perpendicularly 1.5–3 *cun*. Moxibustion may be applied.

Chengshan (BL-57)

Location: On the posterior midline of the leg, between Weizhong (BL-40) and Kunlun (BL-60), when the leg is extended or when the heel is lifted – the acupoint is in the pointed depression directly below the belly of the gastrocnemius muscle.

Applications: Hemorrhoids; constipation; spasm of the low back or leg; beriberi; and paresis of the lower extremities.

Techniques and Notes: Insert the needle perpendicularly 1–2 *cun*. Moxibustion may be applied.

Kunlun (BL-60)

This is the Jing (River) acupoint of the Bladder Meridian.

Location: Posterior to the lateral malleolus, in the depression between the tip of the lateral malleolus and the Achilles tendon.

Applications: Headache; stiff neck; dizziness; difficult labor; lumbosacral pain; heel swelling and pain; and infantile convulsions.

Techniques and Notes: Insert the needle perpendicularly 0.5–0.8 *cun*. Moxibustion may be applied. Acupuncture at this acupoint is **contraindicated for pregnant women**.

Shenmai (BL-62)

This is the Confluence acupoint of the Bladder Meridian with the Yangqiao Meridian.

Location: On the foot, in the depression directly below the lateral malleolus.

Applications: Headache; stiff neck; inflammation of the eye; insomnia; psychosis, epilepsy, pression; low back or leg pain; talipes valgus; drooping of the eyelid; and somnolence.

Techniques and Notes: Insert the needle perpendicularly 0.3–0.5 *cun*. Moxibustion may be applied.

Zhiyin (BL-67)

This is the Jing (Well) acupoint of the Bladder Meridian.

Location: On the lateral aspect of the small toe, 0.1 *cun* posterior to the corner of the nail.

Applications: Malposition of the fetus, difficult labor; headache, eye pain; nasal congestion; and epistaxis.

Techniques and Notes: Insert the needle shallowly 0.1 *cun*. Moxibustion may be applied and is strongly recommended for fetal malposition.

Section 8 Kidney Meridian of Foot-Shaoyin

I Pathway

The Kidney Meridian of Foot-Shaoyin starts at the inferior aspect of the fifth toe and runs obliquely across the sole (Yongquan, KI-1). Emerging from the lower aspect of the tuberosity of the navicular bone and running behind the medial malleolus, it enters the heel. It then ascends along the medial leg to the medial side of the popliteal fossa and continues upward along the posterior-medial thigh toward the vertebral column (Changqiang, GV-1), where it enters the kidney. Here a branch courses to and connects with the bladder (see Fig. 3.8).

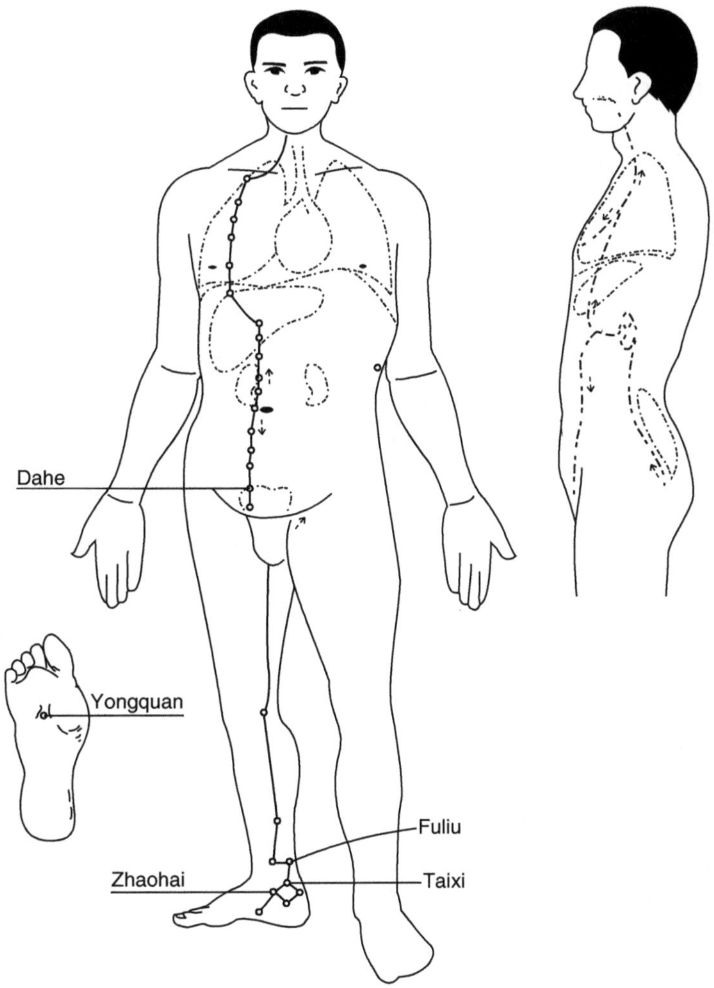

Fig. 3.8 Kidney Meridian of Foot-Shaoyin

The main meridian re-emerges from the kidney. It ascends and passes through the liver and diaphragm, enters the lung, runs along the throat, and terminates at the root of the tongue.

In the lung, a branch arises to join the heart, then runs in the chest to link with the Pericardium Meridian.

II Main Applications

The acupoints of the Kidney Meridian are used mainly in the treatment of urinary, gynecological diseases and diseases of the external genitalia, the kidney, the lung and the throat, as well as other diseases in the regions along its path.

III Commonly Used Acupoints

There are 27 acupoints in all – see Table 3.8. The more useful ones are individually described.

Yongquan (KI-1)

This is the Jing (Well) acupoint of the Kidney Meridian.

Location: On the sole of the foot, in the depression appearing on the anterior part of the sole when the foot is in plantar flexion. The position is at the junction of the anterior one-third and posterior two-thirds of the line connecting the base of the second and third toes and the heel.

Applications: Headache, dizziness; sore throat; loss of voice; constipation; dysuria; epilepsy; syncope; and hotness in the sole.

Techniques and Notes: Insert the needle perpendicularly 0.5–1 *cun*. Moxibustion may be applied.

Taixi (KI-3)

This is the Yuan (Source) and Shu (Stream) acupoints of the Kidney Meridian.

Location: On the medial side of the foot, in the depression between the tip of the medial malleolus and the Achilles tendon.

Table 3.8 Acupoints of Kidney Meridian

Name	Location	Applications
KI-1	Described separately	
KI-2 Rangu	On medial foot, in depression inferior to tuberosity of navicular bone, at border of lighter and darker skin	Irregular menstruation; spermatorrhea; infection of umbilicus in infants; tetanus; spontaneous sweating; diarrhea
KI-3	Described separately	
KI-4 Dazhong	On medial foot, posterior and inferior to medial malleolus, in depression anterior and medial to attachment of Achilles tendon, or in depression 0.5 *cun* below and slightly posterior to KI-3	Hemoptysis; labored breathing; stiffness and pain in low back; psychosis; somnolence; heel pain; irregular menstruation
KI-5 Shuiquan	On medial foot, posterior and inferior to medial malleolus, in depression medial to tuberosity of calcaneus, 1 *cun* directly below KI-3	Irregular menstruation; dysmenorrhea; dysuria; abdominal pain; dizziness
KI-6	Described separately	
KI-7		
KI-8 Jiaoxin Xi (Cleft) acupoint of Yinqiao	On medial leg, posterior to medial border of tibia, 2 *cun* above KI-3, 0.5 *cun* anterior to KI-7	Irregular menstruation; uterine bleeding or prolapse; diarrhea or constipation; pain and swelling of testis; hernia
KI-9 Zhubin Xi (Cleft) acupoint of Yinwei	On medial leg, on line connecting KI-3 to KI-10, 5 *cun* directly above KI-3, medial and inferior to belly of gastrocnemius	Psychosis; epilepsy; vomiting; hernia; leg pain
KI-10 Yingu He (Sea) acupoint	On medial side of popliteal fossa, between tendons of semitendinosus and semimembranosus muscles when knee is flexed	Impotency; hernia; irregular menstruation; metrorrhagia; dysuria; genital pain; psychosis; pain in medial knee and thigh
KI-11 Henggu	On lower abdomen, 0.5 *cun* lateral to Qugu (CV-2), 5 *cun* below center of umbilicus, on superior border of symphysis pubis, 0.5 *cun* from midline	Low abdominal distention and pain; dysuria; enuresis; spermatorrhea; impotence
KI-12	Described separately	
KI-13 Qixue	On lower abdomen, 0.5 *cun* from midline, 3 *cun* below center of umbilicus	Irregular menstruation; diarrhea; dysuria
KI-14 Siman	On lower abdomen, 0.5 *cun* from midline, 2 *cun* below center of umbilicus	Irregular menstruation; constipation; abdominal pain; edema
KI-15 Zhongzhu	On lower abdomen, 0.5 *cun* from midline, 1 *cun* below center of umbilicus	Irregular menstruation; abdominal pain; constipation; diarrhea

(continued)

Table 3.8 (continued)

Name	Location	Applications
KI-16 Huangshu	On middle abdomen, 0.5 *cun* lateral to center of umbilicus	Abdominal pain and distention; vomiting; constipation or diarrhea
KI-17 Shangqu	On upper abdomen, 0.5 *cun* from midline, 2 *cun* above center of umbilicus	Abdominal pain; diarrhea or constipation
KI-18 Shiguan	On upper abdomen, 0.5 *cun* from midline, 3 *cun* above center of umbilicus	Vomiting; abdominal pain; constipation; infertility
KI-19 Yindu	On upper abdomen, 0.5 *cun* from midline, 4 *cun* above center of umbilicus	Abdominal pain; diarrhea; irregular menstruation; infertility; constipation
KI-20 Futonggu	On upper abdomen, 0.5 *cun* from midline, 5 *cun* above center of umbilicus	Abdominal pain and distention; vomiting; indigestion
KI-21 Youmen	On upper abdomen, 0.5 *cun* from midline, 6 *cun* above center of umbilicus	Abdominal pain and distention; vomiting or diarrhea
KI-22 Bulang	On chest, in fifth intercostal space, 2 *cun* from midline	Chest pain; cough, labored breathing; vomiting; mastitis
KI-23 Shenfeng	On chest, in fourth intercostal space, 2 *cun* from midline	Cough, labored breathing; chest and subcostal fullness; vomiting
KI-24 Lingxu	On chest, in third intercostal space, 2 *cun* from midline	Cough, labored breathing; chest tightness; mastitis
KI-25 Shencang	On chest, in second intercostal space, 2 *cun* midline	Cough, labored breathing; chest pain; restlessness
KI-26 Yuzhong	On chest, in first intercostal space, 2 *cun* from midline	Cough, labored breathing; chest and subcostal fullness
KI-27 Shufu	On chest, in depression on lower border of clavicle, or below lower border of clavicle, 2 *cun* midline	Cough, labored breathing; chest pain

Applications: Sore throat; toothache; deafness, tinnitus; insomnia; headache, dizziness, blurred vision; impotency, spermatorrhea; frequent urination; irregular menstruation; low back pain; cough, labored breathing; and diabetes.

Techniques and Notes: Insert the needle perpendicularly 0.5–1 *cun*. Moxibustion may be applied.

Zhaohai (KI-6)

This is the Confluence acupoint between the Kidney and the Yinqiao Meridians.

Location: On the medial foot, in the depression below the tip of the medial malleolus.

Applications: Irregular menstruation, dysmenorrhea; vaginal discharge; dry and sore throat; dysuria or frequent urination; insomnia; and epilepsy.

Techniques and Notes: Insert the needle perpendicularly 0.5–1 *cun*. Moxibustion may be applied.

Fuliu (KI-7)

This is the Jing (River) acupoint of the Kidney Meridian.

Location: On the medial leg, anterior to the Achilles tendon, 2 *cun* directly above Taixi (KI-3).

Applications: Edema; abdominal distention, diarrhea; febrile disease without sweating or with persistent sweating; night sweat; and paresis of the lower extremities.

Techniques and Notes: Insert the needle perpendicularly 0.5–1 *cun*. Moxibustion may be applied.

Dahe (KI-12)

This is the crossing point between the Kidney and the Chong Meridians.

Location: On the lower abdomen, 0.5 *cun* from the anterior midline and 4 *cun* below the umbilicus.

Applications: Spermatorrhea; impotence; uterine prolapse; irregular menstruation; dysmenorrhea, or vaginal discharge.

Techniques and Notes: Insert the needle perpendicularly 1–1.5 *cun*. Moxibustion may be applied.

Section 9 Pericardium Meridian of Hand-Jueyin

I Pathway

The Pericardium Meridian originates in the chest and enters the pericardium. Thence it descends through the diaphragm to connect successively with the upper, middle and lower *jiao* (see Fig. 3.9).

In the chest a branch arises and runs inside the chest before emerging at the acupoint Tianchi (PC-1) 3 *cun* below the axilla. It then ascends to the axilla, then courses along the medial upper arm, running between the Lung and Heart Meridians, to the antecubital fossa and continues downward to the forearm between the tendons of the palmaris longus and the flexor carpi radialis muscles. There it enters the palm and continues along the middle finger to its tip.

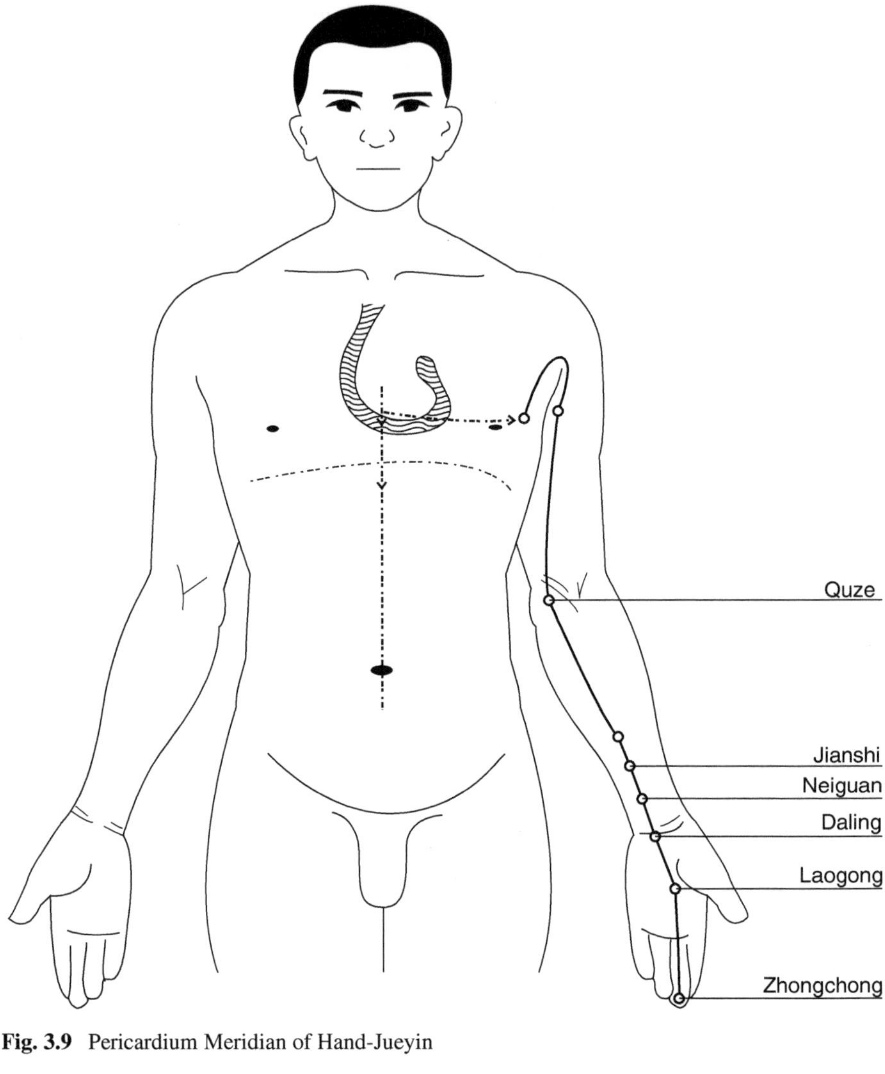

Fig. 3.9 Pericardium Meridian of Hand-Jueyin

In the palm another branch arises at Laogong (PC-8), runs along the fourth finger to its tip and links with the Sanjiao Meridian.

II Main Applications

The acupoints of the Pericardium Meridian are used mainly in the treatment of diseases of the heart, the chest and the stomach, mental diseases, and diseases in the regions along its path.

III Commonly Used Acupoints

There are 9 acupoints in all – see Table 3.9. The more useful ones are individually described.

Quze (PC-3)

This is the He (Sea) acupoint of the Pericardium Meridian.

Location: On the transverse antecubital crease, in the depression medial to the tendon of the biceps muscle.

Applications: Cardiac pain, palpitations of the heart; gastric pain, vomiting, diarrhea; febrile diseases; and spasm in the elbow and arm.

Techniques and Notes: Insert the needle perpendicularly 1–1.5 *cun*, or prick the vein to cause slight bleeding. Moxibustion may be applied.

Jianshi (PC-5)

This is the Jing (River) acupoint of the Pericardium Meridian.

Table 3.9 Acupoints of Pericardium Meridian

Name	Location	Applications
PC-1 Tianchi	On chest, in fourth intercostal space, 1 *cun* lateral to nipple and 5 *cun* from midline	Chest tightness; restlessness; flank and subcostal pain; cough, labored breathing
PC-2 Tianquan	On medial aspect of arm, 2 *cun* below anterior end of axillary fold, between heads of biceps muscle	Cardiac pain; cough; chest and subcostal distention and pain; arm pain
PC-3	Described separately	
PC-4 Ximen Xi (Cleft) acupoint	On palmar aspect of forearm, 5 *cun* above crease of wrist, between tendons of palmaris longus and flexor carpi radialis muscles, on line connecting PC-3 and PC-7	Cardiac pain, chest pain; hematemesis; hemoptysis; epilepsy
PC-5		
PC-6		
PC-7	Described separately	
PC-8		
PC-9		

Location: On the palmar aspect of the forearm, on the line connecting Quze (PC-3) and Daling (PC-7), 3 *cun* above the transverse crease of the wrist and between the tendons of the palmaris longus and flexor carpi radialis muscles.

Applications: Cardiac pain, palpitations; gastric pain, vomiting; epilepsy; febrile diseases; malaria; and arm pain.

Techniques and Notes: Insert the needle perpendicularly 0.5–1 *cun*. Moxibustion may be applied.

Neiguan (PC-6)

This is the Luo (Connecting) acupoint of the Pericardium Meridian as well as the Confluence acupoint between the Pericardium and the Yinwei Meridians.

Location: On the palmar aspect of the forearm, on the line connecting Quze (PC-3) and Daling (PC-7), 2 *cun* above the transverse crease of the wrist and between the tendons of the palmaris longus and flexor carpi radialis muscles.

Applications: Chest tightness; flank pain; heart pain, palpitations of the heart; restlessness; gastric pain, vomiting, eructation; epilepsy; insomnia; depression; dizziness; stroke with hemiplegia; numbness and pain in the upper extremities; cough and labored breathing.

Techniques and Notes: Insert the needle perpendicularly 0.5–1 *cun*. Moxibustion may be applied.

Daling (PC-7)

This is the Shu (Stream) and the Yuan (Source) acupoint of the Pericardium Meridian.

Location: At the center of the transverse crease of the wrist, between the tendons of the palmaris longus and flexor carpi radialis muscles.

Applications: Cardiac pain, palpitations of the heart; pain and flank pain; wrist pain; gastric pain, vomiting; and psychosis.

Techniques and Notes: Insert the needle perpendicularly 0.3–0.5 *cun*. Moxibustion may be applied.

Laogong (PC-8)

This is the Ying (Spring) acupoint of the Pericardium Meridian.

Location: At the center of the palm, between the second and the third metacarpal bones, closer to the latter, where the tip of the middle finger touches when a fist is made.

Applications: Aphthous sores in the mouth; halitosis; cardiac pain; vomiting; psychosis, epilepsy; and stroke with loss of consciousness.

Techniques and Notes: Insert the needle perpendicularly 0.3–0.5 *cun*. Moxibustion may be applied.

Zhongchong (PC-9)

This is Jing (Well) acupoint of the Pericardium Meridian.

Location: In the center on the tip of the middle finger.

Applications: Stroke with loss of consciousness; heat stroke; agitation; cardiac pain; tinnitus; swollen and stiff tongue with pain; and febrile diseases.

Techniques and Notes: Insert the needle shallowly 0.1 *cun* or prick to cause slight bleeding. Moxibustion may be applied.

Section 10 Sanjiao Meridian of Hand-Shaoyang

I Pathway

The Sanjiao Meridian originates at the tip of the fourth finger (Guanchong, SJ-1), runs upward between the fourth and fifth metacarpal bones along the dorsal aspect of the wrist and courses between the radius and ulna. It continues past the olecranon and along the lateral upper arm to reach the shoulder region, where it crosses and passes behind the Gallbladder Meridian. Thence it surmounts the shoulder to reach the supraclavicular fossa, enters the body and proceeds to the pericardium. From the pericardium it descends through the diaphragm to the abdomen and joins the sanjiao organ (see Fig. 3.10).

From the chest a branch arises and runs upward. Emerging from the body in the supraclavicular fossa, somewhat medial to where it entered the body, and ascends along the neck and the posterior border of the ear to the corner of the anterior hairline. Thence it crosses the cheek and terminates in the infra-orbital region.

In the region behind the auricle of the ear a branch enters the ear, emerges in front of the ear and crosses the previous branch at the cheek to reach the outer canthus of the eye. There it links with the Gallbladder Meridian.

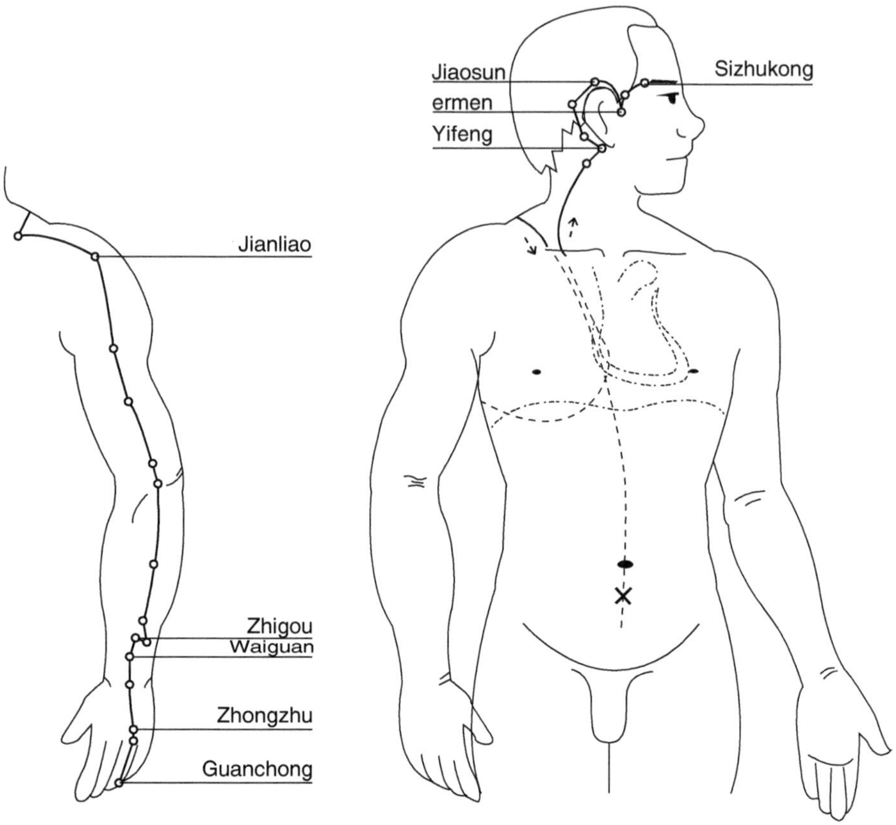

Fig. 3.10 Sanjiao Meridian of Hand-Shaoyang

II Main Applications

The acupoints of the Sanjiao Meridian are used mainly in the treatment of diseases of the ear, the organs on the side of the head, the eye and the throat. They are also used to treat febrile illnesses, malaria and chest or flank pain.

III Commonly Used Acupoints

There are 23 acupoints in all – see Table 3.10. The more useful ones are individually described.

Guanchong (SJ-1)

This is the Jing (Well) acupoint of the Sanjiao Meridian.

Table 3.10 Acupoints of Sanjiao Meridian

Name	Location	Applications
SJ-1	Described separately	
SSJ-2 Yèmén Ying (Spring) acupoint	On dorsum of hand, in depression proximal to margin of web between fourth and fifth fingers	Headache; eye redness; deafness; sore throat; arm pain; malaria
SJ-3		
SJ-4		
SJ-5	Described separately	
SJ-6		
SJ-7 Huizong Xi (Cleft) acupoint	On dorsal forearm, 3 *cun* proximal to dorsal crease of wrist, at ulnar side of SJ-6 and radial side of ulna	Deafness; epilepsy; arm pain
SJ-8 Sanyangluo	On dorsal forearm, 4 *cun* proximal to dorsal crease of wrist, between radius and ulna	Deafness; toothache; acute aphonia; arm pain and numbness
SJ-9 Sidu	On dorsal forearm, 5 *cun* distal to tip of olecranon, between radius and ulna	Edema; difficult with urination; migraine; deafness
SJ-10 Tianjing He (Sea) acupoint	On lateral upper arm, in depression 1 *cun* superior to tip of olecranon, wiith elbow flexed	Migraine; deafness; scrofula; subcostal pain
SJ-11 Qin-glengyuan	On lateral upper arm, elbow flexed, 2 *cun* superior to tip of olecranon	Pain in shoulder and arm; headache; yellowing of eyes
SJ-12 Xiaoluo	On lateral upper arm, at midpoint of line connecting SJ-11 and SJ-13	Headache; toothache; stiff neck; pain in shoulder and back
SJ-13 Naohui	On lateral upper arm, on line joining olecranon and SJ-14, 3 *cun* below SJ-14, on posterior-inferior border of deltoid	Pain in shoulder and arm; scrofula; goiter
SJ-14	Described separately	
SJ-15 Tianliao	On superior angle of scapula, midway between GB-21 and SI-13	Pain in shoulder and arm; stiff neck
SJ-16 Tianyou	On lateral neck, posterior-inferior to mastoid process, at posterior border of sternocleidomastoid muscle, level with angle of mandible	Dizziness; headache; stiff neck; eye pain; deafness
SJ-17	Described separately	
SJ-18 Chimai	On head, at center of mastoid process, at junction of middle and lower third of curve formed by SJ-17 and SJ-20	Headache; tinnitus, deafness; infantile convulsions
SJ-19 Luxi	On head, posterior to ear, at junction of upper and middle third of curve formed by SJ-17 and SJ-20	Headache; tinnitus, deafness; infantile convulsions
SJ-20	Described separately	
SJ-21		
SJ-22 Erheliao	On lateral head, on posterior border of hairline of temple, anterior to root of auricle and posterior to temporal artery	Headache; deafness, tinnitus; ear draining pus; toothache
SJ-23	Described separately	

Location: On the ulnar side of the fourth finger, 0.1 *cun* above the corner of the nail.

Applications: Febrile diseases; syncope; headache; stiffness of the tongue; inflammation of the eye; and sore throat.

Techniques and Notes: Insert the needle shallowly 0.1 *cun*, or prick to cause slight bleeding. Moxibustion may be applied.

Zhongzhu (SJ-3)

This is the Shu (Stream) acupoint of the Sanjiao Meridian.

Location: On the dorsum of the hand, proximal to the fourth metacarpophalangeal joint, in the depression between the fourth and fifth metacarpal bones.

Applications: Headache; eye inflammation; tinnitus, deafness; sore throat; inability to extend or flex the fingers; leg pains; and back pain between the scapulas.

Techniques and Notes: Insert the needle perpendicularly 0.3–0.5 *cun*. Moxibustion may be applied.

Yangchi (SJ-4)

This is the Yuan (Source) acupoint of the Sanjiao Meridian.

Location: In the dorsal crease of the wrist, in the depression at the ulnar side of the tendon of the extensor muscle of the fingers.

Applications: Wrist pain; shoulder and arm pain; deafness; diabetes; sore throat; and malaria.

Techniques and Notes: Insert the needle perpendicularly 0.3–0.5 *cun*. Moxibustion may be applied.

Waiguan (SJ-5)

This is the Luo (Connecting) acupoint as well as the Confluence acupoint of the Sanjiao and the Yangwei Meridians.

Location: On the dorsal forearm, 2 *cun* proximal to the dorsal crease of the wrist, between the radius and ulna.

Applications: Febrile diseases; headache; pain and inflammation of the eye; tinnitus, deafness; pain in the rib cage; and pain and numbness of the arm.

Techniques and Notes: Insert the needle perpendicularly 0.5–1 *cun*. Moxibustion may be applied.

Zhigou (SJ-6)

This is the Jing (River) acupoint of the Sanjiao Meridian.

Location: On the dorsal forearm, 3 *cun* proximal to the dorsal crease of the wrist, between the radius and ulna.

Applications: Constipation; tinnitus, deafness; and pain in the rib cage.

Techniques and Notes: Insert the needle perpendicularly 0.8–1.2 *cun*. Moxibustion may be applied.

Jianliao (SJ-14)

Location: On the shoulder, posterior to Jianyu (LI-15), in the depression posterior and inferior to the acromion when the arm is abducted.

Applications: Inability to raise arm with heaviness in the shoulder joint; arm pain; and inability to move the shoulder and arm.

Techniques and Notes: Insert the needle 1–1.5 *cun* with the tip of the needle aimed toward the shoulder joint. Moxibustion may be applied.

Yifeng (SJ-17)

This is the crossing point between the Sanjiao and the Gallbladder Meridians.

Location: In the depression between the mandibular angle and the mastoid process, posterior to the ear lobe.

Applications: Tinnitus, deafness; cheek swelling; wry mouth and eyes; toothache; and scrofula.

Techniques and Notes: Insert the needle perpendicularly 0.8–1.2 *cun*. Moxibustion may be applied.

Jiaosun (SJ-20)

This is the crossing point of the Sanjiao, the Gallbladder and the Large Intestine Meridians.

Location: On the head, directly above the ear apex, within the hairline.

Applications: Tinnitus; corneal opacity; gingival swelling, toothache; stiff neck; and mumps.

Techniques and Notes: Insert the needle subcutaneously 0.3–0.5 *cun*. Moxibustion may be applied.

Ermen (SJ-21)

Location: On the face, in the depression anterior to the notch above the tragus and slightly superior-posterior to the mandibular condyle – with the mouth open.

Applications: Tinnitus, deafness; ear draining pus; and toothache.

Techniques and Notes: Insert the needle perpendicularly 0.5–1 *cun*. Moxibustion may be applied.

Sizhukong (SJ-23)

Location: On the face, in the depression at the lateral end of the eyebrow.

Applications: Headache; inflammation of the eye; twitching of the eyelid; psychosis; and epilepsy.

Techniques and Notes: Insert the needle subcutaneously 0.5–1 *cun*. Moxibustion may be applied.

Section 11 Gallbladder Meridian of Foot-Shaoyang

I Pathway

The Gallbladder Meridian begins at the outer canthus of the eye (Tongziliao, GB-1), ascends to the corner of the forehead (Hanyan, GB-4), then curves with a broad sweep around the temple to the area behind the ear (Fengchi, GB-20). Thence it runs along the side of the neck, in front of the Sanjiao Meridian, to the shoulder. Turning back, it passes behind the Sanjiao Meridian and proceeds down to the supraclavicular fossa (see Fig. 3.11).

Behind the ear a branch enters the ear, then emerges and passes through the area in front of ear to the posterior aspect of the outer canthus.

A branch (interrupted line in Fig. 3.11) arises at the outer canthus, runs downward to Daying (ST-5) and meets the Sanjiao Meridian in the infra-orbital region. It then passes through Jiache (ST-6) and descends along the neck to enter the supraclavicular fossa, where it meets the main meridian. From the supraclavicular fossa the branch enters the chest, passes through the diaphragm, connects with the liver

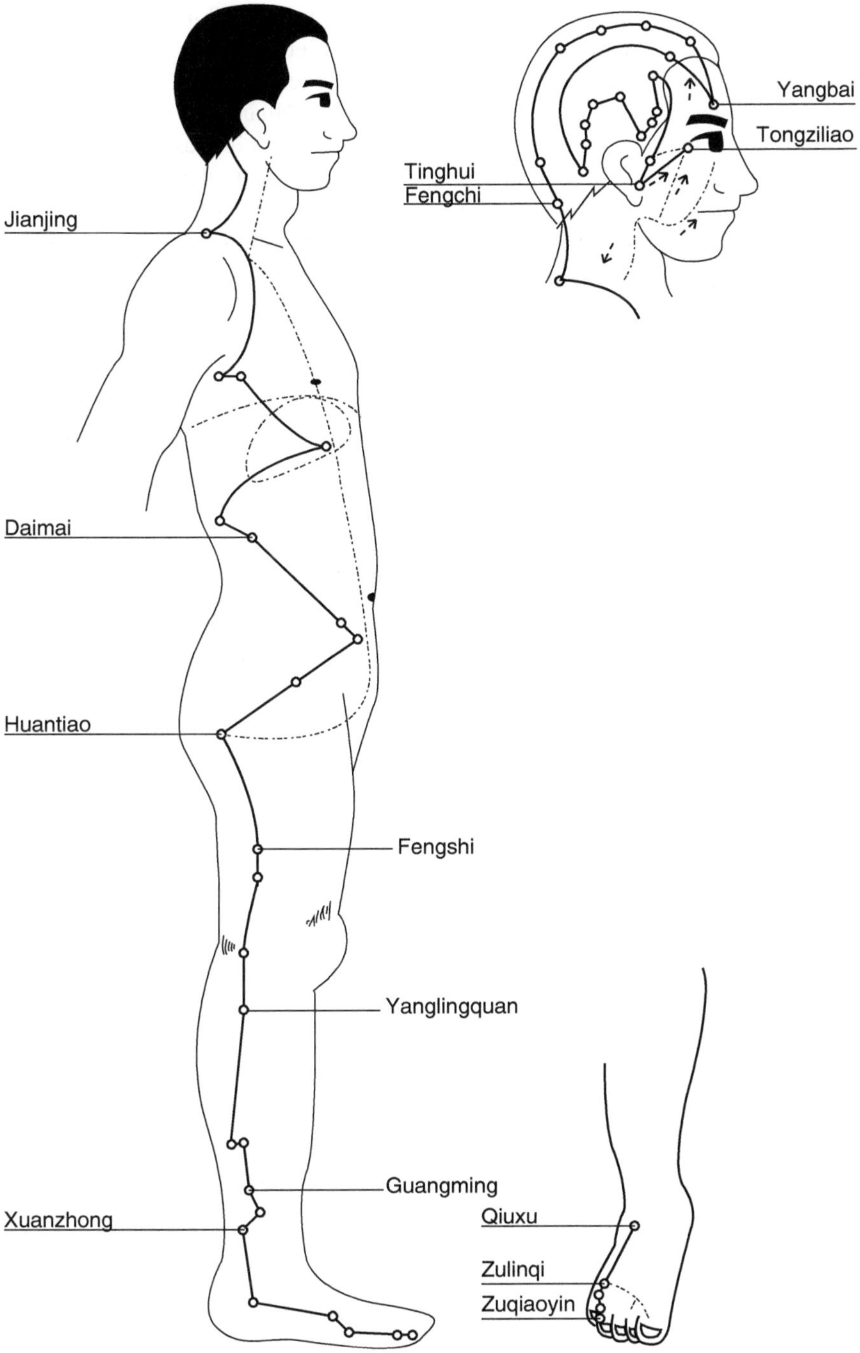

Fig. 3.11 Gallbladder Meridian of Foot-Shaoyang

and continues on to its organ, the gallbladder. It travels within the antero-lateral chest and continues downward in the abdomen to emerge near the femoral artery in the inguinal region. Following emergence it runs superficially along the margin of the pubic hairline, then transversely to the hip region (Huantiao, GB-30).

From the supraclavicular fossa the main meridian (continuous line in Fig. 3.11) runs downward and passes in front of the axilla. It continues along the lateral chest and past the floating ribs to the hip region, where it meets the branch from the outer canthus at Huantiao (GB-30). Thence it descends along the lateral thigh to the lateral side of the knee and continues along the anterior aspect of the fibula to reach the anterior aspect of the external malleolus. From the malleolus it follows the dorsum of the foot to the lateral side of the tip of the fourth toe.

On the dorsum of the foot, a branch takes off at Zulinqi (GB-41) and runs between the first and the second metatarsal bones to the distal portion of the great toe, passes through the nail and terminates at its hairy region, where it links with the Liver Meridian.

II Main Applications

The acupoints of the Gallbladder Meridian are used mainly in the treatment of diseases of the head, eye, ear and throat, mental diseases, and diseases in the regions along its course.

III Commonly Used Acupoints

There are 44 acupoints in all – see Table 3.11. The more useful ones are individually described.

Tongziliao (GB-1)

This is the crossing point of the Gallbladder, the Sanjiao and the Small Intestine Meridians.

Location: On the face, lateral to the outer canthus, on the lateral border of the orbit.

Applications: Headache; inflammation of the eye, corneal opacity, or optic atrophy.

Techniques and Notes: Insert the needle subcutaneously 0.3–0.5 *cun*.

Table 3.11 Acupoints of Gallbladder Meridians

Name	Location	Applications
GB-1	Described separately	
GB-2		
GB-3 Shangguan	Anterior to ear, above ST-7, in Depression above upper border of zygomatic arch	Facial palsy; ear diseases; tooth diseases
GB-4 Hanyan	On head, within temporal hairline, at junction of upper 1/4 and lower 3/4 of line between ST-8 and GB-7	Migraine, vertigo; tinnitus; toothache; epilepsy
GB-5 Xuanlu	On head, within temporal hairline, at midpoint on line connecting ST-8 and GB-7	Migraine; inflammation of eye; toothache
GB-6 Xuanli	On head, within hairline, at junction of lower 1/4 and upper 3/4 of line between ST-8 and GB-7	Migraine; inflammation of eye; tinnitus
GB-7 Qubin	On head, at intersection of vertical line through posterior border of pre-auricular hairline and level line through apex of ear	Temporal headache; toothache; trismus; cheek swelling; sudden hoarseness of voice
GB-8 Shuaigu	On head, superior to ear apex, 1.5 *cun* above hairline, directly above SJ-20	Migraine; dizziness; infantile convulsions
GB-9 Tianchong	On head, directly above posterior border of auricle, 2 *cun* inside hairline, 0.5 *cun* posterior to GB-8	Headache; gingival pain; epilepsy
GB-10 Fubai	On head, posterior-superior to mastoid process, at junction of upper 1/3 and middle 2/3 of curved line from GB-9 to GB-12	Headache; tinnitus, deafness; eye pain; goiter
GB-11 Touqiaoyin	On head, posterior-superior to mastoid process, at junction of middle 2/3 and lower 1/3 of curved line from GB-9 to GB-12	Headache; tinnitus, deafness
GB-12 Wangu	On head, in depression posterior-inferior to mastoid process	Headache; neck stiffness and pain; toothache; facial palsy
GB-13 Benshen	On head, 0.5 *cun* within hairline of forehead, 3 *cun* lateral to GV-24, at junction of medial 2/3 and lateral 1/3 of line from GV-24 to ST-8	Headache; blurred vision; epilepsy; neck spasm; infantile convulsions
GB-14	Described separately	
GB-15 Toulinqi	On head, vertically above pupil, 0.5 *cun* inside hairline, midway between GV-24 and ST-8	Headache; eye diseases; nasal congestion
GB-16 Muchuang	On head, 1.5 *cun* above anterior hairline, 2.25 *cun* lateral to midline	Headache; inflammation of eye; nasal congestion; epilepsy
GB-17 Zhengying	On head, 2.5 *cun* above anterior hairline, 2.25 *cun* from midline	Migraine; vertigo; toothache
GB-18 Chengling	On head, 4 *cun* above anterior hairline, 2.25 *cun* from midline	Headache; vertigo; eye pain; nasal drainage, epistaxis
GB-19 Naokong	On lateral head, superior to occipital protuberance, 2.25 *cun* lateral from midline, level with GV-17	Headache; dizziness; neck pain and stiffness; psychosis; epilepsy
GB-20	Described separately	
GB-21		
GB-22 Yuanye	On lateral chest, on mid-axillary line when arm is raised, 3 *cun* below axilla, in fourth intercostal space	Chest fullness; flank pain; axillary swelling; painful paresis of arm
GB-23 Zhejin	1 *cun* anterior to GB-22, level with nipple, in fourth intercostal space	Chest fullness; flank pain; labored breathing; hiccup; acid regurgitation

(continued)

Table 3.11 (continued)

Name	Location	Applications
GB-24 Riyue Front-Mu acupoint	On upper abdomen, vertically below nipple, in seventh intercostal space, 4 *cun* from midline	Vomiting; acid regurgitation; flank pain; hiccup; jaundice
GB-25 Jingmen Front-Mu acupoint of kidney	On lateral side of waist, 1.8 *cun* posterior to LR-13, below free end of 12th rib	Difficulty with urination; edema; low back pain; abdominal distention, diarrhea
GB-26	Described separately	
GB-27 Wushu	On lateral abdomen, anterior to Anterior-superior iliac spine, 3 *cun* below umbilicus	Abdominal pain; lumbar and thigh pain; hernia; vaginal discharge; constipation
GB-28 Weidao	On lateral abdomen, anterior-inferior to anterior-superior iliac spine, 0.5 *cun* anterior-inferior to GB-27	Abdominal pain; hernia; vaginal discharge; lumbar and thigh pain
GB-29 Juliao	On hip, at midpoint between anterior-superior iliac spine and greater trochanter	Low back pain; atrophy and paresis of lower limbs; hernia
GB-30	Described separately	
GB-31		
GB-32 Zhongdu	On lateral thigh, 2 *cun* below GB-31 or 5 *cun* above transverse popliteal crease, between vastus lateralis and femoral biceps muscles	Numbness, atrophy and paresis of lower limbs; hemiplegia
GB-33 Xiyangguan	On lateral knee, 3 *cun* above GB-34, in depression superior to lateral condyle of femur	Knee swelling, pain, spasticity; leg numbness
GB-34	Described separately	
GB-35 Yangjiao Xi (Cleft) acupoint of Yangwei	On lateral leg, 7 *cun* above tip of lateral malleolus, on posterior border of fibula	Chest and flank tightness; paresis of lower limbs; knee pain; psychosis
GB-36 Waiqiu Xi (Cleft) acupoint	On lateral leg, 7 *cun* above tip of lateral malleolus, on anterior border of fibula, level with GB-35	Pain in neck, chest and flank; paresis of leg
GB-37	Described separately	
GB-38 Yangfu Jing (River) acupoint	On lateral leg, 4 *cun* above tip of lateral malleolus, slightly anterior to anterior border of fibula	Migraine; pain in outer canthus; sore throat; chest and flank pain and fullness; pain in lateral leg; hemiplegia; scrofula
GB-39		
GB-40	Described separately	
GB-41		
GB-42 Diwuhui	On lateral dorsal surface of foot, between fourth and fifth metatarsal bones, proximal to fourth metatarsal head, on medial side of tendon of extensor digiti minimi	Headache; inflammation of eye; flank pain; tinnitus; inflammation of dorsum of foot; mastitis; hematemesis from internal injury
GB-43 Xiaxi Ying (Spring) acupoint	On dorsum of foot, between fourth and fifth toes, at junction of lighter and darker skin, slightly proximal to margin of web	Headache; dizziness; tinnitus, deafness; flank pain; inflammation of eye; mastitis; febrile diseases
GB-44	Described separately	

Tinghui (GB-2)

Location: On the face, anterior to the intertragic notch, in the depression posterior to the mandibular condyle when the mouth is open. (For the intertragic notch, see Volume 2, Part I, Chapter 4, Section 6, Subsection I.)

Applications: Deafness, tinnitus; toothache; wry mouth; and mumps.

Techniques and Notes: Insert the needle perpendicularly 0.5–1 *cun* with the patient's mouth slightly open. Moxibustion may be applied.

Yangbai (GB-14)

This is the crossing point of the Gallbladder and the Yangwei Meridians.

Location: On the forehead, vertically above the pupil, 1 *cun* superior to the center of the eyebrow.

Applications: Wry eye and mouth; drooping of the eyelid, bell's palsy, difficulty in closing the eyes, eye pain, or blurred vision; and dizziness or frontal headache.

Techniques and Notes: Insert the needle subcutaneously 0.3–0.5 *cun*. Moxibustion may be applied.

Fengchi (GB-20)

This is the crossing point of the Gallbladder and the Yangwei Meridians.

Location: On the nape of the neck, inferior to the occipital bone, level with Fengfu (GV-16), in the depression between the upper ends of the sternocleidomastoid and the trapezius muscles.

Applications: Common cold; headache; nasal congestion with discharge, epistaxis; inflammation of the eye; pain and stiffness of the neck; frozen shoulder; dizziness, blurred vision; stroke with hemiplegia; febrile diseases; and epilepsy.

Techniques and Notes: Insert the needle obliquely 0.8–1.2 *cun* toward the tip of the nose, or subcutaneously through Fengfu (GV-16). Caution should be taken to avoid puncturing the medulla. Moxibustion may be applied.

Jianjing (GB-21)

This is the crossing point of the Gallbladder, the Sanjiao, the Stomach and the Yangwei Meridians.

Location: On the shoulder, vertically above the nipple, midway between Dazhui (GV-14) and the acromion, at the highest point on the shoulder.

Applications: Headache; neck pain and stiffness; shoulder and back pain; inability to move the arms; mastitis, difficulty in excreting milk; difficult labor; and scrofula.

Techniques and Notes: Insert the needle perpendicularly 0.5–0.8 *cun*. **Deep insertion is forbidden** so as not to puncture the tip of the lung. **Acupuncture is contraindicated for pregnant women**. Moxibustion may be applied in the absence of pregnancy.

Daimai (GB-26)

This is the crossing point of the Gallbladder and the Dai Meridians.

Location: On the lateral abdomen, 1.8 *cun* below Zhangmen (LR-13), vertically below the free end of the 11th rib, level with the umbilicus.

Applications: Vaginal discharge; abdominal pain; amenorrhea, irregular menstruation; lumbar and flank pain; and hernia.

Techniques and Notes: Insert the needle perpendicularly 1–1.5 *cun*. Moxibustion may be applied.

Huantiao (GB-30)

This is the crossing point of the Gallbladder and the Bladder Meridians.

Location: On the lateral thigh, at the junction of middle two thirds and lateral third of the line connecting the prominence of the great trochanter and the sacral hiatus when the patient is in a lateral recumbent position with the thigh flexed.

Applications: Rheumatic pain; paraplegia; lumbar or leg pain.

Techniques and Notes: Insert the needle perpendicularly 2–3 *cun*. Moxibustion may be applied.

Fengshi (GB-31)

Location: On the median line of the lateral thigh, 7 *cun* above the popliteal crease; or, with the patient standing erect and the arm hanging freely where the tip of the middle finger touches the thigh.

Applications: Painful paraplegia or hemiplegia; beriberi; and total body itch.

Techniques and Notes: Insert the needle perpendicularly 1–2 *cun*. Moxibustion may be applied.

Yanglingquan (GB-34)

This is the He (Sea) acupoint of the Gallbladder Meridian and its Influential acupoint for the tendons.

Location: On the lateral leg, in the depression anterior and inferior to the head of the fibula.

Applications: Paresis of the lower extremities; hemiplegia; knee pain and swelling; chest and flank pain; bitter taste; vomiting; jaundice; and infantile convulsions.

Techniques and Notes: Insert the needle perpendicularly 1–1.5 *cun*. Moxibustion may be applied.

Guangming (GB-37)

This is the Luo (Connecting) acupoint of the Gallbladder Meridian.

Location: On the lateral leg, 5 *cun* above the tip of the lateral malleolus, on the anterior border of the fibula.

Applications: Night blindness; eye pain; reduced visual acuity; knee pain; atrophy and paresis of the lower extremities; and breast pain and swelling.

Techniques and Notes: Insert the needle perpendicularly 1–1.5 *cun*. Moxibustion may be applied.

Xuanzhong (Juegu) (GB-39)

This is the Influential acupoint of the Gallbladder Meridian for the marrow.

Location: On the lateral leg, 3 *cun* above the tip of the lateral malleolus, on the anterior border of the fibula.

Applications: Neck stiffness and pain; distending pain in the chest and flank; atrophy and paresis of the lower extremities; stroke with hemiplegia; beriberi; and hemorrhoids.

Techniques and Notes: Insert the needle perpendicularly 1–1.5 *cun*. Moxibustion may be applied.

Qiuxu (GB-40)

This is the Yuan (Source) acupoint of the Gallbladder Meridian.

Location: Anterior and inferior to the lateral malleolus, in the depression lateral to the tendon of long extensor muscle of the toes.

Applications: Neck pain; paresis of the lower limbs; fullness and pain in the chest and flank; and malaria.

Techniques and Notes: Insert the needle perpendicularly 0.5–0.8 *cun*. Moxibustion may be applied.

Zulinqi (GB-41)

This is the Shu (Stream) acupoint of the Gallbladder Meridian as well as the meridian's Confluence acupoint with the Dai Meridian.

Location: On the lateral-dorsal surface of the foot, in the depression distal to the junction of the fourth and fifth metatarsal bones, on the lateral side of the tendon of the extensor muscle of the little toe.

Applications: Migraine; pain in the outer canthus of the eye; flank pain; swelling and pain of the dorsum of the foot; foot or toe cramps; scrofula; irregular menstruation; mastitis, breast distension; and enuresis.

Techniques and Notes: Insert the needle perpendicularly 0.3–0.5 *cun*. Moxibustion may be applied.

Zuqiaoyin (GB-44)

This is the Jing (Well) acupoint of the Gallbladder Meridian.

Location: On the lateral side of the fourth toe, 0.1 *cun* posterior to the corner of the nail.

Applications: Headache; inflammation of the eye; tinnitus, deafness; sore throat; insomnia; flank pain; irregular menstruation; and stroke with hemiplegia.

Techniques and Notes: Insert the needle shallowly 0.1 *cun*, or prick to cause slight bleeding. Moxibustion may be applied.

Section 12 Liver Meridian of Foot-Jueyin

I Pathway

The Liver Meridian starts on the dorsal great toe, where the hair grows, and runs upward along the dorsal foot to 1 *cun* anterior to the medial malleolus, where it crosses behind the Spleen Meridian. Thence it courses upward past the medial knee and along the medial thigh to the pubic hair region, where it curves around the external genitalia, and continues to the lower abdomen. It then runs upward and curves around the stomach to enter its organ, the liver, and connects with the gallbladder. From the gallbladder it passes through the diaphragm and spreads into the region of the ribs. It then ascends along the posterior throat to the nasopharynx and connects with the "eye system" (the area where the eyeball links with the brain). It continues upward, emerges from the forehead and meets the Du Meridian at the vertex of the head (see Fig. 3.12).

A branch arises from the liver, passes through the diaphragm and links with the Lung Meridian.

Another branch arises in the "eye system," courses to the cheek and curves around the inner surfaces of the lips.

II Main Applications

The acupoints of the Liver Meridian are used mainly in the treatment of diseases of the liver, gynecological diseases, diseases of the external genitalia and diseases in the regions along its pathway.

III Commonly Used Acupoints

There are 14 acupoints in all – see Table 3.12. The more useful ones are individually described.

Dadun (LR-1)

This is the Jing (Well) acupoint of the Liver Meridian.

Location: On the lateral side of the great toe, 0.1 *cun* lateral to the corner of the nail.

Applications: Hernia; enuresis; amenorrhea; metrorrhagia; prolapse of the uterus; and epilepsy.

Techniques and Notes: Insert the needle obliquely 0.1–0.2 *cun*, or prick to cause slight bleeding. Moxibustion may be applied.

Xingjian (LR-2)

This is the Ying (Spring) acupoint of the Liver Meridian.

Location: On the dorsal foot between the first and second toes, at the junction of the lighter and darker skin, proximal to the margin of the web.

Applications: Inflammation of the eye; optic atrophy; irregular menstruation, dysmenorrhea, or vaginal discharge; difficulty with urination, dysuria; insomnia; and epilepsy.

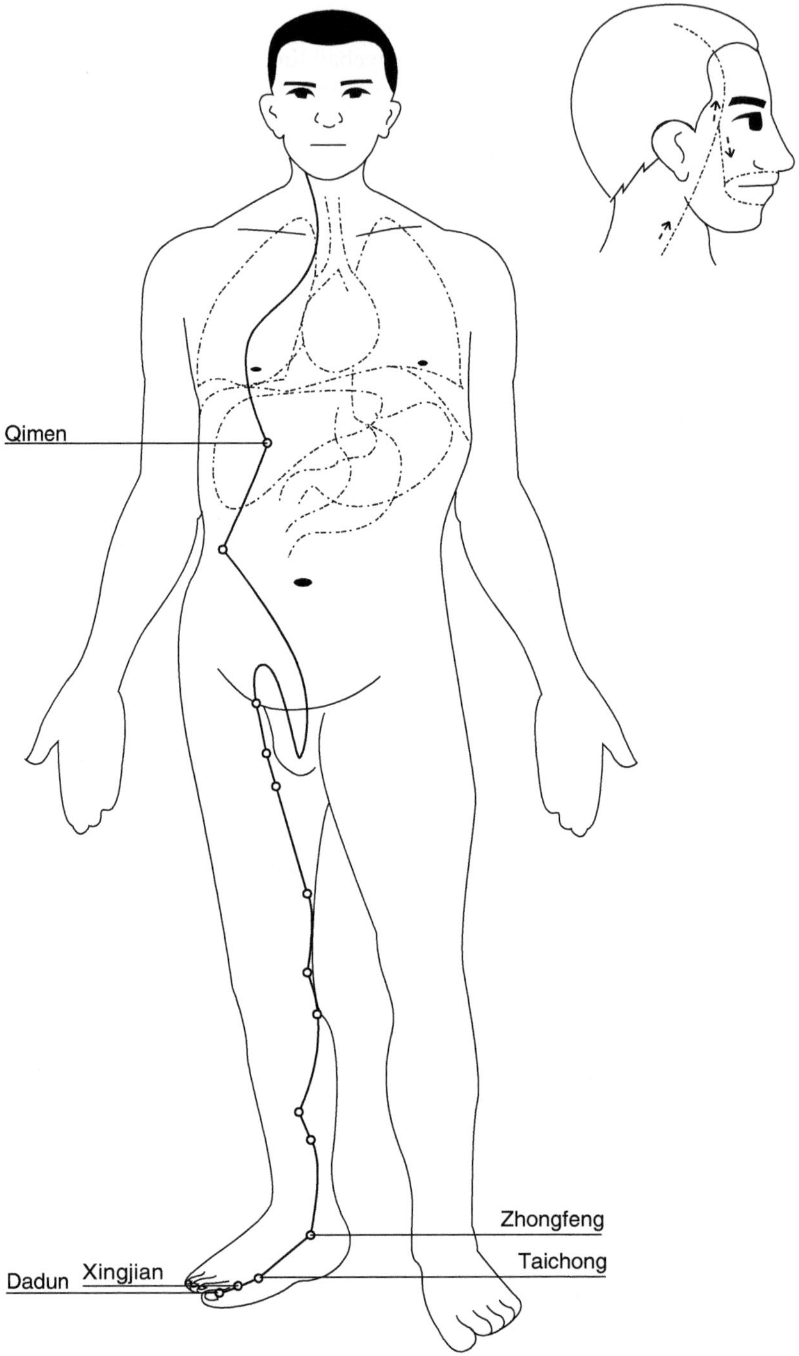

Fig. 3.12 Liver Meridian of Foot-Jueyin

Table 3.12 Acupoints of Liver Meridian

Name	Location	Applications
LR-1		
LR-2	Described separately	
LR-3		
LR-4		
LR-5 Ligou Luo (Connecting) acupoint	On medial leg, 5 *cun* above tip of medial malleolus, on midline of medial aspect of tibia	Difficulty with urination; enuresis; vulvar itch; irregular Menstruation; vaginal discharge; hernia; testicular swelling and pain
LR-6 Zhongdu Xi (Cleft) acupoint	On medial leg, 7 *cun* above tip of medial malleolus, on midline of medial aspect of tibia	Hernia; metrorrhagia; abdominal pain; persistent lochia
LR-7 Xiguan	On medial leg, posterior-inferior to medial tibial condyle, 1 *cun* posterior to SP-9, in upper portion of medial head of gastrocnemius muscle	Knee swelling and pain; paresis of the lower limbs
LR-8 Ququan He (Sea) acupoint	On medial knee, at medial end of popliteal crease when knee is flexed, posterior to medial epicondyle of femur, in depression of anterior border of insertions of semimem-branosus and semitendinosus muscles	Irregular menstruation, dysmenorrhea, vaginal discharge; vulvar itch; knee pain; spermatorrhea; difficulty with urination; abdominal pain
LR-9 Yinbao	On medial thigh, 4 *cun* above medial epicondyle of femur, between vastus medialis and sartorius muscles	Irregular menstruation; difficulty with urination; abdominal pain; enuresis
LR-10 Zuwuli	On medial thigh, 3 *cun* below ST-30, at proximal end of thigh, below pubic tubercle and on lateral border of long abductor muscle	Low abdominal pain; anuria; prolapse of uterus; testicular swelling and pain; somnolence
LR-11 Yinlian	On medial thigh, 2 *cun* below ST-30, at proximal end of thigh, below pubic tubercle and on lateral border of long abductor muscle	Irregular menstruation; vaginal discharge; low abdominal pain
LR-12 Jimai	Lateral to pubic tubercle, 2.5 *cun* from midline, at inguinal groove where femoral artery is palpable, lateral-inferior to ST-30	Hernia; pain in the external genitalia; prolapse of uterus
LR-13 Zhangmen[a]	On lateral abdomen, below free end of 11th rib	Abdominal pain and distention; diarrhea; flank pain; abdominal masses
LR-14	Described separately	

[a] lR-13 zhangmen is also the front-mu acupoint of the spleen and the influential acupoint of the *zang* organs

Techniques and Notes: Insert the needle obliquely 0.5–0.8 *cun*. Moxibustion may be applied.

Taichong (LR-3)

This is the Shu (Stream) and the Yuan (Source) acupoints of the Liver Meridian.

Location: On the dorsal foot, in the depression distal to the junction of the first and second metatarsal bones.

Applications: Headache; dizziness; inflammation of the eye; wry eye and mouth; irregular menstruation, dysmenorrhea, metrorrhagia, or vaginal discharge; enuresis; hernia; insomnia; depression; epilepsy; infantile convulsion; atrophy, numbness and pain of the lower extremities.

Techniques and Notes: Insert the needle perpendicularly 0.5–0.8 *cun*. Moxibustion may be applied.

Zhongfeng (LR-4)

This is the Jing (River) acupoint of the Liver Meridian.

Location: On the dorsal foot, anterior to the medial malleolus, between Shangqiu (SP-5) and Jiexi (ST-41), in the depression medial to the tendon of the anterior tibialis muscle.

Applications: Hernia; abdominal pain; difficulty with urination; and spermatorrhea.

Techniques and Notes: Insert the needle perpendicularly 0.5–0.8 *cun*. Moxibustion may be applied.

Qimen (LR-14)

This is the Front-Mu acupoint of the Liver Meridian and the crossing point of the Liver Meridian with the Spleen and the Yinwei Meridians.

Location: On the chest, vertically below the nipple, in the sixth intercostal space, 4 *cun* from the midline.

Applications: Mastitis; depression; chest tightness; abdominal distention; vomiting; and acid regurgitation.

Techniques and Notes: Insert the needle obliquely or subcutaneously 0.5–0.8 *cun*. Moxibustion may be applied.

Section 13 Du Meridian

I Pathway

The Du Meridian arises within the lower abdomen. It courses to the perineum, then runs along the interior of the spinal column to Fengfu (GV-16) at the nape of the neck, where it enters the brain (not shown in Fig. 3.13). Thence it ascends to the vertex and winds along the forehead to the septal cartilage of the nose (see Fig. 3.13). (Note: the alphanumeric code of acupoints on the Du Meridian is GV-xx.)

II Main Applications

The acupoints of the Du Meridian are used mainly in the treatment of mental diseases, febrile diseases, local diseases of the lumbosacral region, back, head and neck, as well as diseases of the corresponding visceral organs.

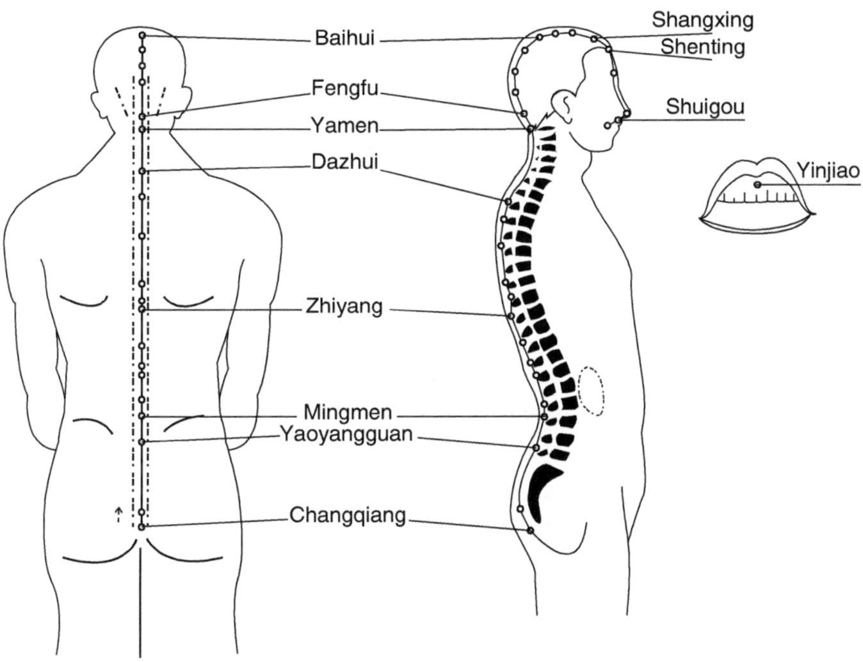

Fig. 3.13 Du Meridian

III Commonly Used Acupoints

There are 28 acupoints in all – see Table 3.13. The more useful ones are individually described.

Changqiang (GV-1)

This is the crossing point of the Du Meridian with the Gallbladder and the Kidney Meridians. It is also the Luo (Connecting) acupoint of the Du Meridian.

Location: Below the tip of the coccyx, midway between the tip of the coccyx and the anus.

Applications: Diarrhea, hematochezia, constipation, hemorrhoids, prolapse of the rectum; back pain; and epilepsy.

Techniques and Notes: Insert the needle obliquely 0.8–1 *cun* in front of the coccyx. Moxibustion is not advisable.

Yaoyangguan (GV-3)

Location: On the midline of the back, in the depression below the spinous process of the fourth lumbar vertebra.

Applications: Spermatorrhea, impotence; irregular menstruation; lumbosacral pain; and paresis of the lower extremities.

Techniques and Notes: Insert the needle slightly obliquely upward 0.5–1 *cun*. Moxibustion may be applied.

Mingmen (GV-4)

Location: On the midline of the back, in the depression below the spinous process of the second lumbar vertebra.

Applications: Spermatorrhea, impotence; irregular menstruation, vaginal discharge; diarrhea; lumbosacral stiffness and pain.

Techniques and Notes: Insert the needle obliquely upward 0.5–1 *cun*. Moxibustion may be applied.

Zhiyang (GV-9)

Location: On the midline of the back, in the depression below the spinous process of the seventh thoracic vertebra.

Table 3.13 Acupoints of Du Meridian

Name	Location	Applications
GV-1	Described separately	
GV-2 Yaoshu	On sacrum and on posterior midline, at sacral hiatus	Irregular menstruation; lumbar stiffness and pain; hemorrhoids; paresis of lower extremities
GV-3	Described separately	
GV-4		
GV-5 Xuansu	On midline of back, in depression below spinous process of first lumbar vertebra	Diarrhea, abdominal pain; lumbar pain and stiffness
GV-6 Jizhong	On midline of back, in depression below spinous process of 11th thoracic vertebra	Diarrhea; hemorrhoids; epilepsy; lumbar pain and stiffness
GV-7 Zhongshu	On midline of back, in depression below spinous process of tenth thoracic vertebra	Jaundice; vomiting; abdominal distention; lumbar pain and stiffness
GV-8 Jinsuo	On midline of back, in depression below spinous process of ninth thoracic vertebra	Epilepsy; tetany; back stiffness; gastric pain
GV-9	Described separately	
GV-10 Lingtai	On midline of back, in depression below spinous process of sixth thoracic vertebra	Cough; labored breathing; furuncles; back pain and stiffness
GV-11 Shendao	On midline of back, in depression below spinous process of fifth thoracic vertebra	Palpitations of heart; forgetfulness; cough; back pain and stiffness
GV-12 Shenzhu	On midline of back, in depression below spinous process of third thoracic vertebra	Cough, labored breathing; epilepsy; back stiffness and pain
GV-13 Taodao	On midline of back, in depression below spinous process of first thoracic vertebra	Headache; malaria; febrile diseases; back stiffness
GV-14		
GV-15	Described separately	
GV-16		
GV-17 Naohu	On head, 2.5 *cun* above midpoint of posterior hairline, 1.5 *cun* above GV-16, in depression above external occipital protuberance	Headache; dizziness; stiff neck; loss of voice; epilepsy
GV-18 Qiangjian	On head, 4 *cun* above midpoint of posterior hairline and 1.5 *cun* above GV-17	Psychosis; headache; dizziness, stiff neck
GV-19 Houding	On head, 5.5 *cun* above midpoint of posterior hairline and 3 *cun* above GV-17	Headache; dizziness; psychosis; epilepsy
GV-20	Described separately	
GV-21 Qianding	On head, 3.5 *cun* above to midpoint of the anterior hairline and 1.5 *cun* anterior to GV-20	Headache; dizziness; nasal discharge; epilepsy
GV-22 Xinhui	On head, 2 *cun* above to midpoint of anterior hairline and 3 *cun* anterior to GV-20	Headache; dizziness; nasal discharge; epilepsy
GV-23	Described separately	
GV-24		
GV-25 Suliao	On face, at center of apex of nose	Nasal discharge; epistaxis; labored breathing; coma; syncope
GV-26	Described separately	
GV-27 Duiduan	On anterior midline of face, at junction of philtrum and upper lip	Psychosis; gingival pain and swelling; epistaxis; wry mouth
GV-28 Yinjiao	Inside upper lip, at junction of upper gum and labial frenulum	Psychosis; gingival swelling and pain; nasal discharge

Applications: Jaundice; chest and flank fullness and pain; cough, labored breathing; back pain and stiffness.

Techniques and Notes: Insert the needle slightly obliquely upward 0.5–1 *cun*. Moxibustion may be applied.

Dazhui (GV-14)

This is the crossing point of the Du Meridian with the six Yang meridians (the Large Intestine, the Small Intestine, the Stomach, the Bladder, the Sanjiao and the Gallbladder).

Location: On the midline of the back, in the depression below the spinous process of the seventh cervical vertebra.

Applications: Common cold, cold-aversion; pain and stiffness of the head and neck; malaria; febrile diseases, high fever with night sweats; cough, labored breathing; and epilepsy.

Techniques and Notes: Insert the needle slightly obliquely upward 0.5–1 *cun*. Moxibustion may be applied.

Yamen (GV-15)

Location: On the nape, 0.5 *cun* directly above the midpoint of the posterior hairline, below the first cervical vertebra.

Applications: Acute hoarseness of the voice; stroke; stiffness of the tongue with inability to speak; psychosis; epilepsy; stiffness and pain in the head and neck; and epistaxis.

Techniques and Notes: Insert the needle perpendicularly or obliquely downward 0.5–1 *cun*. **Do not aim the needle upward or insert it deeply**. Moxibustion may be applied.

Fengfu (GV-16)

This is the crossing point of the Du Meridian with the Yangwei Meridian.

Location: On the nape, on the posterior midline, 1 *cun* directly above the midpoint of the posterior hairline and directly below the external occipital protuberance.

Applications: Stroke; stiffness of the tongue with difficulty to speak; hemiplegia; psychosis; epilepsy; stiffness and pain in the head and neck; vertigo; sore throat; and epistaxis.

Techniques and Notes: Insert the needle perpendicularly or obliquely downward 0.5–1 *cun*. Deep puncture is not advisable. Moxibustion may be applied.

Baihui (GV-20)

This is the crossing point of the Du and the Bladder Meridians.

Location: On the midline of the head, 5 *cun* directly above the midpoint of the anterior hairline, at the midpoint of the line connecting the apexes of the two auricles.

Applications: Headache; dizziness; stroke with aphasia; hemiplegia; syncope; forgetfulness; insomnia; diarrhea, prolapse of the rectum; enuresis; and psychosis.

Techniques and Notes: Insert the needle subcutaneously 0.5–0.8 *cun*. Moxibustion may be applied.

Shangxing (GV-23)

Location: On the midline of the head, 1 *cun* directly above the midpoint of the anterior hairline.

Applications: Headache; eye pain; epistaxis or nasal discharge; stroke with hemiplegia; and psychosis.

Techniques and Notes: Insert the needle subcutaneously 0.5–1 *cun*. Moxibustion may be applied.

Shenting (GV-24)

This is the crossing point of the Du Meridian with the Bladder and the Stomach Meridians.

Location: On the midline of the head, 0.5 *cun* directly above the midpoint of the anterior hairline.

Applications: Headache; dizziness; insomnia; palpitations of the heart; nasal discharge; and epilepsy.

Techniques and Notes: Insert the needle subcutaneously 0.5–1 *cun*. Moxibustion may be applied.

Shuigou (Renzhong) (GV-26)

This is the crossing point of the Du Meridian with the Large Intestine and the Stomach Meridians.

Location: On the face, at the junction of the upper 1/3 and lower 2/3 of the philtrum.

Applications: Psychosis; coma; syncope; infantile convulsions; acute low back pain; and wry mouth and eye.

Techniques and Notes: Insert the needle obliquely upward 0.3–0.5 *cun*. Moxibustion may be applied.

Section 14 Ren Meridian

I Pathway

The Ren Meridian arises within the lower abdomen and courses to the perineum, where it emerges. It runs to the pubic region and ascends along the abdomen and chest to arrive at the throat. It then continues upward, curves around the lips, passes through the cheek and enters the infra-orbital region (see Fig. 3.14).

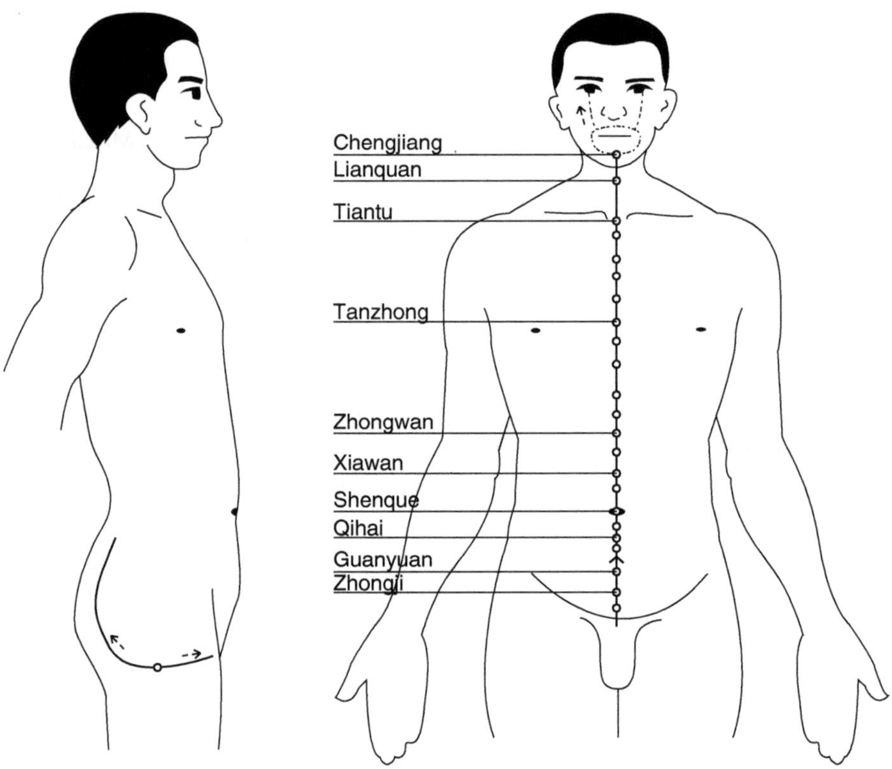

Fig. 3.14 Ren Meridian

II Main Applications

The acupoints of the Ren Meridian are used mainly in the treatment of diseases of the genitourinary system and the intestinal tract. A few of the acupoints have tonic effects, and some others can be used to treat mental diseases.

III Commonly Used Acupoints

There are 24 acupoints in all – see Table 3.14. The more useful ones are individually described.

Zhongji (CV-3)

This is the Front-Mu acupoint of the Bladder Meridian and the crossing point of the Ren, the Spleen, the Kidney and the Liver Meridians.

Location: On the midline of the abdomen, 4 *cun* below the center of the umbilicus.

Applications: Spermatorrhea; impotence; enuresis; anuria; irregular menstruation; metrorrhagia; vaginal discharge; and hernia.

Techniques and Notes: Insert the needle perpendicularly 0.5–1 *cun*. Moxibustion may be applied.

Guanyuan (CV-4)

This is the Front-Mu acupoint of the Small Intestine Meridian and the crossing point of the Ren, the Spleen, the Kidney and the Liver Meridians.

Location: On the midline of the abdomen, 3 *cun* below the center of the umbilicus.

Applications: Spermatorrhea; impotence; polyuria; enuresis; difficulty with urination; irregular menstruation, amenorrhea; metrorrhagia; vaginal discharge; a weak constitution from deficiency or excessive physical labor; and the flaccid type of stroke.

Techniques and Notes: Insert the needle perpendicularly 1–2 *cun*. Moxibustion may be applied.

Qihai (CV-6)

Location: On the midline of the abdomen, 1.5 *cun* below the center of the umbilicus.

Table 3.14 Acupoints of Ren Meridian

Name	Location	Applications
CV-1 Huiyin	On perineum, midpoint between anus and root of scrotum or midpoint between anus and posterior commissure of major lips of vulva	Hemorrhoids; genital itch or pain; prolapse of uterus; irregular menstruation; difficulty with urination; spermatorrhea; psychosis
CV-2 Qugu	On midline of abdomen, at midpoint of upper border of pubic symphysis	Difficulty with urination; enuresis; spermatorrhea; impotence; dysmenorrhea
CV-3	Described separately	
CV-4		
CV-5 Shimen Front-Mu acupoint of sanjiao	On midline of abdomen, 2 *cun* below center of umbilicus	Abdominal distention; edema; difficulty with urination; amenorrhea; vaginal discharge; metrorrhagia; diarrhea; hernia
CV-6	Described separately	
CV-7 Yinjiao	On midline of abdomen, 1 *cun* below center of umbilicus	Abdominal pain; hernia; edema; irregular menstruation; vaginal discharge
CV-8	Described separately	
CV-9 Shuifen	On midline of abdomen, 1 *cun* above center of umbilicus	Edema; anuria; diarrhea; abdominal pain; vomiting
CV-10	Described separately	
CV-11 Jianli	On midline of abdomen, 3 *cun* above center of umbilicus	Gastric pain; vomiting; anorexia; abdominal distention; edema
CV-12	Described separately	
CV-13 Shangwan	On midline of abdomen, 5 *cun* above center of umbilicus	Gastric pain; vomiting; hiccup; abdominal distention; epilepsy
CV-14 Juque Front-Mu acupoint of heart	On midline of abdomen, 6 *cun* above center of umbilicus	Chest pain; heart pain; palpitations of heart; vomiting; psychosis; epilepsy
CV-15 Jiuwei Luo (Connecting) acupoint	On anterior midline, 1 *cun* below symphysis of xiphisternum	Chest pain; hiccup; abdominal distention; psychosis; epilepsy
CV-16 Zhongting	On anterior midline, level with fifth intercostal space, on symphysis of xiphisternum	Chest and flank fullness; heart pain; vomiting
CV-17	Described separately	
CV-18 Yutang	On anterior midline, at level of third intercostal space	Cough; labored breathing; chest pain; vomiting
CV-19 Zigong	On anterior midline, at level of second intercostal space	Cough; labored breathing; chest pain
CV-20 Huagai	On anterior midline, at level of first intercostal space	Cough; labored breathing; chest and flank pain and fullness
CV-21 Xuanji	On anterior midline, in center of manubrium of sternum, 1 *cun* below CV-22	Cough, asthma, chest pain, sore throat
CV-22		
CV-23	Described separately	
CV-24		

Applications: Low abdominal pain; enuresis; spermatorrhea; impotence; irregular menstruation; amenorrhea; metrorrhagia; diarrhea; a weak constitution from deficiency or excessive physical labor; and the flaccid type of stroke.

Techniques and Notes: Insert the needle perpendicularly 1–2 *cun*. Moxibustion may be applied.

Shenque (CV-8)

Location: On the middle abdomen at the center of the umbilicus.

Applications: The flaccid type of stroke; coldness of all four limbs; diarrhea with rectal prolapse; abdominal pain with borborygmus; sweating on one side of the body; and edema.

Techniques and Notes: Needling of this acupoint is prohibited. Moxibustion, often with ginger or salt, may be applied.

Xiawan (CV-10)

This is the crossing point of the Ren and Spleen Meridians.

Location: On the midline of the abdomen, 2 *cun* above the center of the umbilicus.

Applications: Epigastric pain; abdominal pain and distention; borborygmus; diarrhea, vomiting; and hiccup.

Techniques and Notes: Insert the needle perpendicularly 1–2 *cun*. Moxibustion may be applied.

Zhongwan (CV-12)

This is the Front-Mu acupoint of the stomach, the Influential acupoint for the *fu* organs, and the crossing point of the Ren, the Small Intestine, the Sanjiao and the Stomach Meridians.

Location: On the midline of the abdomen, 4 *cun* above the center of the umbilicus.

Applications: Gastric pain; abdominal distention; borborygmus; vomiting; hiccup; diarrhea; jaundice; cough with much sputum; and insomnia.

Techniques and Notes: Insert the needle perpendicularly 1–2 *cun*. Moxibustion may be applied.

Tanzhong (CV-17)

This is the Front-Mu acupoint of the pericardium and the Influential acupoint for Qi.

Location: On the anterior midline, at the level of the fourth intercostal space, midway between the nipples.

Applications: Labored breathing; chest pain; chest tightness; palpitations of the heart; heart pain; insufficient lactation; hiccup; and difficulty in swallowing.

Techniques and Notes: Insert the needle subcutaneously 0.3–0.5 *cun*. Moxibustion may be applied.

Tiantu (CV-22)

This is the crossing point between the Ren and the Yinwei Meridians.

Location: On the anterior midline, at the center of the sternal notch.

Applications: Cough; labored breathing; chest pain; sore throat; sudden hoarseness of the voice; difficulty in swallowing; and goiter.

Techniques and Notes: Insert the needle perpendicularly 0.2 *cun*, then continue the insertion with the needle tip aimed downward along the posterior surface of the sternum 0.5–1 *cun*. Moxibustion may be applied.

Lianquan (CV-23)

This is the crossing point between the Ren and the Yinwei Meridians.

Location: On the neck and on the anterior midline, above the laryngeal prominence, in the depression above the upper border of the hyoid bone.

Applications: Sublingual swelling and pain; excessive salivation; tongue stiffness with difficulty to speak; sudden hoarseness of voice; and difficulty in swallowing.

Techniques and Notes: Insert the needle obliquely 0.5–0.8 *cun* toward the tongue root.

Chengjiang (CV-24)

This is the crossing point of the Ren and the Stomach Meridians.

Location: On the face, in the depression at the center of chin-lip groove.

Applications: Wry eye and mouth; gingivitis; excessive salivation; sudden hoarseness of the voice; psychosis; and enuresis.

Techniques and Notes: Insert the needle obliquely 0.3–0.5 *cun*. Moxibustion may be applied.

Section 15 Extra-Meridian Acupoints

In addition to the acupoints on the 12 regular meridians, the Du and the Ren Meridians, there are 22 commonly used acupoints not affiliated with any of the meridians. In the following they are loosely grouped by the region of the body where they are found.

I Acupoints on Head and Neck

Sishencong (EX-HN-1)

There are actually four acupoints under this name.

Location: On the vertex of the head, respectively 1 *cun* anterior, posterior, left and right of Baihui (GV-20).

Applications: Headache; dizziness; insomnia; forgetfulness; and epilepsy.

Techniques and Notes: Insert the needle perpendicularly 0.5–0.8 *cun*. Moxibustion may be applied.

Yintang (EX-HN-3)

Location: On the forehead, midway between the medial ends of the two eyebrows.

Applications: Headache; heaviness in the head; dizziness; insomnia; nasal discharge, epistaxis; infantile convulsions.

Techniques and Notes: Insert the needle subcutaneously 0.3–0.5 *cun*. Moxibustion may be applied.

Yuyao (EX-HN-4)

Location: On the forehead, within the eyebrow, vertically above the pupil when looking straight.

Applications: Drooping or twitching of the eyelids; inflammation of the eye; supra-orbital pain; wry mouth and eyes; and corneal opacity.

Techniques and Notes: Insert the needle subcutaneously 0.3–0.5 *cun*. Moxibustion is not applicable.

Taiyang (EX-HN-5)

Location: On the temple, in the depression the breadth of one finger behind the lateral end of the eyebrow and the outer canthus.

Applications: Headache; dizziness; inflammation of the eye; wry mouth and eyes; and facial pain.

Techniques and Notes: Insert the needle perpendicularly or obliquely 0.3–0.5 *cun* or prick to cause bleeding. Moxibustion may be applied.

Shangyinxiang (EX-HN-8)

Location: On the face, at the highest point of the nasolabial groove.

Applications: Nasal discharge, and boils on the nose.

Techniques and Notes: Insert the needle subcutaneously upward 0.3–0.5 *cun*. **Moxibustion is not applicable**.

Anmian

Location: On the nape of the neck, midway between Yifeng (SJ-17) and Fengchi (GB-20).

Applications: Insomnia; dizziness; headache; palpitations of the heart; psychosis; and epilepsy.

Techniques and Notes: Insert the needle perpendicularly 0.8–1.2 *cun*. Moxibustion may be applied.

II Acupoint on Chest and Abdomen

Zigong (EX-CA-1)

Location: On the lower abdomen, 4 *cun* below the center of the umbilicus and 3 *cun* lateral to Zhongji (CV-3).

Applications: Prolapse of the uterus, irregular menstruation, metrorrhagia, dysmenorrhea, or amenorrhea; infertility; hernia; and low back pain.

Techniques and Notes: Insert the needle perpendicularly 0.8–1.2 *cun*. Moxibustion may be applied.

III Acupoints on Back

Dingchuan (EX-B-1)

Location: On the back, below the spinous process of the seventh cervical vertebra, 0.5 *cun* from the posterior midline.

Applications: Labored breathing; cough; chest tightness; shortness of breath; and sore throat.

Techniques and Notes: Insert the needle perpendicularly 0.3–0.5 *cun*. Moxibustion may be applied.

Jiaji (EX-B-2)

There are actually 34 acupoints under this name, arranged along the two sides of the spinal column.

Location: Each acupoint is 0.5 *cun* from the midline, just below the lower border of each spinous process of a vertebra, from the first thoracic to the fifth lumbar vertebra.

Applications: Jiaji on the upper back: diseases of the heart, the lung and the upper limbs. Acupoints on the mid back: diseases of the stomach and the intestines. Acupoints on lower (lumbar) back: diseases in the lumbar and abdominal regions and in the lower limbs.

Techniques and Notes: Insert the needle perpendicularly 0.3–0.5 *cun*, or tap with the plum-blossom-needle (Volume 1, Part I, Chapter 4). Moxibustion may be applied.

Yaoyan (EX-B-7)

Location: On the lower back, below the lower border of the spinous process of the fourth lumbar vertebra, in the depression about 3.5 *cun* from the midline.

Applications: Irregular menstruation; vaginal discharge; and lumbar pain.

Techniques and Notes: Insert the needle perpendicularly 1–1.5 *cun*. Moxibustion may be applied.

IV Acupoints on Upper Extremities

Jianqian

Location: On the shoulder, midway between the end of the anterior axillary fold and Jianyu (LI-15) when sitting with the arm adducted.

Applications: Pain in the shoulder and arm; and inability to raise the arms.

Techniques and Notes: Insert the needle perpendicularly 1–1.5 *cun*. Moxibustion may be applied.

Yaotongdian (EX-UE-7)

There are two acupoints under this name on each hand, four in all.

Location: On the dorsum of the hand, midway between the transverse wrist crease and the metacarpophalangeal joint, between the second and third metacarpal bones and between the fourth and fifth metacarpal bones.

Applications: Acute lumbar sprain.

Techniques and Notes: Insert the needle obliquely 0.5–0.8 *cun* toward the center of the metacarpus from both sides.

Baxie (EX-UE-9)

There are four acupoints under this name.

Location: Four points on the dorsum of each hand, one each at the junction of the lighter and darker skin proximal to the margin of the web between each pair of adjacent fingers.

Applications: High fever; eye pain; finger numbness; and swelling and pain of the dorsum of the hand.

Techniques and Notes: Insert the needle obliquely 0.5–0.8 *cun*, or prick to cause slight bleeding.

Sifeng (EX-UE-10)

There are four acupoints on each hand.

Location: On the palmar surface of the second to the fifth fingers, one acupoint at the midpoint of the transverse creases of each of the proximal interphalangeal joints.

Applications: Malnutrition and indigestion syndrome in children; and whooping cough.

Techniques and Notes: Prick to cause slight bleeding, or following the pricking squeeze out a small amount of yellowish viscous fluid locally.

Shixuan (EX-UE-11)

There are ten acupoints in all on both hands.

Location: In the center of the tips of each of the ten fingers, about 0.1 *cun* from the free margin of the nails.

Applications: Coma; stroke; epilepsy; high fever; and sore throat.

Techniques and Notes: Puncture shallowly 0.1–0.2 *cun*, or prick to cause slight bleeding.

V Acupoints of Lower Extremities

Heding (EX-LE-2)

Location: In the depression proximal to the midpoint of the upper border of the patella.

Applications: Knee pain; weakness of the foot and leg; and paralysis.

Techniques and Notes: Insert the needle perpendicularly 1–1.5 *cun*. Moxibustion may be applied.

Dannang (EX-LE-6)

Location: On the upper part of the lateral side of the leg, in the depression 2 *cun* directly anterior-inferior to the head of the fibula (Yanglingquan, GB-34).

Applications: Acute or chronic cholecystitis; cholelithiasis; and paresis of the lower extremities.

Techniques and Notes: Insert the needle perpendicularly 1–2 *cun*. Moxibustion may be applied.

Lanwei (EX-LE-7)

Location: On the upper part of the lateral side of the leg, about 2 *cun* below Zusanli (ST-36), the breadth of one finger lateral to the anterior crest of the tibia.

Applications: Acute or chronic appendicitis; indigestion; paresis of the lower extremities.

Techniques and Notes: Insert the needle perpendicularly 1.5–2 *cun*. Moxibustion may be applied.

Bafeng (EX-LE-10)

There are all together eight acupoints, four on each foot.

Location: On the dorsum of the foot, at the junction of the lighter and darker skin proximal to the margin of the web between each pair of adjacent toes.

Applications: Beriberi; toe pain; snake or insect bites; swelling and pain of the dorsum of the foot.

Techniques and Notes: Insert the needle obliquely 0.5–0.8 *cun*, or prick to cause slight bleeding.

Guidance for Study

I Aim of Study

To acquire familiarity with the location and the main applications of the acupoints commonly used in acupuncture. This is the foundation for the clinical application of acupuncture.

II Objectives of Study

After completing this chapter the learners will

1. Be familiar with the pathways of the 14 meridians and their connections with the related *zang–fu* organs;
2. Be familiar with the acupoints of the 14 meridians, especially with every first and last acupoint;
3. Know the location and main applications of the commonly used acupoints.

III Exercises for Review

1. Describe the pathway and main applications of each of the 12 regular meridians.
2. Describe the pathways and main applications of the Du and the Ren Meridians.
3. Describe the pathways of the branches of the Bladder meridian on the back?
4. When the stomach meridian runs to its end, which meridian does it connect to?
5. Which meridian does the Gallbladder Meridian connect to on the foot?
6. How many acupoints does each meridian have? Name the first and the last acupoints of each meridian.
7. Describe the location and main applications of the following five acupoints of the Lung Meridian: LU-1 (Zhongfu), LU-5 (Chize), LU-7 (Lieque), LU-9 (Taiyuan) and LU-11 (Shaoshang).
8. Locate the following acupoints of the Large Intestine Meridian: LI-1 (Shangyang), LI-4 (Hegu), LI-11 (Quchi), and LI-15 (Jianyu).
9. How many commonly used acupoints does the Stomach Meridian have on the head? Describe their locations and main applications.
10. What are the main applications of ST-36 (Zusanli) and ST-25 (Tianshu)?
11. What kind of specific points are the following acupoints: ST-45 (Lidui), ST-44 (Neiting), ST-41 (Jiexi), ST-40 (Fenglong), ST-39 (Xiajuxu), ST-37 (Shangjuxu), ST-36 (Zusanli), ST-34 (Liangqiu), and ST-25 (Tianshu)?
12. For what kinds of conditions can ST-44 (Neiting), LI-4 (Hegu) be used to treat? For what kinds of conditions can ST-40 (Fenglong) be used to treat?
13. Locate the following acupoints: SP-1 (Yinbai), SP-4 (Gongsun), SP-6 (Sanyinjiao) and SP-9 (Yinlingquan). What kind of conditions can they used to treat?
14. Describe the location and main applications of the following acupoints: HT-1 (Jiquan), HT-3 (Shaohai), HT-5 (Tongli), HT-7 (Shenmen) and HT-9 (Shaochong).
15. For what kinds of conditions can SI-1 (Shaoze) and SI-3 (Houxi) be used to treat?
16. How many commonly used points of the Small Intestine Meridian are found on the face? Describe their locations and main applications.
17. What cautions must be taken when applying acupuncture on BL-1 (Jingming)?
18. For what conditions is BL-67 (Zhiyin) mainly used to treat?
19. Describe the locations and main applications of all the Back-Shu acupoints.
20. Describe the locations and main applications of the following acupoints: BL-40 (Weizhong), BL-54 (Zhibian), BL-57 (Chengshan) and BL-60 (Kunlun).
21. Describe the locations and main applications of the following acupoints: KI-1 (Yongquan), KI-3 (Taixi), KI-6 (Zhaohai) and KI-7 (Fuliu).
22. Describe the locations and main applications of the following acupoints: PC-3 (Quze), PC-5 (Jianshi), PC-6 (Neiguan), PC-7 (Daling), PC-8 (Laogong) and PC-9 (Zhongchong).
23. What are the main applications of SJ-5 (Waiguan) and SJ-6 (Zhigou) respectively?
24. Which acupoints of the Gallbladder Meridian can be used to treat disorders of the ear? Describe their locations.

25. What cautions must be taken when applying acupuncture on GB-21 (Jianjing)?
26. What are the main applications of GB-20 (Fengchi) and what cautions must be taken when applying acupuncture on it?
27. How many of the acupoints of the Gallbladder Meridian are useful for treating eye disorders?
28. Describe the locations and main applications of the following acupoints: GB-30 (Huantiao), GB-31 (Fengshi), GB-34 (Yanglingquan), and GB-40 (Qiuxu).
29. Describe the locations and main applications of the following acupoints: LR-1 (Dadun), LR-2 (Xingjian), and LR-3 (Taichong).
30. Which of the commonly used acupoints of the Ren Meridian are distributed on the abdomen? Describe their locations and main applications.
31. Which of the commonly used acupoints of the Du Meridian are distributed on the head? Describe their locations and main applications.
32. Describe the location and main applications of GV-14 (Dazhui)?
33. Describe the location of GV-20 (Baihui)? For what conditions is it useful for treating?
34. Which of the commonly used extra-meridian acupoints are distributed on the head? Describe their main applications.
35. Describe the conditions for which each of the following extra-meridian acupoints is useful in treatment: Sifeng (EX-UE-10), Shixuan (EX-UE-11), Baxie (EX-UE-9), Bafeng (BE-10), Jiaji (EX-B-2), and Danangxue (EX-LE-6).
36. At which acupoints is acupuncture contraindicated or not advisable in pregnant women?
37. At which acupoints is moxibustion contraindicated or not advisable?

Chapter 4
Techniques of Acupuncture and Moxibustion

Section 1 Filiform Needle

I Structure and Selection of Needle

The filiform needle is one of nine kinds of needles used in acupuncture in ancient China. Most of the filiform needles used at present are made of stainless steel. The structure of the filiform needle may be described in five parts (Fig. 4.1):

Tip: the sharp point of the needle.
Shaft: the part between the handle and the tip.
Root: the connecting part between the shaft and the handle.
Handle: the part above the shaft, which is held in the hand.
Tail: the part at the end of the handle.

Carefully inspect the needles before use. In general, the tip must not be too sharp but must not be dull – like a pine needle. The shaft must be straight, round and smooth, flexible and resilient. If the shaft is eroded, rusted or bent, the needle should be discarded. The root must not be eroded or loose, since it may break.

In addition, select a needle of appropriate size – whether long or short, thick or thin – in accordance with the patient's sex, age, body type, constitution, the thickness or thinness of the acupoint where acupuncture is to be applied and the depth to which the needle is to be inserted.

II Preparations Prior to Acupuncture Treatment

1 Patient's Posture

In acupuncture treatment the patient's posture is important for the correct location of the acupoints, for the manipulation of the needles during insertion, for prolonged needle retention in place, for moxibustion, and for avoiding fainting during the

Z.W. Liu and L. Liu (eds.), *Essentials of Chinese Medicine: Volume 2*,

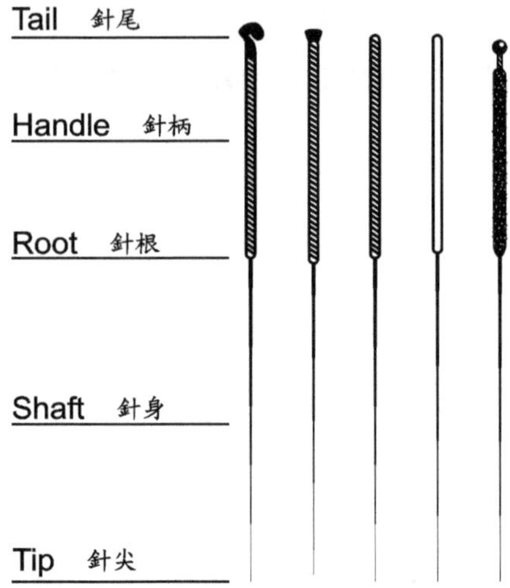

Fig. 4.1 Structure of filiform needle

procedure. It is also important for avoiding the bending or breaking of the needles or their becoming stuck.

The commonly used postures are as follows.

i Recumbent Postures

In general, use the recumbent postures as much as possible for new, nervous, aged or weak, or seriously ill patients to avoid fainting.

Supine Posture (Fig. 4.2): Suitable for needling the acupoints on the head and face, chest and abdominal region, the medial side of the upper limbs, the anterior side of the lower limbs, and the hands and feet.

Prone Posture (Fig. 4.3): Suitable for needling the acupoints on the posterior head and neck, back, lumbar and buttock regions, and the posterior part of the lower limbs.

Lateral Recumbent (Fig. 4.4): Suitable for needling the acupoints on the posterior-lateral head, neck and back.

ii Upright Postures

Leaning Back Posture (Fig. 4.5): Suitable for needling the acupoints on the forehead, face, neck and the upper portion of the chest.

Leaning Forward Posture (Fig. 4.6): Suitable for needling the acupoints on the vertex, posterior head, posterior neck, shoulder and back.

Lateral Sitting Posture (Fig. 4.7): Sitting with one side of the face resting on a table: suitable for needling the acupoints on the lateral side of the face, side of the head, neck, and for some of the acupoints around the ear.

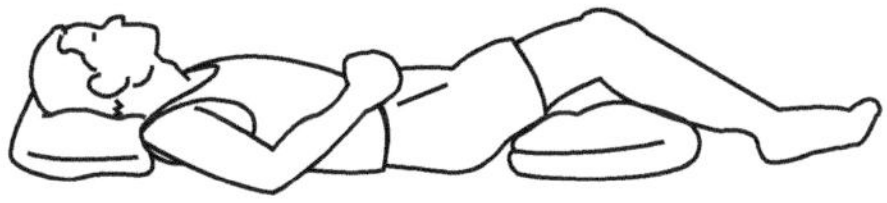

Fig. 4.2 Supine posture

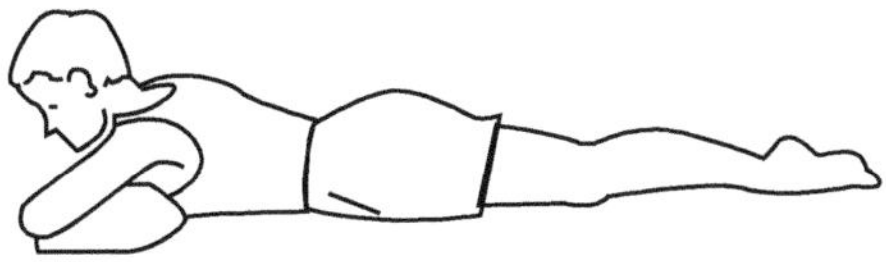

Fig. 4.3 Prone posture

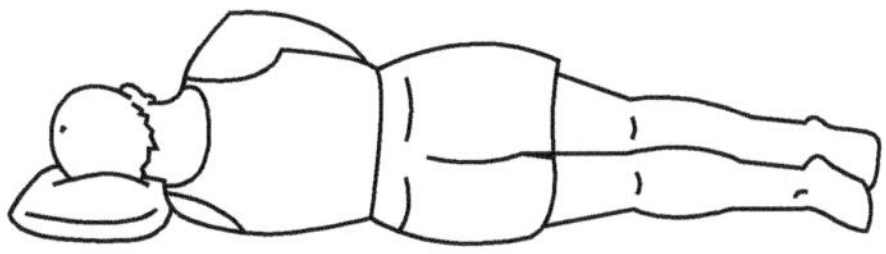

Fig. 4.4 Lateral recumbent

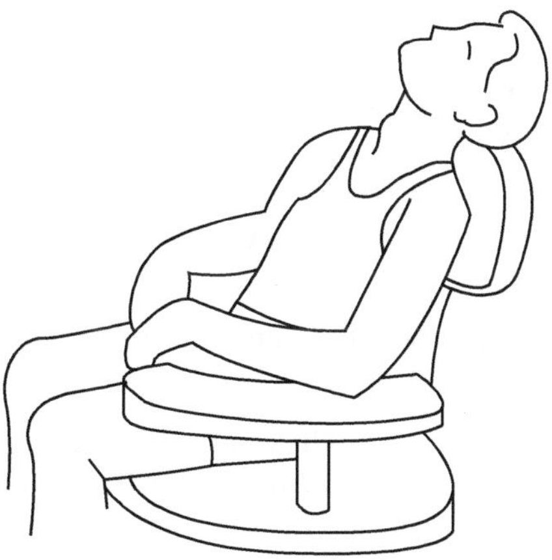

Fig. 4.5 Leaning back posture

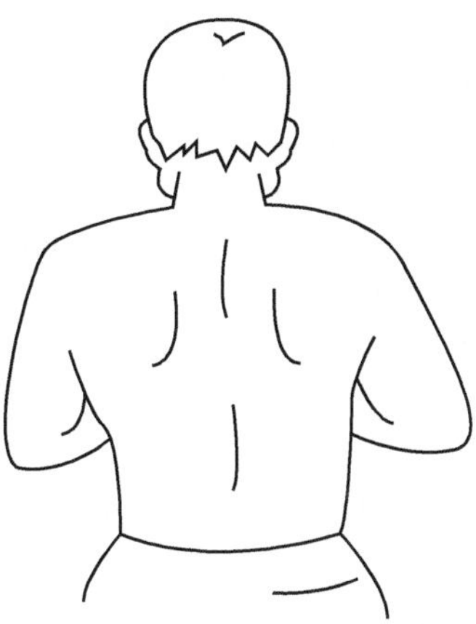

Fig. 4.6 Prone sitting posture

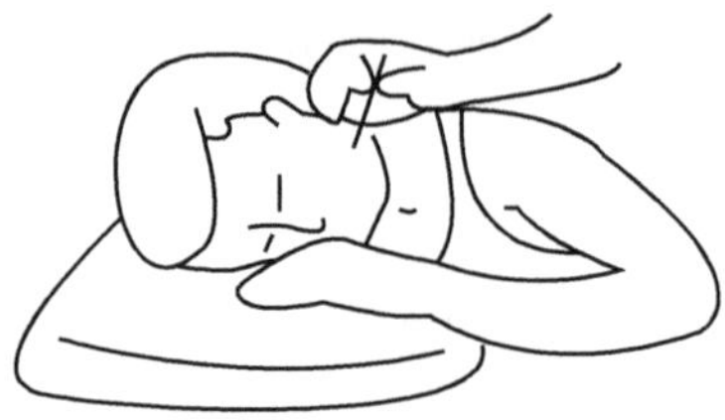

Fig. 4.7 Lateral sitting posture

2 *Sterilization*

Nowadays, pre-sterilized and disposable acupuncture needles are used. Where these are not available, reusable needles may be sterilized by the following procedures.

Sterilization refers to the sterilization of the needles and other instruments, the physicians' hands and the area where acupuncture is applied.

Sterilizing Instruments: The following techniques may be chosen, depending on circumstances.

Autoclave Sterilization: Cleaned needles and other instruments wrapped in gauze are sterilized in an autoclave at 1.5 atmospheric pressure and 120°C for 15 min or longer.

Boiling Sterilization: Cleaned needles and other instruments are boiled in water for 15–20 min.

Chemical Sterilization: Cleaned needles are soaked in 70% alcohol for at least 30 min. Wipe off the liquid from the needles for use, using sterile wipes. Glass instruments and instruments that are less heat-resistance should be soaked in bromogeramine (1:1,000) for 1–2 h.

Disinfecting Practitioners' Hands: Before acupuncture treatment, the practitioner's hands should be cleansed with water and soap or with alcohol.

Disinfecting Area of Acupoint: The area on the body surface selected for needling should be clean and disinfected with a cotton swab soaked in 70% alcohol, or with 2.5% tincture of iodine (remove the iodine with 70% alcohol). Do not touch the disinfected area with articles that have not been sterilized or disinfected, to avoid contaminating it.

III Techniques of Needling

The selection among the following techniques depends on the anatomic features of the area where the acupoints are located and on the required depth and manipulation. Choose a technique that tends to produce the least amount of pain.

1 Inserting Needle

In general, use the right hand, the "needling hand," to hold the needle and the left hand, the "assisting hand," to press the area or support the shaft of the needle. (For left-handed physicians, the left hand may be the "needling hand" and the right the "assisting hand.") The function of the needling hand is to hold and manipulate the needle, and the function of the assisting hand is to fix the location of an acupoint and to grip the needle shaft in assisting the needling hand to insert the needle. At present the commonly used techniques of insertion are as follows.

i One Handed Insertion

The handle of the needle is held between the thumb and index finger of the needling hand and the lower portion of the shaft is steadied with the tip of the middle finger (Fig. 4.8). Insert the needle after the acupoint has been massaged for a few seconds so that the patient experiences numbness, slight soreness or a comfortable feeling in the area. This method is suitable for the insertion of a filiform needle that is 0.5–1 *cun* long.

ii Two Handed Insertion

The needle is inserted using both hands acting in unison.

Finger-Press Insertion (Fig. 4.9): Gently press on the acupoint with the nail of the thumb or another finger of the assisting hand. Insert the needle with the needling hand, using the fingernail of the assisting hand as guide. This method is suitable for puncturing with short needles.

Pinched-Needle Insertion (Fig. 4.10): Hold a dry sterile cotton ball around the needle tip with the assisting hand so that the needle tip is directly on the selected acupoint and hold the needle handle with the needling hand. As the needling hand

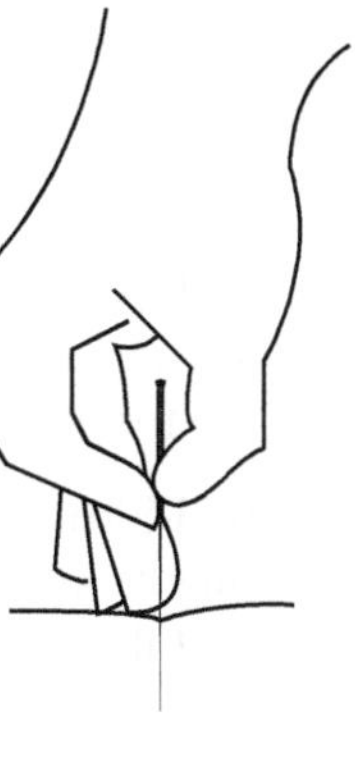

Fig. 4.8 One-handed insertion

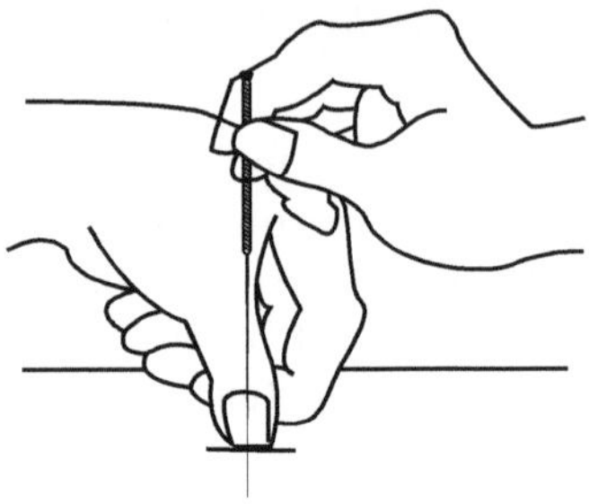

Fig. 4.9 Finger-press insertion

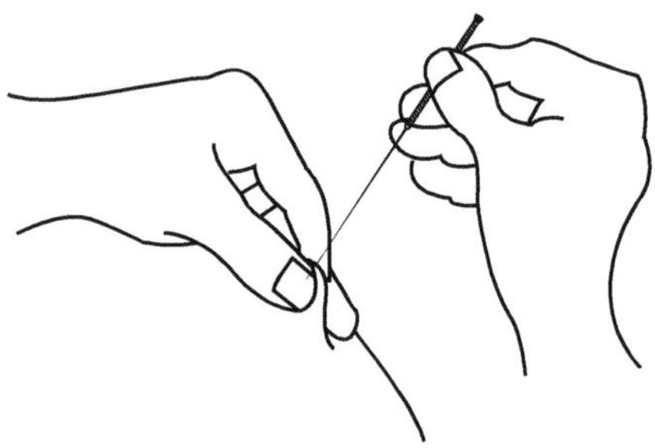

Fig. 4.10 Pinched-needle insertion

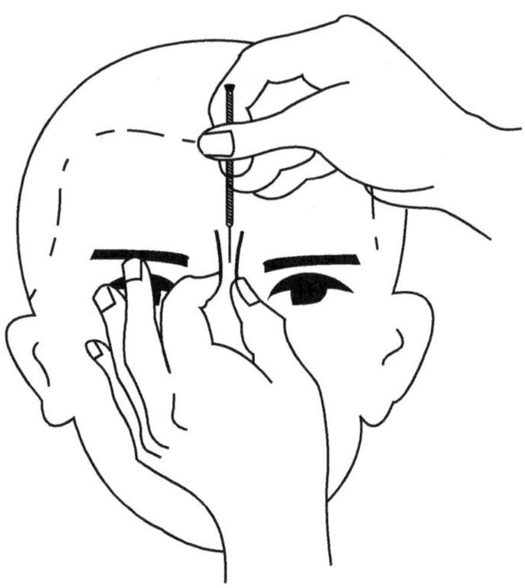

Fig. 4.11 Pinched-skin insertion

presses the needle downward, the assisting hand guides the needle tip into the skin. (Be sure the needle tip does not carry any cotton fiber into the skin.) This method is suitable for puncturing with long needles.

Pinched-Skin Insertion (Fig. 4.11): Pinch the skin around the acupoint with the assisting hand and hold the needle with the needling hand. Insert the needle into the acupoint through the pad of skin formed by the pinching. This method is suitable for puncturing acupoints in areas where the muscle and skin are thin.

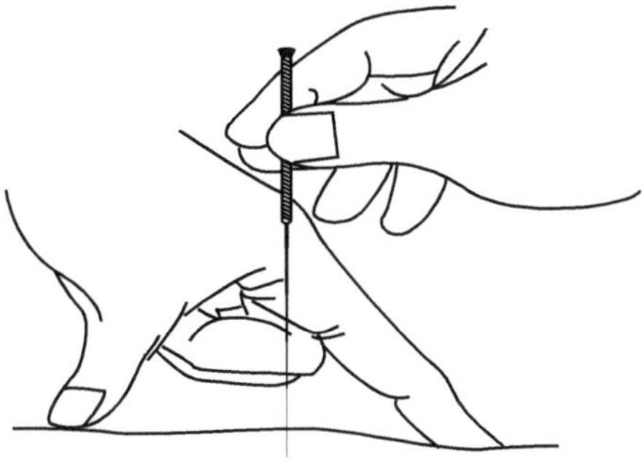

Fig. 4.12 Stretched-skin insertion

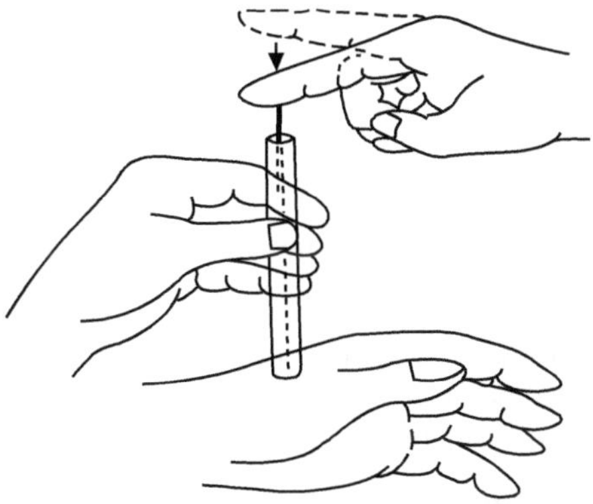

Fig. 4.13 Insertion using tube

Stretched-Skin Insertion (Fig. 4.12): With the assisting hand stretch the skin taut over the acupoint and insert the needle into the acupoint with the needling hand. This method is suitable for puncturing acupoints in an area where the skin is loose.

iii Insertion Using a Tube

Select a sterile metal or glass tube with a bore of appropriate size (just big enough for the needle to pass through easily) and about 2 in. in length. Apply pressure on the needle tail with the index finger, but using wrist action. When the correct depth is attained remove the tube over the top while grasping the exposed part of the shaft (see Fig. 4.13).

2 *Angle and Depth of Insertion*

The angle and depth of insertion of the acupuncture needle are especially important. Using the correct angle and depth facilitates the induction of the "needle sensation" (see below, Sub-subsection 3), brings about the desired therapeutic result and ensures safety.

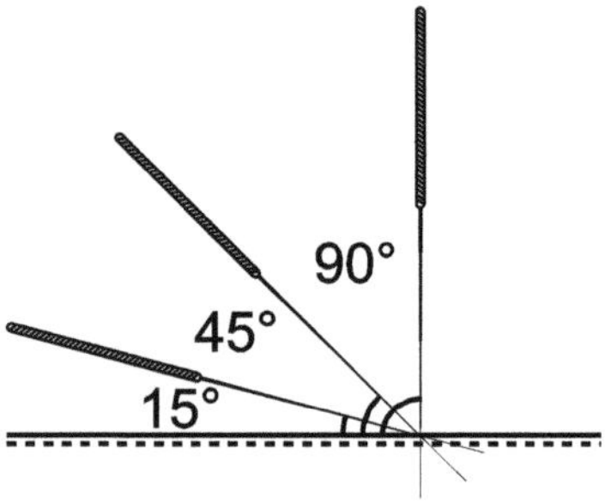

Fig. 4.14 Angles of insertion

i Angle of Insertion

The angle of insertion refers to the angle formed between the needle and the skin surface as the needle is inserted. In general, acupuncture uses three angles (see Fig. 4.14).

Perpendicular: The needle is inserted perpendicularly, forming a 90° angle with the skin surface. This is appropriate for most of the acupoints.

Oblique: The needle is inserted at an angle of 45° with the skin surface. This method is used for acupoints in which deep insertion is not advisable, or used to avoid puncturing blood vessels or scars.

Subcutaneous (Horizontal, Transverse): The needle is inserted at an angle of 15–25° with the skin surface. This method is suitable for acupoints on the skin or muscle.

ii Depth of Insertion

In general, the depth of insertion of the acupuncture needle depends on the pathological condition and the location of the acupoints. Patients with different constitutions and body types have different needling sensations; therefore, the depth of insertion must be determined with full consideration of the actual conditions, location of acupoints and the specific traits of each patient. Only by doing so will the physician obtain better therapeutic results.

3 *Manipulations and Arrival of Qi (Needling Sensation)*

When the acupuncture needle is inserted correctly, meridian Qi arrives at the needle and produces the needling sensation. To the patient the needling sensation may be soreness, numbness, a feeling of distention or heaviness around the acupoint, sometimes a feeling of coldness, warmth, itch, pain, a feeling of electric shock, or a feeling of ants crawling. At the same time, to the physician it may be a sensation of tenseness or dragging around the needle.

Many factors influence the arrival of Qi, hence the needling sensation. The main ones are related to the constitution of the patient, the severity of the illness, the location of the acupoint, and the needling manipulations. In general, it develops quickly in a patient with abundant meridian Qi, or Qi and blood. Conversely, it may develop slowly or not at all in a patient with excessive Yin or deficient Yang.

The needling sensation does not come easily if the location is not accurate. In such cases, manipulation of the needle may be necessary to induce the arrival of meridian Qi and the needling sensation.

The techniques of manipulation can be divided into two general types: fundamental and auxiliary.

i Fundamental Manipulations

These are the basic manipulations in acupuncture. The two commonly used techniques are as follows. They may be used either alone or in combination, depending upon the diagnosis of the patient's condition.

Lifting and Thrusting (Fig. 4.15): When the needle has been inserted to an appropriate depth it is alternately pulled back slightly (lifting) and pushed in slightly (thrusting).

Twisting or Rotating (Fig. 4.16): The needle is twisted or rotated back and forth when it has been inserted to the desired depth. The manipulation is performed with the thumb and the index and middle fingers of the needling hand on the handle of the needle.

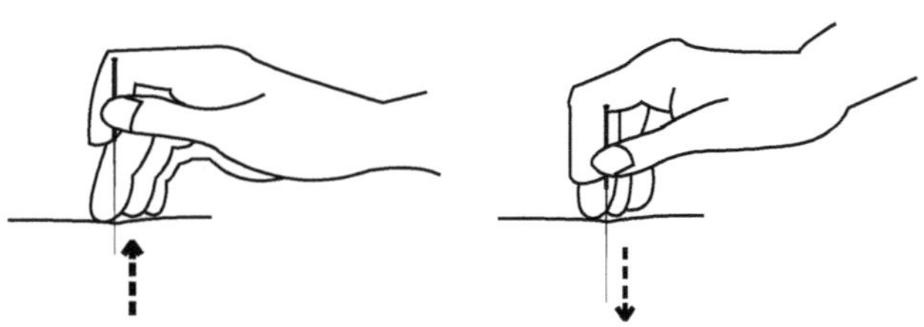

Fig. 4.15 Thrusting and lifting

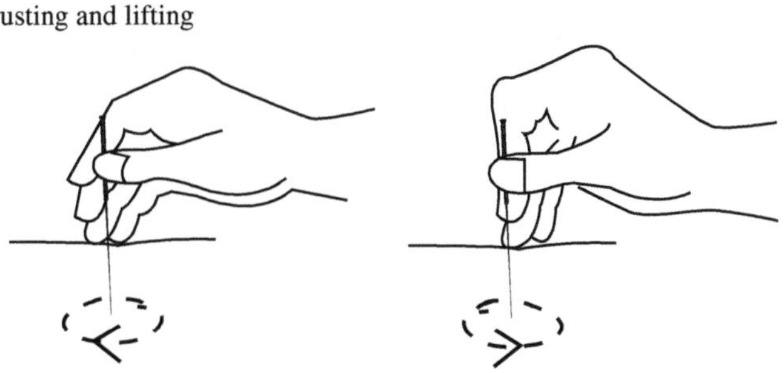

Fig. 4.16 Twisting and rotating

ii Auxiliary Manipulations

The auxiliary manipulations include massaging, flicking, scraping, shaking and flying.

Massaging (Fig. 4.17): Press or tap along the course of the meridian toward the needle from either direction. This manipulation promotes the circulation of Qi and blood so that meridian Qi can reach the needle.

Flicking (Fig. 4.18): With the needle in position gently flick the needle handle to make it vibrate slightly. This magnifies the stimulation to induce the arrival of Qi.

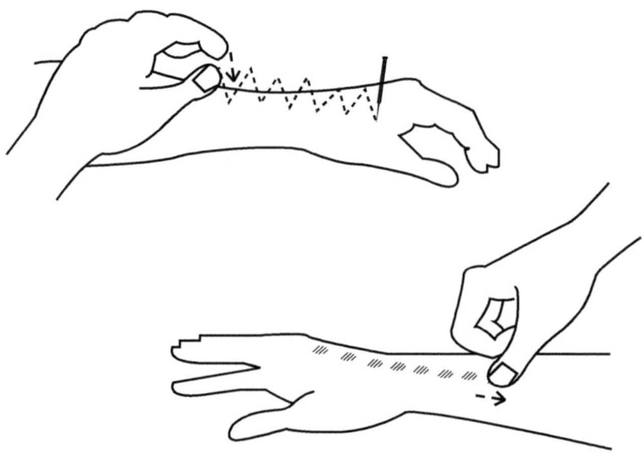

Fig. 4.17 Massaging

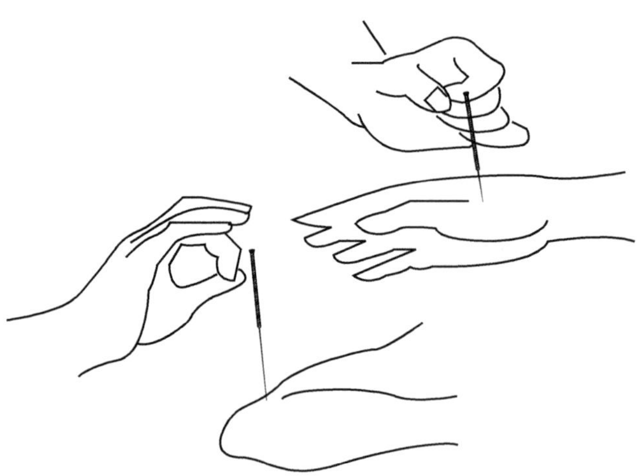

Fig. 4.18 Flicking

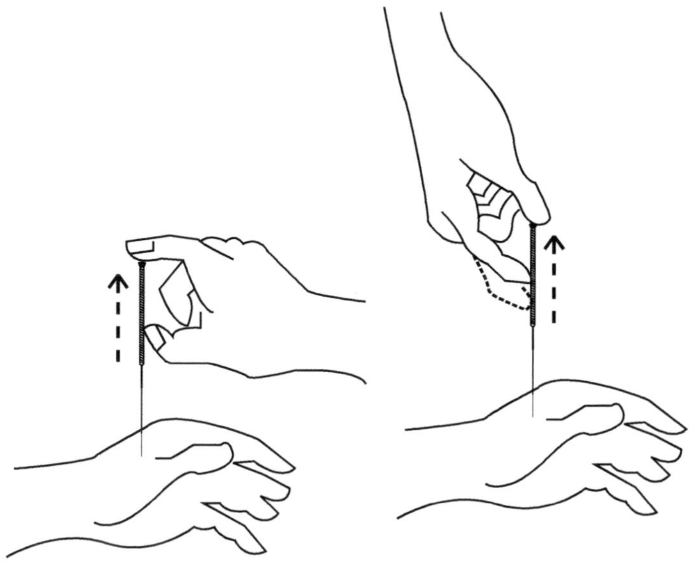

Fig. 4.19 Scraping

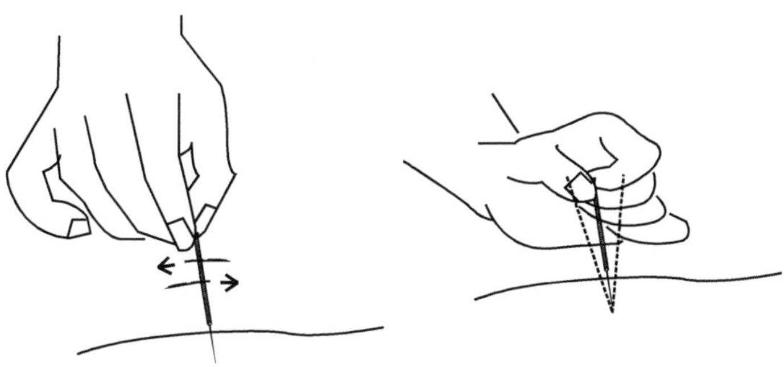

Fig. 4.20 Shaking

Scraping (Fig. 4.19): After the needle has been inserted to an appropriate depth, gently scrape its handle with a fingernail. This maneuver also promotes the arrival of Qi, and it spreads the needling sensation.

Shaking (Fig. 4.20): After the needle has been inserted to an appropriate depth, gently shake the needle at its handle. Shaking conducts the flow of Qi and the needling sensation in a desired direction.

Flying: After the needle has been inserted to an appropriate depth, twirl the needle and release it, moving the fingers away like the spreading wings of a bird taking flight. This manipulation can induce the spread of the meridian Qi and enhance the therapeutic result.

4 *Reinforcing and Reducing Techniques*

The fundamental manipulations of acupuncture are capable of reinforcing what is deficient and reducing what is excessive in the body. The basic reinforcing and reducing techniques are as follows. They may be used in combination in clinical practice.

i By Twisting or Rotating Needle

Twisting or rotating the needle to the left (counterclockwise) is reinforcing, whereas twisting or rotating to the right (clockwise) is reducing (see Fig. 4.21).

ii By Direction of Insertion

Inserting the needle in the direction of the course of its meridian is reinforcing. Conversely, inserting the needle in the opposite direction is reducing (see Fig. 4.22).

For example, take the three Yin meridians of the hand. These meridians run from the chest to the hand. Hence, when applying acupuncture to an acupoint along any of these meridians, inserting the needle aimed toward the hand is reinforcing, whereas inserting the needle aimed away from the hand is reducing.

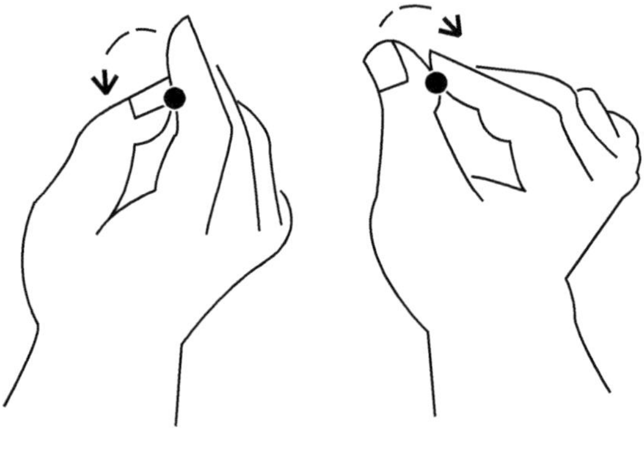

Fig. 4.21 Reinforcing and reducing

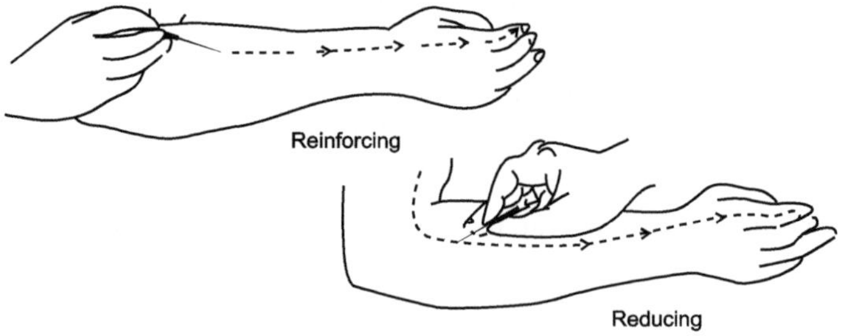

Fig. 4.22 By direction of insertion

iii By Speed of Insertion and Withdrawal

Slow insertion and rapid withdrawal of the needle is reinforcing. Conversely, rapid insertion and slow withdrawal of the needle is reducing.

iv By Lifting and Thrusting

After the needle has been inserted to an appropriate depth and the needling sensation appeared, heavy thrusting and gentle lifting, with more thrusting than lifting, is reinforcing. Conversely, gentle thrusting and heavy lifting, with more lifting than thrusting, is reducing.

v By Respiratory Cycle

Insertion of the needle during exhalation and withdrawal during inhalation is reinforcing. Conversely, insertion of the needle during inhalation and withdrawal during exhalation is reducing.

vi By Rapidity of Blockage of Hole

Slow withdrawal of the needle followed by immediate blockage of the hole is reinforcing. Conversely, rapid withdrawal of the needle followed by delayed blockage of the hole is reducing.

vii Even Reinforcing–Reducing

After the needle has been inserted and the needling sensation has appeared, lift, thrust and rotate the needle evenly, then withdraw it at a moderate speed. This is known as even reinforcing–reducing (neither reinforcing nor reducing).

5 *Complex Reinforcing and Reducing Techniques*

In addition to the techniques in the previous subsection, there are the following complex reinforcing and reducing techniques.

i Setting Mountain on Fire (Reinforcing)

First determine the depth to which the acupoint is to be punctured. Divide this depth into three equal portions – superficial, medium and deep.

After the needle has been slowly inserted beneath the skin, thrust the needle heavily and lift it slightly, keeping the tip in the superficial portion of the depth. Repeat this cycle 9 times.

Then insert the needle to the medium portion of the depth. Again, thrust heavily and lift slightly for nine cycles, keeping the tip in the medium portion of the depth.

Finally insert the needle to the deep portion of the depth. Repeat the heavy thrusting and slight lifting for nine cycles, keeping the tip within the deep portion of the depth.

Upon completing these cycles lift the needle directly from the deep to the superficial portion of the depth and repeat the process.

The entire process may be repeated, several times as needed, until a warm sensation develops. When the needling sensation has appeared, quickly withdraw the needle and block the hole.

This operation may be performed in combination with the reinforcing technique of inserting the needle during exhalation and withdrawing it during inhalation.

ii Penetrating Heavenly Cold (Reducing)

Insert the needle into the acupoint to the deep portion of the required depth. Lift the needle quickly and thrust slowly, and repeat this cycle for 6 times.

Then lift the needle to the medium portion of the depth and repeat the quick-lift and slow-thrust cycle for 6 times.

Further life the needle to the superficial portion of the depth, and again repeat the quick-lift and slow-thrust cycle for 6 times.

The entire process may be repeated several times until a cold sensation appears. Then shake the needle while withdrawing it to enlarge the hole.

The operation may be performed in combination with the reducing technique of inserting the needle during inhalation and withdrawing it during exhalation.

6 *Retention and Withdrawal of Needle*

Retention of the needle means to keep it in place after it has been inserted into an acupoint. The purpose of leaving it in place is to strengthen the needling sensation and to facilitate the manipulation of the needle. In general, the needle is left in place for 10–20 min, but this may be adjusted as appropriate for the circumstances. Meanwhile, the needle may be manipulated at intervals to maintain a certain level of stimulation to the patient and to strengthen the therapeutic effect. For patients with a dull needling sensation, retaining the needle serves as a way of waiting for Qi to arrive.

When the needle no longer needs to be retained it should be withdrawn. Press the skin around the acupoint with the thumb and index finger of the assisting hand, rotate the needle gently while lifting it slowly to the superficial level, then withdraw it quickly and press the punctured acupoint with a sterilized cotton ball for a while to stop bleeding.

IV Management of Possible Accidents

1 Fainting

This is due to improper positioning, nervous tension, a delicate constitution or too forceful manipulation techniques.

The symptoms are sudden dizziness, nausea and vomiting, pallor, palpitations of the heart, shortness of breath, a drop of blood pressure, cold extremities, and a thin and rapid or deep pulse. In severe cases, there may be loss of consciousness, sudden cyanosis of lips and fingernails or fecal and urinary incontinence.

In case of fainting, stop needling immediately and withdraw all the needles. Comfort the patient and help him/her to lie down, and offer him/her some tepid water. The symptoms will disappear after a short rest.

In severe cases, press hard with fingernail or needle on Renzhong (DU-26) and Suliao (DU-25), and apply moxibustion at Zusanli (ST-36) and Guanyuan (RN-4) to wake the patient. If the patient does not respond to the above measures, other emergency measures should be taken. (Consult a standard textbook on Emergency Medicine. The student must learn how to manage fainting before attempting to apply acupuncture.)

2 Stuck Needle

If the needle is stuck because of muscle spasm, leave the needle in place for a while. Ask the patient to relax or gently talk the patient into relaxing. Then remove the needle by rotating it and massaging the skin around the acupoint. Another way is to insert another needle nearby to induce relaxation of the muscle.

If the needle is stuck due to excessive rotation in one direction, the condition will be overcome when the needle is rotated in the opposite direction to loosen the bound muscle fibers and then gentle lifting and thrusting alternately.

3 Bent Needle

This may result from unskillful or too forceful manipulation, the needle striking some hard tissue, a change of the patient's posture after insertion, striking of the handle or improper management of a stuck needle.

Do not rotate or twist the needle, since that may cause the needle to break. If the bending is due to a change in posture, move the patient to the original posture to remove the needle. If the bend is slight the needle may be removed slowly. If the bend is more severe, attempt to withdraw it by following the course of the bend.

4 Broken Needle

This may arise from too strong manipulation of the needle after insertion, from strong muscle spasm, or a sudden movement of the patient with the needle in place, or especially because of poor quality or erosion of the needle. When a needle breaks, the practitioner must remain calm and ask the patient not to move to prevent shifting of the broken part. If the broken part protrudes from the skin, remove it with forceps. If the broken part is at the same level of the skin or slightly beneath the skin, press the skin around the site to expose it, then remove it with forceps. If the broken part is completely under the skin, surgical removal may be necessary.

5 Hematoma

A mild hematoma caused by subcutaneous bleeding will usually disappear by itself. If the local swelling and pain are bothersome or the hematoma is large, use the following measures. First apply a cold compress to the area of the hematoma to stop further bleeding. When bleeding has definitely stopped, apply a warm compress and local pressure or light massage to help disperse and reabsorb the blood. On very rare occasions, the hematoma may be so large that it presses on the nerves or blood vessels, affecting motor functions or circulation. In such a circumstance it may require surgical evacuation.

6 Pneumothorax

Certain acupoints are located where the distance from the skin surface to the lung is quite short. These include the following:

Acupoints in or near the supraclavicular fossa
Acupoints in or near the supra-sternal notch
Acupoints on both sides of the 11th thoracic vertebra
Acupoints above the eighth intercostal space on the mid-axillary line
Acupoints above the sixth intercostal space on the mid-clavicular line

Occasionally, because of improper direction, angle or depth of the needle, the pleura and lung may be injured and air may enter the thoracic cavity causing pneumothorax.

When a pneumothorax develops, the patient may suddenly feel chest pain, shortness of breath or dyspnea, or chest distention. There may also be shock with cyanosis, sweating and a drop in blood pressure. (The student must learn how to recognize this complication and how to stabilize and treat the patient before attempting to apply acupuncture. Consult a standard textbook on Emergency Medicine.)

7 *Unanticipated Complications*

On very rare occasions, under the stress of acupuncture some patients may develop a heart attack or stroke. (The student must learn how to recognize these complications and how to stabilize and treat such patients before attempting to apply acupuncture. Consult a standard textbook on Emergency Medicine.)

V Cautions and Precautions

1. For patients who are weak, nervous or new to acupuncture, choose a recumbent posture.
2. **Pregnancy**: For female patients who are pregnant acupuncture is contraindicated at certain acupoints, as follows: during the first 3 months, all acupoints on the lower abdomen; and beyond the first 3 months, all acupoints on the entire abdomen and the lumbosacral region. The following acupoints must be completely avoided during any stage of pregnancy: Sanyinjiao (SP-6), Hegu (LI-4), Zhiyin (BL-67) and Kunlun (BL-60).
3. **Menstruation**: If a female patient is menstruating, postpone all acupuncture treatment until menses have ended, except for disorders related to menstruation.
4. **Infants**: If the anterior fontanel of the head has not yet closed acupuncture at acupoints on the vertex is contraindicated. In children who may not be cooperative, needles must not be left in place after insertion.
5. **Blood vessels**: Unless bleeding is part of the therapy, the physician must avoid all blood vessels, especially arteries, during acupuncture. **Bleeding disorders**. In all patients with a bleeding disorder acupuncture is contraindicated.
6. **Skin lesions**: In a patient with skin infections, ulcers, scars, or tumors, acupuncture is not applied except where the skin is normal.
7. When applying acupuncture to acupoints around the **eye** or on the **neck**, such as Fengfu (DU-16) and Yamen (DU-15), and on the back, the physician must pay special attention to the angle and depth of insertion. Do not rotate, lift or thrust more than minimally. It is permissible, however, to retain the needle for a prolonged period of time.
8. Pay special attention when applying acupuncture to acupoints on the **chest, flank, subcostal region, back and loin**, where important viscera are located. Overly deep puncture of these acupoints may injure the corresponding internal viscera, leading to accidents and bad results. The physician must know well the anatomy of acupoints and strictly control the angle and depth of puncture.

Section 2 Three-Edged Needles

I Structure

The three-edged needle is used to prick the skin to cause bleeding. It is made of stainless steel with a cylindrical handle, a triangular prismatic shaft up to about 2.4 in. long and a sharp tip. There are three general sizes: large, medium and small (see Fig. 4.23).

II Applications

Acupuncture with the three-edged needle is applicable to various diseases of Heat, diseases of evil strength, and various pain syndromes. Examples include heat stroke, acute tonsillitis and other inflammatory conditions of the throat, conjunctivitis, various sprains, furuncles, lymphangitis, and neurodermatitis. Additional applications are listed under each technique.

III Techniques

The following three techniques are used with the three-edged needle. All are carried out using standard sterilization and antiseptic techniques. In general, this technique is applied once a day, once every other day, or once every 3–7 days. Each therapeutic course consists of 3–5 such treatments.

1 Spot Pricking

This was known as "collateral pricking" in ancient times.

Massage the site to cause local congestion. Hold the needle to expose approximately a tenth of an inch of the tip and direct the tip precisely at the spot to be punctured. Swiftly prick it to a depth of 1/3 to 1/2 of the exposed tip (1 to 2 mm),

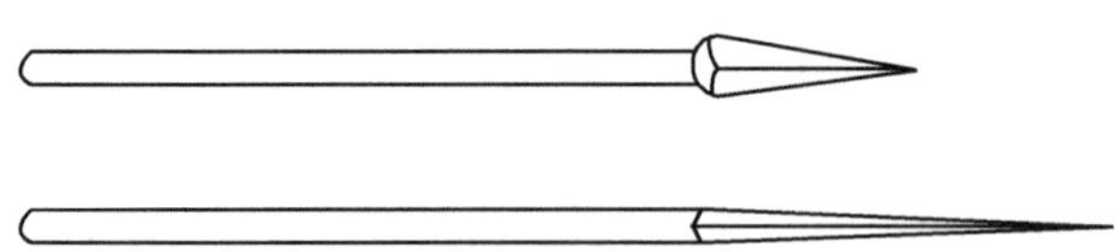

Fig. 4.23 Three-edged needles

withdraw the needle immediately and squeeze out a few drops of blood. Then press over the punctured hole with a sterile swab to stop the bleeding.

This technique is mainly used for treating apoplexy with coma, heatstroke, acute tonsillitis, or acute lumbar sprain.

2 *Scattered Pricking*

This technique is also termed "surrounding needling."

Hold the needle as for spot pricking. Stretch the skin over the area to be treated and prick the skin repeatedly around the affected area, perpendicularly and rapidly. Then gently press the skin to obtain a little bloodletting.

This technique is mainly used for treating traumatic pain due to stagnant blood, erysipelas, carbuncles or sores.

3 *Tissue-Breaking Pricking*

With one hand, press down on opposite sides of the acupoint or sensitive spot to fix the location. The sensitive spot is usually recognizable as a rash, 1 to 1.5 in. in diameter, which often has a dark yellow, greenish dark yellow, reddish or white color, and which blanches on pressure. Hold the needle with the thumb above the other fingers, exposing about a tenth inch of the tip. Aim the needle at an angle of 15–30° from the skin surface, quickly break the skin of the acupoint or affected area and insert the needle deep into the subcutaneous tissue. Then gently move upward to break some of the fibrous tissue.

When pricking and breaking it is advisable to use wrist action. Upon completion of the procedure apply topical antisepsis and cover with sterile dressing.

This technique is applicable to painful and red swellings of the eye, erysipelas, hemorrhoids and other conditions.

IV Cautions and Precautions

1. Strictly observe standard sterilization and antisepsis to prevent iatrogenic infection.
2. Perform the manipulation gently and swiftly. No more than a few drops of blood should be squeezed out. Never injure an artery.
3. Do not use this technique in a patient with a bleeding disorder. It should be used with great care in pregnant or postpartum patients. It should also be used with care in those patients who are famished or overly fatigued or who have over-eaten.

Section 3 Plum Blossom Needle

I Structure of Plum Blossom Needle

The plum blossom needle, also known as the skin needle or seven star needle, consists of the following three parts (see Fig. 4.24).

The handle is the part to be held by the hand. About 7–10 in. long it is usually made of plastic, Plexiglas, Bakelite or water buffalo horn, and is quite elastic.

The head is the part where the needles are inlaid and is 0.1–0.4 in. in diameter. It may be inlaid with needles on one or both sides.

There are seven stainless needles. They are arranged to form a circular (cylindrical) or a plum blossom pattern.

II Applications

The plum blossom needle is used in acupuncture treatment of high blood pressure, headache, myopia, neurasthenia, gastrointestinal disorders, alopecia areata (hair loss in a circumscribed area), dysmenorrhea, joint pains, lumbar back pain, numbness of skin, intercostal neuralgia, facial paralysis, neurodermatitis, and other conditions.

III Technique

Apply standard sterilization and antisepsis. Hold the end of the handle against the thenar prominence with the fourth and fifth fingers and hold the handle with the thumb and third fingers, with the second finger pressing on the middle of the handle (Fig. 4.25).

Tap quickly and perpendicularly on the skin using wrist action (Fig. 4.26), so that there is no oblique or slipping motion (Fig. 4.27). If light tapping is indicated, tap until the local area appears red and slightly swollen. If heavy tapping is indicated,

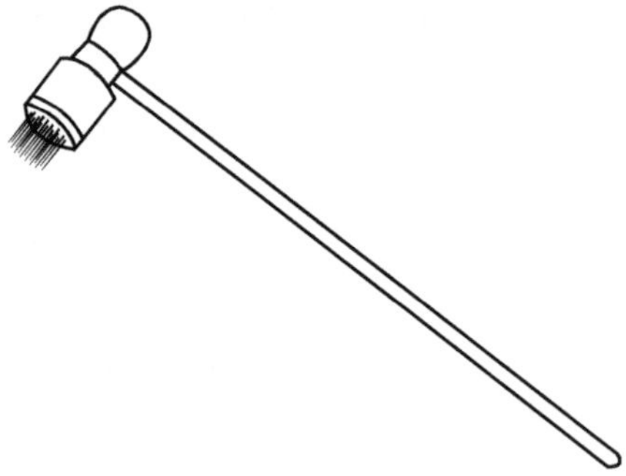

Fig. 4.24 Plum blossom needle

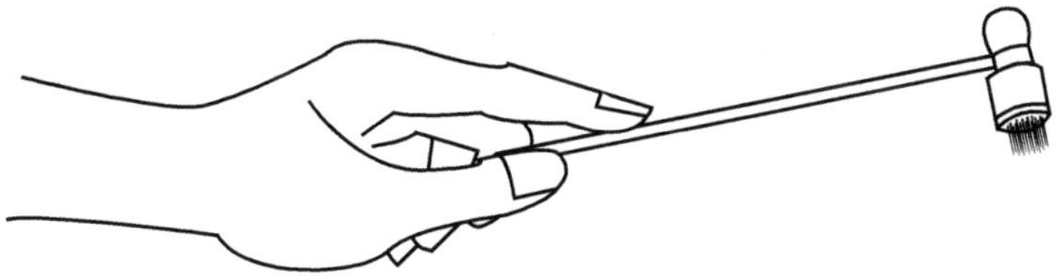

Fig. 4.25 Holding plum blossom needle

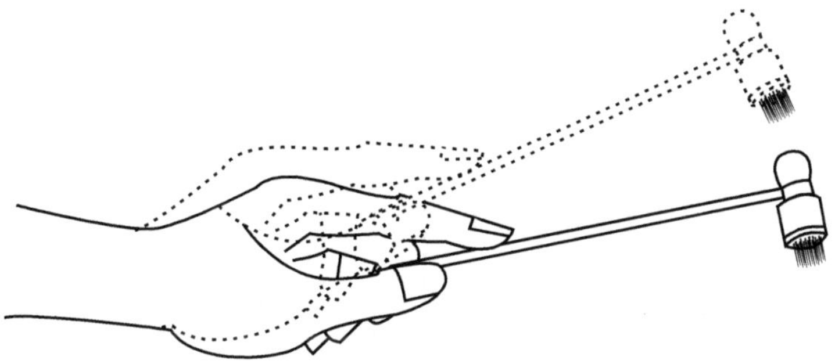

Fig. 4.26 Correct way to tap

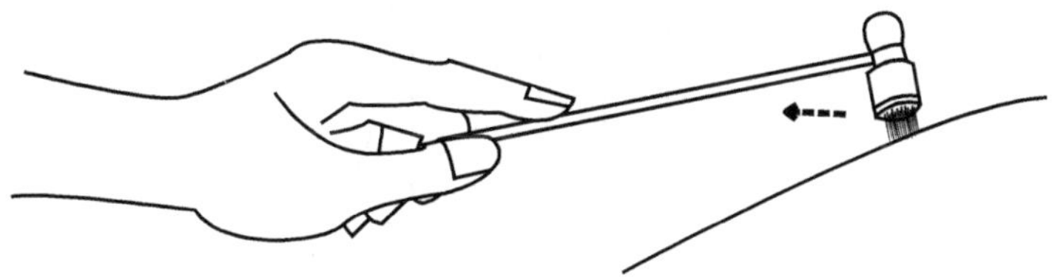

Fig. 4.27 Incorrect way to tap

tap until the local area begins to bleed. In general, in each treatment session 5–7 taps are performed, at a rate of about 80 per min and at an interval space of 0.4–0.8 in.

Whether the tapping should be light or heavy depends upon the pathological condition and the patient's physical constitution.

IV Areas of Application

There are four types of location for the application of plum blossom needling.

1. Plum blossom needling is applied along five parallel lines on the back (Fig. 4.28). The middle line is the posterior median line over the spinal column (the Du Meridian). The others are 1.5 and 3 *cun* respectively from the median line, on both sides (branches of the Bladder Meridian on the back).

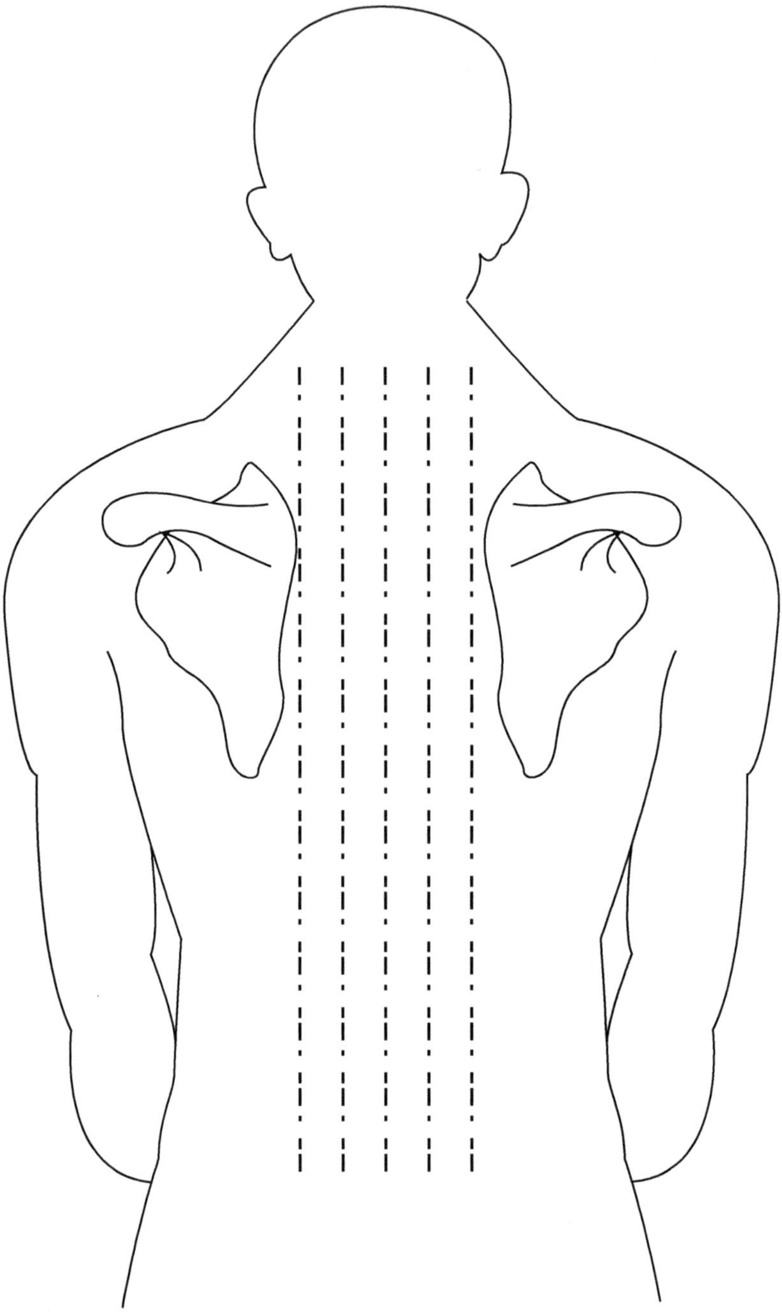

Fig. 4.28 Routine stimulating area in plum blossom needling

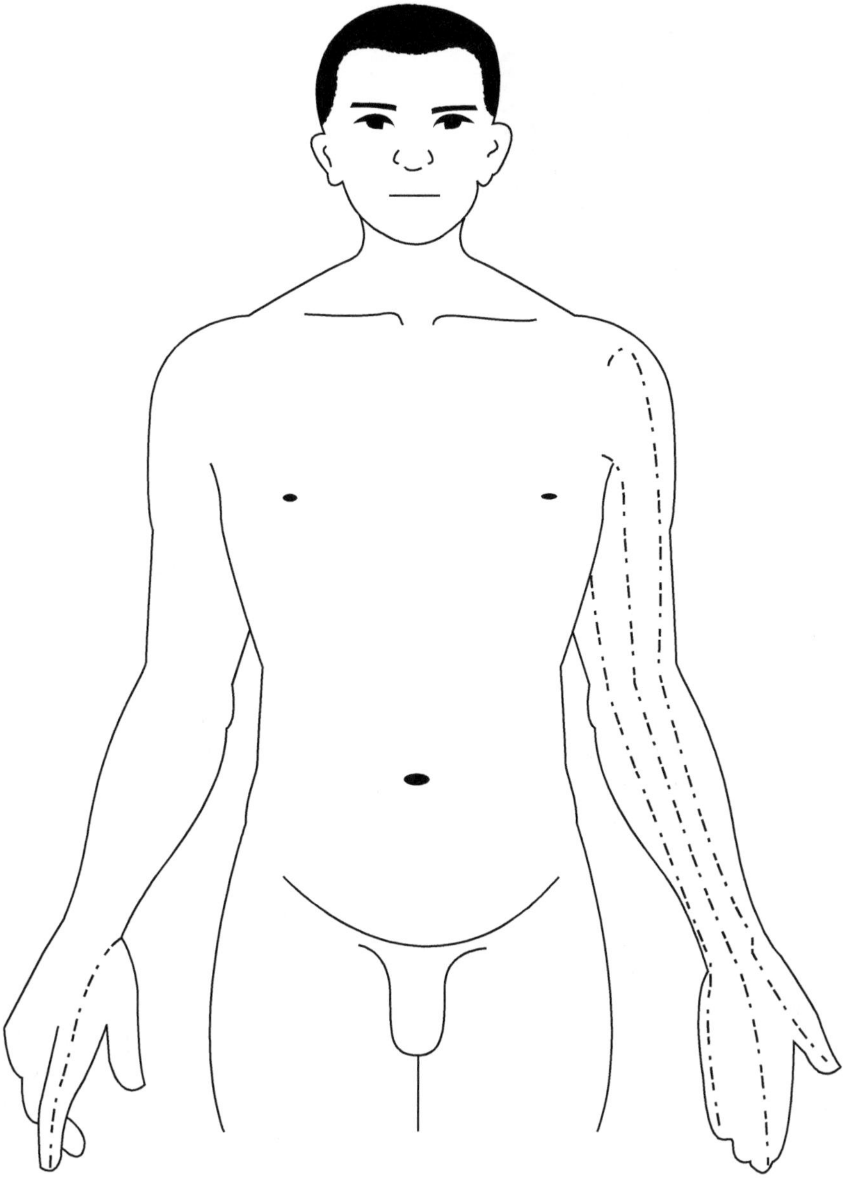

Fig. 4.29 Tapping along meridian

2. Plum blossom needling is also applied along the course of the meridian that corresponds to the diseased *zang–fu* organ (Fig. 4.29). For example, to treat labored breathing and cough tap along the course of the Lung Meridian of Hand-Taiyin. For migraine, tap along the courses of the Gallbladder Meridian of Foot-Shaoyang and the Sanjiao Meridian of Hand-Shaoyang.

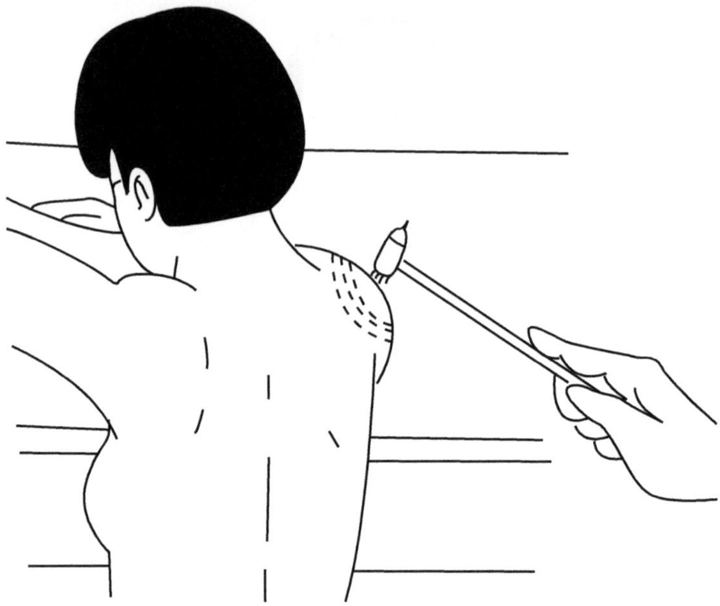

Fig. 4.30 Tapping of affected area

3. Acupoints appropriate to the disease are also tapping locations. For example, for labored breathing due to failure of the kidney to receive Qi tapping may be performed on the following acupoints: Zhongfu (LU-1), Feishu (BL-13), Gaohuang (BL-43), Shenshu (BL-23), Taixi (KI-3), and Fuliu (KI-7).
4. The affected area may be tapped, in either a linear or a circular pattern. For example, in the treatment of pain in the shoulder joint, tapping is applied in a circular pattern (Fig. 4.30) around the shoulder joint. In alopecia areata, the local affected area and the area around it may be tapped.
5. Sometimes, proper treatment requires tapping using more than one location. In treating neurasthenia, for example, tapping may be applied first along the line on the back as in paragraph (1) followed by tapping at such acupoints as Xinshu (BL-15), Shenmen (HT-7) BL23), Ganshu (BL-18). In treating intercostal neuralgia, tapping is applied to some acupoints along the course of the Liver Meridian as well as the painful intercostal area along a line from the medial to the lateral side.

V Cautions and Precautions

1. Prior to treatment check the apparatus to ensure that the needles are even and free of bends or hooks.

2. Ensure sterilization and antisepsis before and after the treatment so as to avoid iatrogenic infection.
3. Tapping is not recommended in areas of local trauma or ulcers. It is also contraindicated in those patients with bleeding disorders.

Section 4 Electro-Acupuncture

Electro-acupuncture is a therapeutic modality that combines needling and electrical stimulation. It is accomplished by applying a small amount of electric current to the needle after its insertion and arrival of Qi.

The instrument used in electro-acupuncture is composed of two parts: the filiform needle and the electric stimulator. There are different models of electroacupuncture stimulators available on the market. Most of them are designed to deliver biphasic pulse stimulation at low voltage. The three commonly available output patterns are continuous pulses, dense-disburse pulses, and intermittent pulses.

I Technique

Insert needles at the chosen acupoints. When the needling sensation has appeared, adjust the electric output of the stimulator to zero ("0") and connect the output leads to the handles or shafts of the needles. Turn on the power supply and select the required waveform and frequency.

High frequency (50–100 Hz) continuous stimulation inhibits the excitability of sensory and motor nerves. It may be used for analgesia, sedation and relaxation of muscle spasm.

Low frequency (2–5 Hz) continuous stimulation is more suitable for improvement of muscle contraction, and is commonly used in paralytic conditions as well as for soft tissue injury.

Dense-disburse pulse stimulation (e.g., an alternation of 4 and 50 Hz each lasting 1.5 s) has an excitatory effect, overcoming sensory adaptation frequently associated with continuous stimulation. It may be used for paralysis, soft tissue injury, frostbite and sciatica.

Intermittent pulse stimulation (e.g., 1.5-s trains of high frequency pulses separated by 1.5 s without stimulation) also has a powerful excitatory effect. It is often used for paralytic conditions.

The intensity of electrical stimulation should be increased in steps. After each increase, allow the patient 1–2 min to adapt. The patient will first feel a slight tingling sensation, at which point the intensity of stimulation is the sensory threshold. As the intensity increases, the stimulation will become painful, reaching the pain threshold. The intensity for treatment should be set between the sensory threshold and the pain threshold. To avoid electrical shock, always increase the intensity slowly. In general, the time of electrical stimulation is 10–20 min for each treatment, after finishing intensity adjustment. But this may be prolonged depending on the requirements of the pathological condition.

II Applications

All diseases that respond to acupuncture with the filiform needle can be treated with electro-acupuncture. Clinically, this method is mainly used to treat a variety of pain conditions, epilepsy, palsy, joint pain, neurasthenia, and high blood pressure.

III Cautions and Precautions

1. The electric current should be increased gradually, in small steps, in order to avoid intense muscular contraction that may result in bent or broken needles.
2. For an electric stimulator with the maximum output voltage over 40 V its maximum current output must not exceed 1 mA in order to avoid electric shock.
3. For a patient with heart disease, avoid the electric current passing through the heart.
4. For a patient with a weak constitution or nervousness, too much electric current is not advisable as it may cause the patient to faint.
5. Do not use needles that have been used in moxibustion, as the surface of the needle may have become oxidized.

Section 5 Scalp Acupuncture

While the theory of the meridians serves to guide the use of traditional acupuncture, some new theories have been put forward for applying acupuncture at specific regions of the body. This section describes scalp acupuncture. Section 6 describes ear acupuncture.

Scalp acupuncture is the twentieth-century discovery of a physician of Western medicine working in China. It is a method designed for treating and preventing diseases. In clinical practice it is often applied in the treatment of brain diseases.

I Stimulation Zones and Main Applications

The scalp is divided into a number of stimulation zones. Two principal lines are used for reference in this division. One is the antero-posterior midline over the vertex, connecting the midpoint between the eyebrows to the lower border of the occipital

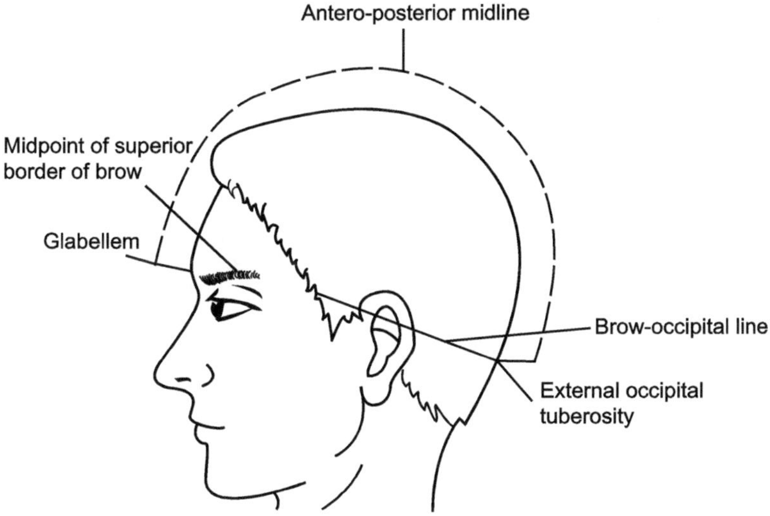

Fig. 4.31 Lines defining stimulation zones

tuberosity. The other connects the midpoint of the superior border of the eyebrows to the tip of the occipital tuberosity, but courses laterally across the temple, one on each side (see Fig. 4.31).

1 Motor Zone

The motor zone is defined by the following two points. The first is 0.5 cm posterior to the midpoint of the antero-posterior midline over the vertex. The second is the intersection of the lateral eyebrow-occiput line with the anterior border of the hairline at the temple. The motor zone is the zone defined by the line connecting these two points (see Fig. 4.32).

The motor zone can be subdivided. The upper 1/5 is the motor zone for the lower limbs and the trunk. The middle 2/5 is the motor zone for the upper limbs. The lower 2/5 is the motor zone for the face.

The lower limb motor zone is used in the treatment of paralysis of the contra-lateral lower limb. The upper limb motor zone is used in the treatment of paralysis of the contra-lateral upper limb. The facial motor zone is used in the treatment of contra-lateral facial paralysis, motor aphasia, excessive salivation and dysphonia.

2 Sensory Zone

The sensory zone is defined by a line that is parallel to the line defining the motor zone but is 1.5 cm posterior to it. The sensory zone is similarly subdivided: the

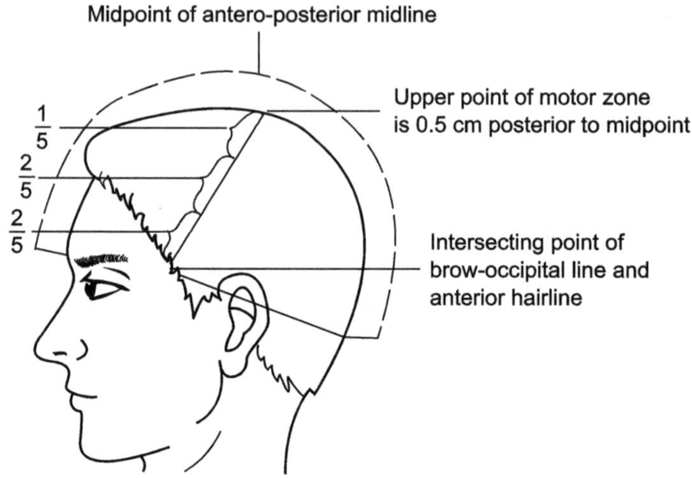

Fig. 4.32 Motor zones

upper 1/5 is the zone for the lower limbs, the head and the trunk; the middle 2/5 is the zone for the upper limbs; and the lower 2/5 is the zone for the face (see Fig. 4.33).

The upper 1/5 is used in the treatment of pain, numbness or paresthesia of the contra-lateral flank or lower limb, occipital headache, pain in the nape of the neck, or tinnitus. The middle 2/5 is used in the treatment of pain, numbness or paresthesia of the contra-lateral upper limb. The lower 2/5 is used in the treatment of contra-lateral facial numbness, trigeminal neuralgia, toothache or arthritis of the temporomandibular joint.

In scalp-acupuncture anesthesia employed in surgical operations on the corresponding parts of the body, the sensory zone is used in combination with the thoracic, stomach and reproduction zones (see below).

3 Chorea-Tremor Zone

The chorea-tremor zone is defined by a line parallel to the line defining the motor zone, but is 1.5 cm anterior to it. It is used in the treatment of chorea, Parkinson's disease, and other conditions. If the symptoms are limited to one side of the body, the needle is applied to the zone on the opposite side of the body. If they are bilateral, then needle both sides (see Fig. 4.33).

4 Vertigo-Auditory Zone

This zone is located 1.5 cm directly above the auricular apex and extends horizontally about 2 cm in each direction. It is used in the treatment of tinnitus, impaired hearing, dizziness and vertigo (see Fig. 4.33).

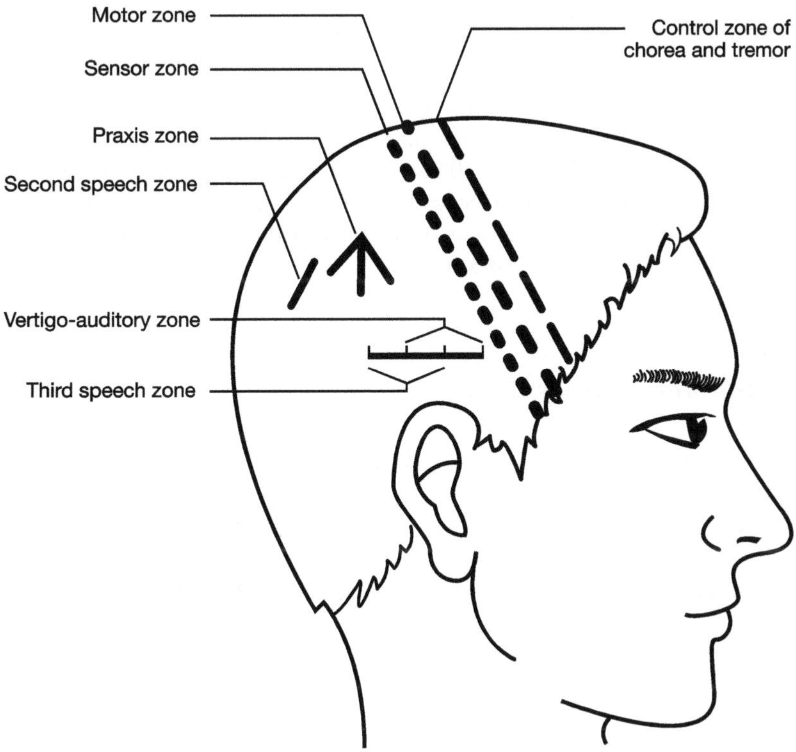

Fig. 4.33 Lateral stimulation zones

5 *Second Speech Zone*

This zone is a vertical line 3 cm in length, starting from a point 2 cm posterior-inferior to the parietal tubercle and running parallel to the antero-posterior midline. It is used in the treatment of nominal aphasia (inability to express the names of objects; see Fig. 4.33).

6 *Third Speech Zone*

This zone partially overlaps the vertigo-auditory zone. It begins at the midpoint of the vertigo-auditory zone and extends horizontally 4 cm posteriorly. It is used in the treatment of sensory aphasia (inability to understand the meaning of speech symbols, whether written, spoken or tactile; see Fig. 4.33).

7 Praxis Zone

This is the zone that is shaped like the symbol of an arrowhead. The tip of the point is over the parietal tubercle. The three lines are each 3 cm long. The middle line is vertical and the other two make a 40° angle with the vertical line. The entire zone is just anterior and slightly superior to the second speech zone. The praxis zone is used in the treatment of apraxia (loss of the previously acquired ability to perform intricate or skilled acts; see Fig. 4.33).

8 Foot-Motor-Sensory Zone

The foot-motor-sensory zone on each side begins at a point 1 cm lateral of the mid-point of the antero-posterior midline and runs for 3 cm parallel to the midline. This zone is used in the treatment of contra-lateral lower limb pain, numbness, paralysis, acute lumbar sprain, polyuria due to disease of the cerebral cortex, nocturia, prolapse of the uterus, and other conditions (see Figs. 4.34 and 4.35).

9 Visual Zone

The visual zone on each side is 4 cm long and runs parallel to the antero-posterior midline and overlies the occipital protuberance about 1 cm from the midline. The visual zone is used in the treatment of cortical visual disturbances (see Fig. 4.35).

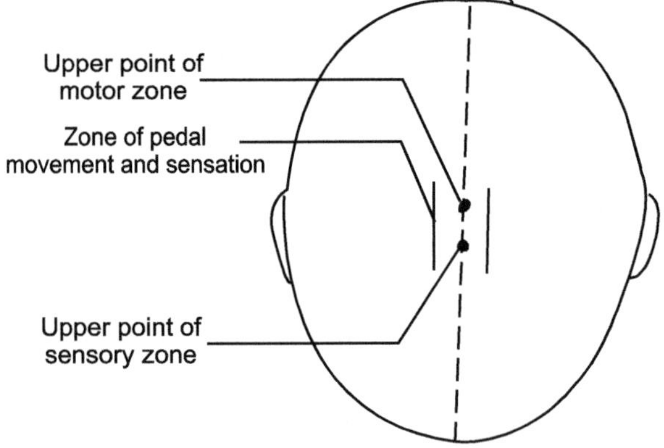

Fig. 4.34 Vertical view

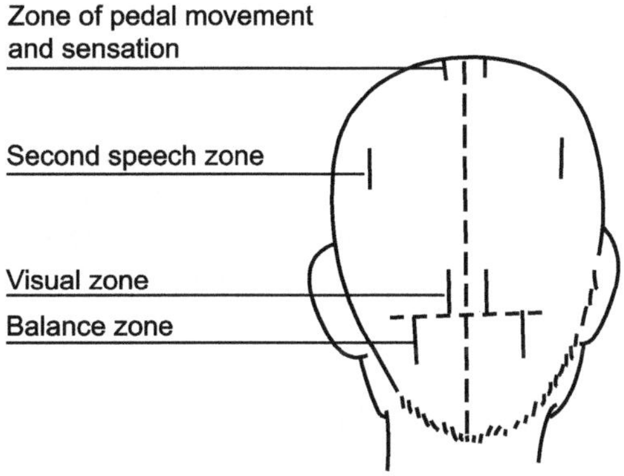

Fig. 4.35 Posterior stimulation zones

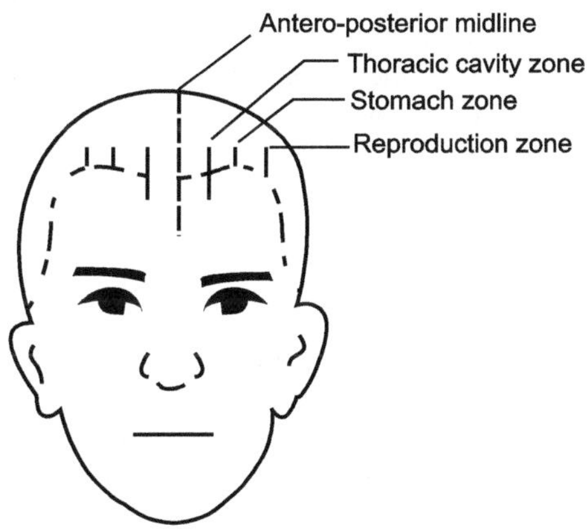

Fig. 4.36 Anterior stimulation zones

10 Balance Zone

The balance zone on each side is about 4 cm long and runs parallel to the antero-posterior midline. It overlies the lower part of the occipital protuberance at 3.5 cm from the midline. It is used in the treatment of equilibrium disturbances caused by diseases in the cerebellum (see Fig. 4.35).

11 Stomach Zone

The stomach zone on each side begins at the point of the hair margin vertically above the pupil and runs upward as a 2-cm long straight line parallel to the antero-posterior midline. It is used in the treatment of gastric pain, epigastric discomfort and related conditions (see Fig. 4.36).

12 Thoracic-Cavity Zone

The thoracic-cavity zone on each side is a 4-cm long straight line that runs parallel to the antero-posterior midline. Its midpoint is at the hair margin and it is midway between the stomach zone and the midline. It is used in the treatment of chest pain, chest congestion, palpitations of the heart, coronary artery insufficiency, asthma, hiccup, and other conditions (see Fig. 4.36).

13 Reproduction Zone

The reproduction zone on each side begins at the angle of the frontal hairline and runs as a 2-cm straight line upward, parallel to the midline. It is used in the treatment of functional uterine bleeding, pelvic inflammation, and vaginal discharge. It is also used in conjunction with the foot-motor-sensory zone to treat prolapse of the uterus and other organs (see Fig. 4.36).

II Technique

Place the patient in a sitting or recumbent posture. Select the appropriate stimulation zone and apply standard sterilization and antisepsis procedures (see Fig. 4.37).

Select a No. 26–28 filiform needle that is 2–3 *cun* long. At an angle of 30° with the skin surface insert the needle quickly under the skin or into the underlying muscle to the appropriate depth, using a twisting motion. Following insertion continue to twist the needle for 2–3 min and leave the needle in place for 5–10 min. Repeat the twisting manipulation 2 or 3 times, then withdraw the needle.

For a patient with hemiplegia, while the needle is in place exercise the limbs, passively if necessary, for motion and strengthening. The results will be better if the patient develops a sensation of heat, numbness, distention, cold or tremor in the affected limbs during treatment.

Alternately, electro-acupuncture may be applied, using alternating current with a frequency of 200–300 cycles per min. The intensity of the electrical stimulation is adjusted as appropriate. Electro-acupuncture should be applied once daily or once every other day. Each course of treatment consists of 10–15 treatments. If necessary, the course of treatment may be repeated after a week or so of rest.

III Cautions and Precautions

1. The physician must diagnose the disease correctly and choose the stimulation zone accurately.

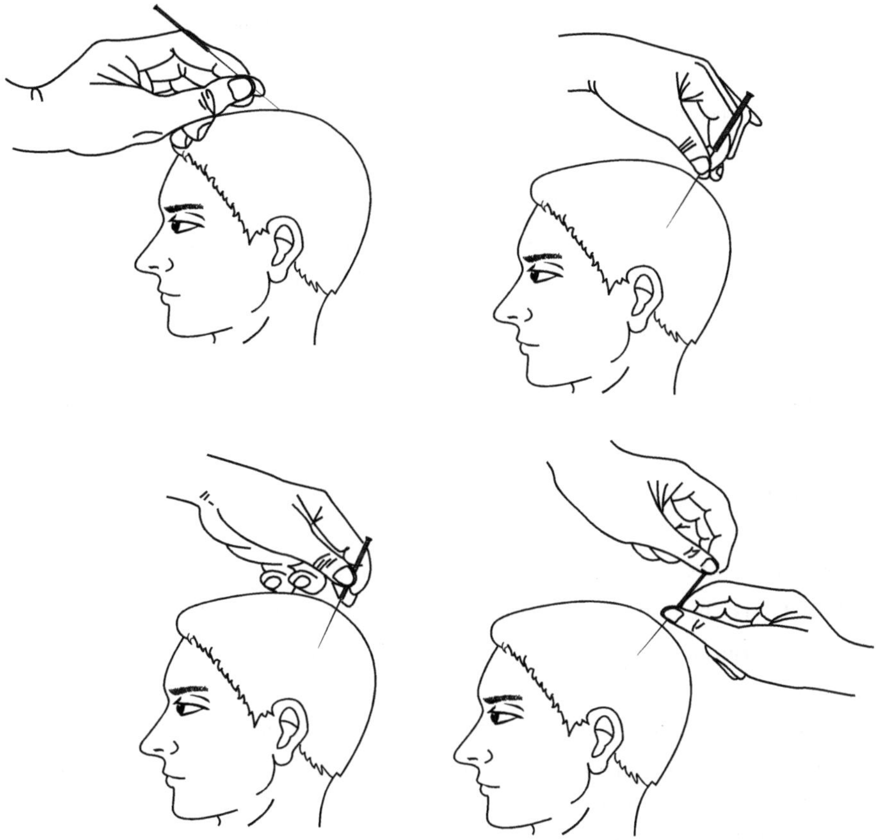

Fig. 4.37 Scalp acupuncture techniques

2. To avoid fainting from the needling, place the patient in a recumbent posture or a sitting posture in an armchair.
3. Strict sterilization and antisepsis procedures must be observed.
4. If a patient has a high fever, an acute inflammation or heart failure, scalp acupuncture is not advisable until these conditions have improved.
5. For a patient with hemiplegia caused by cerebral hemorrhage, wait until the bleeding has stopped and the condition is stable before applying scalp acupuncture.

Section 6 Ear Acupuncture

As in the case of scalp acupuncture, ear acupuncture is a modern development, the work of a physician in France. The features of ear acupuncture are easy manipulation, broad applicability, fewer side effects, economical treatment, and good results.

For surface anatomy of ear, please refer to Fig. 4.38.

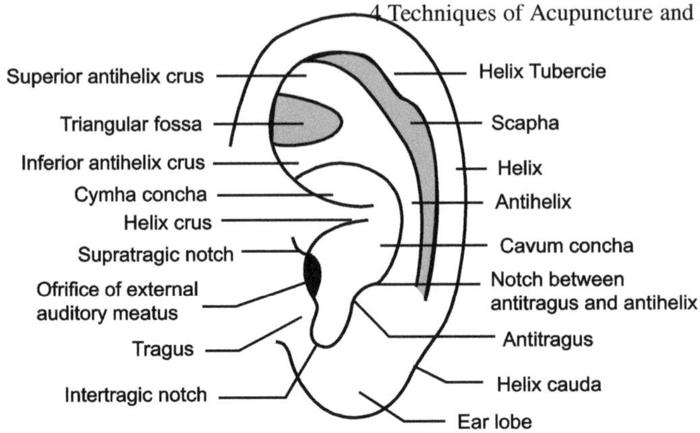

Fig. 4.38 Surface anatomy of ear

I Surface Anatomy of Ear

Helix: the curved rim of the outer border of the auricle.

Helix Crus: the transverse terminus of the helix near the middle of the auricle.

Helix Tubercle: a small tubercle at the posterior-superior aspect of the helix.

Helix Cauda: the inferior part of the helix where it merges into the earlobe.

Antihelix: the ridge inside and more or less parallel with the helix; its upper end bifurcates into the superior and the inferior antihelix crura.

Triangular Fossa: the triangular depression between the two crura of the antihelix.

Scapha: the narrow curved depression between the helix and the antihelix. It is also known as "the scaphoid fossa."

Tragus: the protruding and curved cartilaginous flap that forms part of the anterior wall of the ear canal.

Supratragic Notch: the depression between the upper border of the tragus and the helix crus.

Antitragus: a small tubercle opposite to the tragus; it is superior to the earlobe and anterior to the end of the helix cauda.

Intertragic Notch: the depression between the tragus and antitragus.

Antihelix Notch: the shallow depression between the antitragus and antihelix.

Earlobe: the lowest part of the auricle where there is no cartilage.

Cymba Conchae: the depression superior to the helix crus.

Cavum Conchae: the depression inferior to the helix crus.

Orifice of the External Auditory Meatus: the opening of the ear canal.

II Distribution of Ear Acupoints

The shape of the auricle resembles that of the upside down fetus. Acupoints located on the earlobe are related to the head and facial region. Those on the scapha are related to the upper limbs. Those on the antihelix and its two crura are related to the trunk and lower limbs. Those in the cavum and cymba conchae are related to the internal organs. Those arranged in a ring pattern around the helix crus are related to the digestive tract (see Fig. 4.39).

III Commonly Used Auricular Acupoints

There are 68 of these acupoints, organized by the regions of the auricle. For the purposes of directionality, assume that the auricle lies flat against the head. The numbering of these acupoints is for convenience only (see Fig. 4.40).

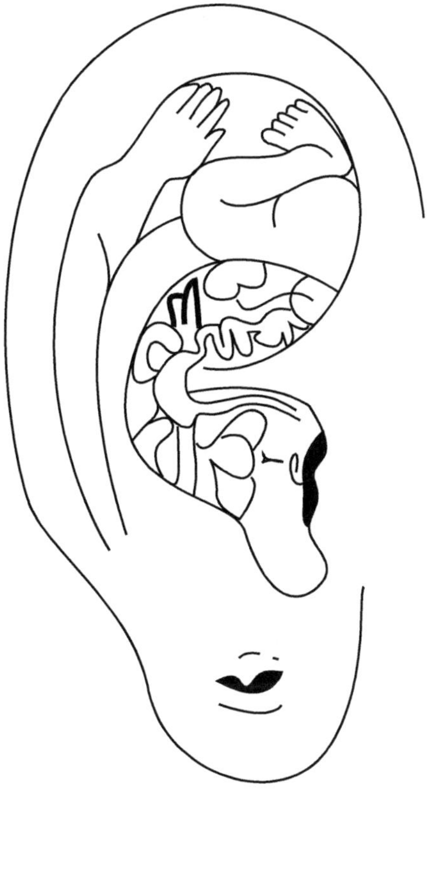

Fig. 4.39 Pattern of ear acupoints

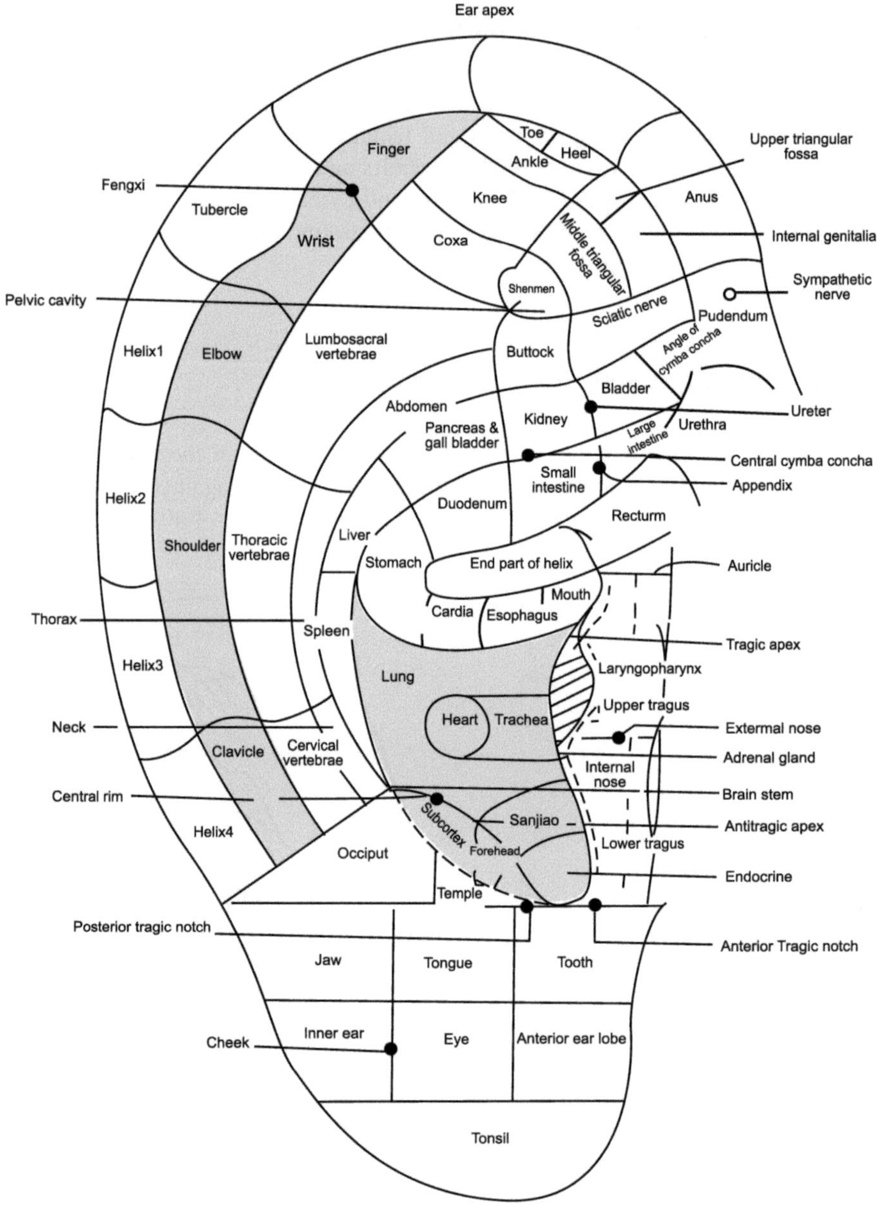

Fig. 4.40 Commonly used ear acupoints

1 Helix Crus and Helix

(1) Acupoint Ear Center (Diaphragm)
Location: on the helix crus.
Applications: hiccup, jaundice, digestive tract diseases, skin disorders, and childhood enuresis.

(2) Acupoint Rectum (Lower Rectum)
Location: next to the helix crus, near the supratragic notch.
Applications: constipation or diarrhea, prolapse of the rectum, internal and external hemorrhoids, and tenesmus.

(3) Acupoint Urethra
Location: on the helix at the level of the lower border of the inferior antihelix crus.
Applications: enuresis, urinary frequency, urgency and pain, and retention of urine.

(4) Acupoint External Genitalia
Location: on the helix at the level of the upper border of the inferior antihelix crus.
Applications: impotence and inflammatory diseases of the external genital organs.

(5) Acupoint Front Ear Apex (Hemorrhoid)
Location: on the helix at the level of the lower border of the superior antihelix crus.
Applications: internal and external hemorrhoids.

(6) Acupoint Ear Apex
Location: at the superior tip of the helix.
Applications: fever, high blood pressure, and acute conjunctivitis.

(7) Acupoint Liver Yang
Location: at the helix tubercle.
Applications: dizziness, headache, and high blood pressure.

2 Scapha

(8) Acupoint Finger
Location: at the apex of the scapha.
Applications: disorders of the fingers, such as pain or numbness.

(9) Acupoint Fengxi (Allergic or Urticaria Acupoint)
Location: at the midpoint between the Finger and the Wrist acupoints.
Applications: urticaria, skin itch, asthma, and allergic rhinitis.

(10)–(13) Acupoints Wrist, Elbow, Shoulder, Shoulder Joint
Location: divide the scapha between from the beginning of Acupoint Finger to the beginning of Acupoint Clavicle into five equal parts. These

then are the Acupoints Finger, Wrist, Elbow, Shoulder and Shoulder Joint, in sequence from superior to inferior.
Applications: diseases affecting the corresponding areas of the body.

(14) Acupoint Clavicle
Location: in the scapha at the level of the antihelix notch.
Applications: inflammation around the shoulder joint and pulse-less disease.

3 *Superior Antihelix Crus*

(15) Acupoint Toe
Location: at the lateral-superior angle of the superior antihelix crus.
Applications: toe pain and paronychia (inflammation of tissue folds around a nail).

(16) Acupoint Heel
Location: at the medial-superior angle of the superior antihelix crus.
Applications: heel pain.

(17) Acupoint Ankle
Location: midway between Acupoints Heel and Knee.
Applications: diseases affecting the ankle, and ankle sprain.

(18) Acupoint Knee
Location: in the middle portion of the superior antihelix crus.
Applications: disorders of the knee, such as swelling and pain of the knee joint.

(19) Acupoint Hip
Location: at the inferior 1/3 of the superior antihelix crus.
Applications: hip joint pain and sciatica.

4 *Inferior Antihelix Crus*

(20) Acupoint Buttocks
Location: in the posterior 1/3 of the inferior antihelix crus.
Applications: pain in the buttocks area or the lumbosacral region, and sciatica.

(21) Acupoint Sciatica Nerve
Location: in the middle 1/3 of the inferior antihelix crus.
Applications: sciatica.

(22) Acupoint Sympathetic Nerve
Location: at the terminus of the inferior antihelix crus.
Applications: palpitations, spontaneous sweating, autonomous nervous system disorders, gastrointestinal pain and spasm, heart pain, and ureteral stones or colic.

5 Antihelix

(23) Acupoint Cervical Vertebrae
Location: divide the region of the antihelix from the antihelix notch to the bifurcation into the antihelix crura into five equal segments. The lower 1/5 is Acupoint Cervical Vertebrae, the middle 2/5 Acupoint Thoracic Vertebrae and the upper 2/5 Acupoint Lumbosacral Vertebrae.
Applications: stiff neck, and disorders of the cervical vertebrae.
(24) Acupoint Thoracic Vertebrae
Location: see Acupoint Cervical Vertebrae.
Applications: chest and flank pain, mastitis, insufficient lactation, and premenstrual mammary distention and pain.
(25) Acupoint Lumbosacral Vertebrae
Location: see Acupoint Cervical Vertebrae.
Applications: lumbosacral pain, abdominal pain, leg pain, and peritonitis.
(26) Acupoint Neck
Location: on the border of the cavum conchae next to Acupoint Cervical Vertebrae.
Applications: stiff neck, wryneck, swelling and pain of the neck.
(27) Acupoint Thorax
Location: on the border of the cavum conchae next to Acupoint Thoracic Vertebrae.
Applications: chest pain and tightness, and insufficient lactation.
(28) Acupoint Abdomen
Location: on the border of the cavum conchae next to Acupoint Lumbosacral Vertebrae.
Applications: abdominal pain and distention, diarrhea, and acute lumbar sprain.

6 The Triangular Fossa

(29) Acupoint Shenmen
Location: at the point where the antihelix bifurcates into the superior and inferior antihelix crus, in the posterior 1/3 of the triangular fossa.
Applications: insomnia, dream-disturbed sleep, and pain.
(30) Acupoint Pelvic Cavity
Location: slightly inferior to the medial side of the bifurcating point between the superior and inferior antihelix crus.
Applications: inflammation of the pelvic organs and their adnexa, irregular menstruation, lower abdominal pain, and abdominal distention.
(31) Acupoint Internal Genitalia (Acupoint Uterus or Acupoint Seminal Palace)
Location: in the depression in the midpoint of the bottom of the triangular fossa.

Applications: irregular menstruation, dysmenorrhea, vaginal discharge, metrorrhagia, spermatorrhea, premature ejaculation, and inflammation of the prostate gland.

7 The Tragus

(32) Acupoint Auricle
Location: on the supratragic notch close to the helix.
Applications: inflammation of the external auditory canal, otitis media, tinnitus, and dizziness.

(33) Acupoint External Nose
Location: at the center of the tragus.
Applications: nasal furuncle, congestion or inflammation of the nose, and simple obesity.

(34) Acupoint Tragic Apex
Location: at the tip of the upper protuberance on the border of the tragus.
Applications: fever and pain.

(35) Acupoint Adrenal
Location: at the tip of the protuberance at the lower tragus.
Applications: rheumatoid arthritis, mumps, mandibular lymphadenitis, severe itch, dizziness, pain, and deafness.

(36) Acupoint Pharynx-Larynx
Location: in the upper half of the medial aspect of the tragus.
Applications: hoarseness, acute and chronic pharyngitis and tonsillitis.

(37) Acupoint Internal Nose
Location: in the lower half of the medial aspect of the tragus.
Applications: rhinitis, sinusitis, and epistaxis.

8 The Antitragus

(38) Acupoint Antitragus Apex (Acupoint Asthma-Soothing)
Location: at the tip of the antitragus.
Applications: asthma, bronchitis, mumps, skin itch, and epididymitis.

(39) Acupoint Middle Border (Acupoint Brain)
Location: at the midpoint between the apex of the antitragus and antihelix notch.
Applications: arrested mental development, enuresis, and auditory vertigo.

(40) Acupoint Occiput
Location: at the posterior-superior corner of the lateral aspect of the antitragus.
Applications: dizziness, vertigo, headache, insomnia, asthma, epilepsy, and neurasthenia.

(41) Acupoint Temple (Acupoint Taiyang)
Location: at the midpoint of the lateral aspect of the antitragus.
Application: migraine.

(42) Acupoint Forehead
Location: at the anterior-inferior corner of the lateral aspect of the antitragus.
Applications: headache, dizziness, insomnia, and dream-disturbed sleep.

(43) Acupoint Brain (Acupoint Subcortex)
Location: on the medial aspect of the antitragus.
Applications: arrested mental development, insomnia, dream-disturbed sleep, tinnitus due to kidney deficiency, pseudo-myopia, and neurasthenia.

9 *Helix Crus*

(44) Acupoint Mouth
Location: close to the posterior-superior border of the orifice of the external auditory meatus.
Applications: facial paralysis, stomatitis, cholecystitis and cholelithiasis.

(45) Acupoint Esophagus
Location: at the middle 2/3 of the inferior aspect of the helix crus.
Applications: inflammation of the esophagus, and spasm of the esophagus.

(46) Acupoint Cardia
Location: at the lateral 1/3 of the inferior aspect of the helix crus.
Applications: spasm of the gastric cardia, and nervous vomiting.

(47) Acupoint Stomach
Location: around the terminus of the helix crus.
Applications: spasm of the stomach, gastritis, gastric ulcer, indigestion, insomnia, and toothache.

(48) Acupoint Duodenum
Location: in the posterior 1/3 of the superior aspect of the helix crus.
Applications: duodenal ulcer, spasm of the pylorus of the stomach, cholecystitis and cholelithiasis.

(49) Acupoint Small Intestine
Location: in the middle 1/3 of the superior aspect of the helix crus.
Applications: indigestion, and palpitations of the heart.

(50) Acupoint Large Intestine
Location: in the anterior 1/3 of the superior aspect of the helix crus.
Applications: diarrhea or constipation, cough, and acne.

(51) Acupoint Appendix
Location: between Acupoint Small Intestine and Acupoint Large Intestine.
Applications: appendicitis, and diarrhea.

10 Cymba Conchae

(52) Acupoint Kidney
Location: on the lower border of the inferior antihelix crus, directly above Acupoint Small Intestine.
Applications: diseases of the urinary and genital systems, gynecological diseases, lumbar pain, tinnitus, insomnia, and dizziness.
(53) Acupoint Ureter
Location: between Acupoint Kidney and Acupoint Bladder.
Applications: colicky pain of the ureter due to stones.
(54) Acupoint Bladder
Location: on the anterior-inferior border of the inferior antihelix crus.
Applications: diseases of the Bladder Meridian of Foot-Taiyang, low back pain, cystitis, retention of urine, and occipital headache.
(55) Acupoint Cymba Conchae Angle (Acupoint Prostate)
Location: at the anterior-superior angle of the cymba conchae.
Applications: inflammation of the prostate gland or the urethra.
(56) Acupoint Liver
Location: on the posterior-inferior border of the cymba conchae.
Applications: subcostal pain, dizziness, eye diseases, irregular menstruation and dysmenorrhea.
(57) Acupoint Pancreas-Gallbladder
On the left side is Acupoint Pancreas, and on the right side is Acupoint Gallbladder.
Location: between Acupoint Liver and Acupoint Kidney.
Applications: inflammation of the pancreas, diabetes mellitus, and diseases of the bile duct.

11 Cavum Conchae

(58) Acupoint Heart
Location: in the central depression of the cavum conchae.
Applications: palpitations of the heart, insomnia, hysteria, heart pain, irregular pulse, neurasthenia, and stomatitis.
(59) Acupoint Lung
Location: around the central depression of the cavum conchae.
Applications: cough, chest congestion, skin itch, constipation, and simple obesity.
(60) Acupoint Trachea
Location: between the orifice of the external auditory meatus and Acupoint Heart.
Application: cough.

(61) Acupoint Spleen
Location: at the posterior-superior aspect of the cavum conchae.
Applications: abdominal distention, chronic diarrhea, indigestion, anorexia, and irregular menstruation.

(62) Acupoint Endocrine
Location: at the base of the cavum conchae in the intertragic notch.
Applications: dysmenorrhea, impotence, irregular menstruation, climacteric syndrome, and endocrine dysfunction.

(63) Acupoint Sanjiao
Location: at the base of the cavum conchae, superior to the intertragic notch.
Applications: constipation, edema, abdominal distention, lateral arm pain, and simple obesity.

12 Earlobe

(64) Acupoint Eye-1
Location: on the anterior-inferior side of the intertragic notch.
Applications: glaucoma and pseudo-myopia.

(65) Acupoint Eye-2
Location: on the posterior-inferior aspect of the intertragic notch.
Applications: imperfect refraction and pseudo-myopia.

(66) Acupoint Lower Tragic Notch (Blood Pressure-Elevating Acupoint)
Location: on the inferior aspect of the intertragic notch.
Applications: low blood pressure and collapse.

(67) Acupoint Tooth
Location: the earlobe below the level of the lower border of the intertragic notch is partitioned into nine equal sections. The sequence of these sections is as follows: top row, from anterior to posterior; then middle row, from anterior to posterior; and finally, bottom row, from anterior to posterior. The acupoints are as follows: Acupoint Tooth (Section 1), Acupoint Tongue (Section 2), Acupoint Jaw (Section 3), Acupoint Anterior Earlobe (Acupoint Neurasthenia; Section 4), Acupoint Eye (Section 5), Acupoint Inner Ear (Section 6), Acupoint cheek (on the border between Acupoints Eye and Inner Ear), and Acupoint Tonsil (covering Section 7–9).
Applications: toothache, and diseases of the face.

13 Back Surface of Auricle

(68) Acupoint Anti-Hypertension
Location: in the Y-shaped depression between the backside of the antihelix crura.
Applications: high blood pressure, and skin itch.

IV Clinical Application of Ear Acupuncture

1 *Selection of Acupoints*

i Guidelines

1. Select the acupoints corresponding to the diseased area or organ. For example, select Acupoint Eye (64–65) for diseases of the eye. Select Acupoint Stomach (47) for diseases of the stomach.
2. Select acupoints in accordance with the theories of zang–fu organs or of the meridians. For example, select Acupoint Lung (59) for skin diseases. Select Acupoint Small Intestine (49) for irregular heart rhythm.
3. Select acupoints in accordance to the principles of physiology and pathology of modern medicine. For example, select Acupoint Endocrine for irregular menstruation. Select Acupoint Sympathetic Nerve (22) for gastrointestinal diseases.
4. Select acupoints on the basis of clinical experience. For example, select Acupoint Ear Apex (6) for inflammation of the eye. Select Acupoint Anti-Hypertension for high blood pressure.

ii Examples

The following are examples of selected acupoints for some common conditions.

Gastric Pain: Acupoints Stomach (47), Sympathetic Nerve (22), Shenmen (29), Spleen (61), or Brain (43).
Constipation: Acupoint Large Intestine (50), Rectum (2), or Sympathetic Nerve (22).
Parenteral Fluid Reaction: Acupoint Adrenal (35) or Antitragus Apex (38).
Carsickness or Seasickness: Acupoint Brain (43), Middle Border (39), Occiput (40), or Stomach (47).
Neurasthenia: Acupoint Shenmen (29), Kidney (52), Stomach (47), Heart (58), Occiput (40), Anterior Earlobe (67), or Brain (43).

2 *Techniques of Ear Acupuncture*

i Searching for Sensitive Spot

Following the diagnosis of the condition and the selection of acupoint to use, find the sensitive spot in the area of the selected ear acupoint. The sensitive spot is where there is some change from normal, such as a color change, a swelling or tubercle, the appearance of ridges, depressions, folding or vascular changes. When found, the sensitive spot is the spot for needling.

The sensitive spot can also be found by using a probe, a matchstick or the handle of a filiform needle to press gently for tenderness. In addition, today the physician can measure the electrical resistance in the area of the selected acupoint. The sensitive spot is where the electrical resistance is reduced from normal.

ii Techniques of Stimulation

Sterilize the area as described in Section 1, Subsection II, Sub-subsection 2. Follow standard aseptic practice. Select an appropriate acupuncture needle, usually the short-handle filiform needle of 0.5 *cun* or a special thumbtack needle.

Needling (Fig. 4.41): Stabilize the auricle with the assisting hand. Hold the filiform needle in the needling hand and insert it into the acupoint, penetrating the cartilage but avoiding pushing it through the ear. The filiform needle is usually left in place for 20–30 min, but in a case of chronic disease it may be kept in place for 1–2 h or even longer. While the needle is in place it may be manipulated at intervals.

If the thumbtack needle is employed, after insertion immobilize it in the acupoint with adhesive tape and keep it in place for 2–3 days.

Following the insertion of the needle, most patients feel a sensation of pain, heat or distention in the local area where the needle is inserted. A few patients also feel a sensation of soreness or heaviness, or a special sensation of cold, numbness or heat. These sensations may radiate along the course of the main meridian and its collateral meridians. In general, patients who experience these sensations obtain more satisfactory therapeutic results.

After the needle is removed, press on the puncture hole with a dry sterile cotton ball for a while to avoid bleeding. If necessary, swab with alcohol or iodine at once to avoid infection.

Patients with acute diseases are treated once or twice a day. Patients with chronic diseases are treated once a day or every other day. A course of treatment lasts

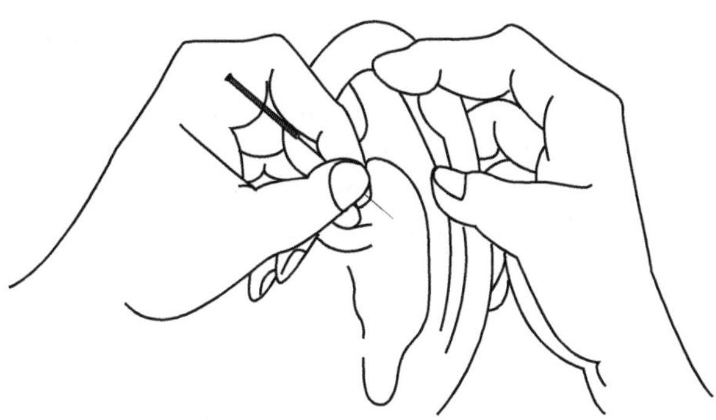

Fig. 4.41 Ear acupuncture with filiform needle

10 successive days. After each course stop treatment for 5–7 days. Treatment may be repeated, as needed.

Seed-Pressing Therapy: This technique is devised as an alternative to needling in order to reduce the risk of infection. The procedure is as follows. After standard sterilization, place a hard pellet, such as a seed of the cowherd plant (*Vaccaria segetalis*) or radish (*Raphanus sativus*), on the sensitive spot of the selected ear acupoint and secure it in place tightly against the acupoint with a small piece of adhesive plaster (0.5 cm by 0.5 cm). Press the pellet by hand to produce a sensation of soreness, distention, pain, or heat in the acupoint. Instruct the patient to press the pellet in a similar manner for 2–3 min, 3–5 times a day.

In general, leave the pellet in place for 3–5 days. Five to ten treatments constitute a course.

3 Cautions and Precautions

1. Observe strict antisepsis to avoid infection.
2. Needling is contraindicated if there is frostbite or inflammation on the auricle.
3. For an elderly patient or one with a weak constitution, instruct the patient to rest properly before and after the needling procedure.
4. Needling is contraindicated in pregnant women with a history of habitual abortion.

4 Management of Accidents During Ear Acupuncture

i Dizziness

If the patient feels mildly dizzy or faint, it is not necessary to withdraw the needle. Instruct the patient to lie down and rest. A drink of water may help. If the dizziness or fainting sensation is severe, stop needling immediately and withdraw the needle. Instruct the patient to lie down, then gently stimulate the Acupoints Adrenal (35), Brain (43) and Occiput (40). This will usually make the condition disappear. If there is actual loss of consciousness, place the patient in the recumbent position. In addition to gentle stimulation of these acupoints, apply moxibustion to the acupoint Baihui (DU-20). This will quickly restore consciousness to the patient.

ii Infection of Auricle

Swab the area with 2.5% tincture of iodine 3 times daily. In general, the infection will resolve after 2–3 days.

Alternatively, physicians today may prefer to cleanse the infected area with hydrogen peroxide and apply an antibiotic ointment. (Be sure to ask if the patient is allergic to the antibiotic in the ointment.)

iii Perichondritis

Apply an ignited moxa stick to the diseased area, with the degree of heat determined by the patient's maximal tolerance. Each treatment lasts 15–30 min. Treat 3 times per day until the infection is no longer fluctuant. If suppuration has taken place it may be necessary to drain it. After draining the pus, begin the moxibustion treatment.

Section 7 Moxibustion and Cupping Therapy

I Moxibustion

Moxibustion is a method of treating and preventing diseases by using the heat from burning moxa to stimulate the acupoints. Moxa comes from the mugwort *Artemisia vulgaris*. It is prepared by grinding the dry leaves and sifting it to remove stalks and other matter. The moxa leaf is fragrant and is easy to ignite. It has been used for thousands of years by acupuncturists to warm the meridians and expel Cold, to induce the smooth flow of Qi and blood, and to reduce swelling and disperse accumulated pathogens.

1 Commonly Used Moxibustion

There are many types of moxibustion. The following sections introduce the most common types of moxibustion using moxa cones, moxa sticks and the warming needle.

i Moxibustion with Moxa Cones

Knead and shape moxa into a cone or cylinder. These may vary in size from that of a grain of wheat to that of a half-olive. One unit of treatment is the use of one cone or cylinder at one acupoint. Moxibustion with moxa may be direct or indirect (see Figs. 4.42 and 4.43).

Direct Moxibustion: In direct moxibustion place the moxa cone directly on the skin and ignite (Fig. 4.44). Direct moxibustion is further classified as non-scarring and scarring moxibustion, depending on the degree of skin burn.

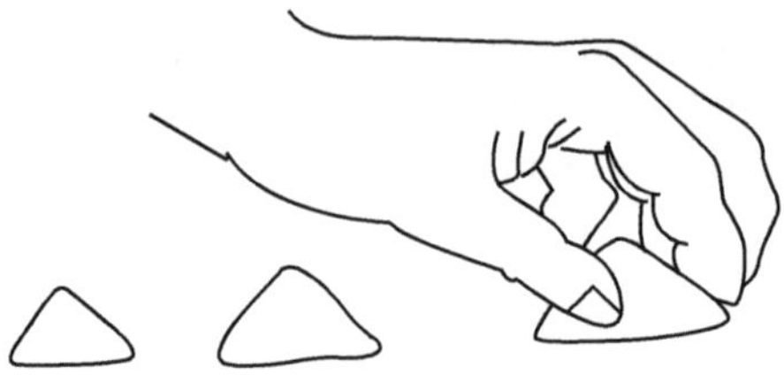

Fig. 4.42 Moxa cones

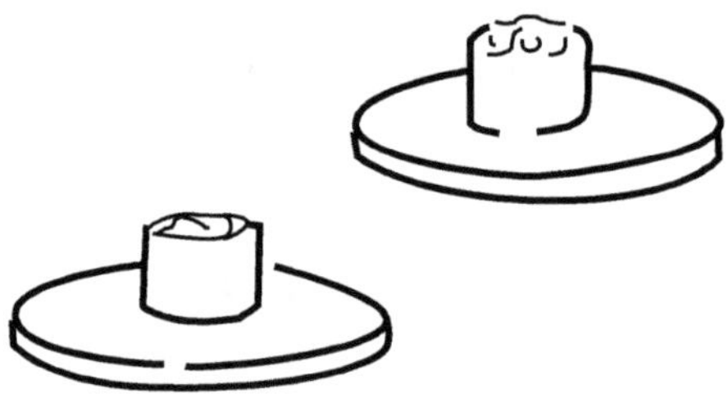

Fig. 4.43 Moxa cylinders

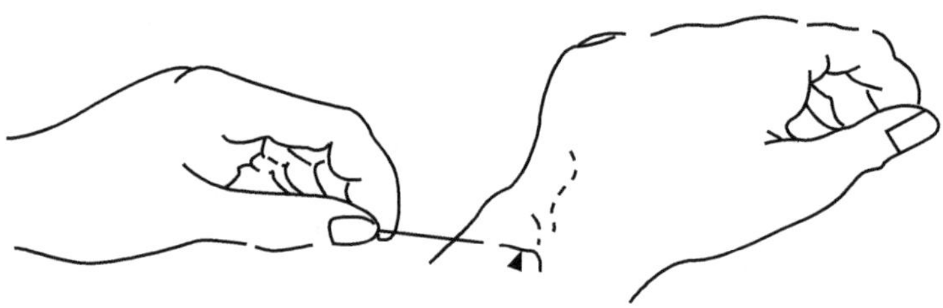

Fig. 4.44 Direct moxibustion

In **non-scarring** (or non-festering) moxibustion, first apply a small amount of vaseline to the area of the acupoint. Place the moxa over the acupoint and ignite. When 3/5 or 3/4 of it is burnt or the patient feels pain, remove the cone or cylinder and replace it with another one. Continue until the skin becomes ruddy but without blistering. Upon healing, the skin does not form a scar. Non-scarring moxibustion is used to treat diseases of chronic, deficiency or Cold nature.

In **scarring** (or festering) moxibustion, first apply some garlic juice to the area of the acupoint. Place the moxa on the acupoint and ignite it. Allow the moxa to burn up completely. Remove the ash and repeat (garlic juice and moxa) until the required units of moxa have been used. During moxibustion, if the patient feels a burning pain pat gently on the skin around the acupoint to alleviate the pain. Following a proper amount of moxibustion festering will appear and a post-moxibustion sore will be formed a week later. After 45 days or so, the post-moxibustion sore will usually heal and the scab will fall off by itself, leaving a scar on the skin. Some of the conditions for which scarring moxibustion is employed are asthma, pulmonary tuberculosis, and epilepsy. Direct scarring moxibustion may also be used to prevent apoplexy.

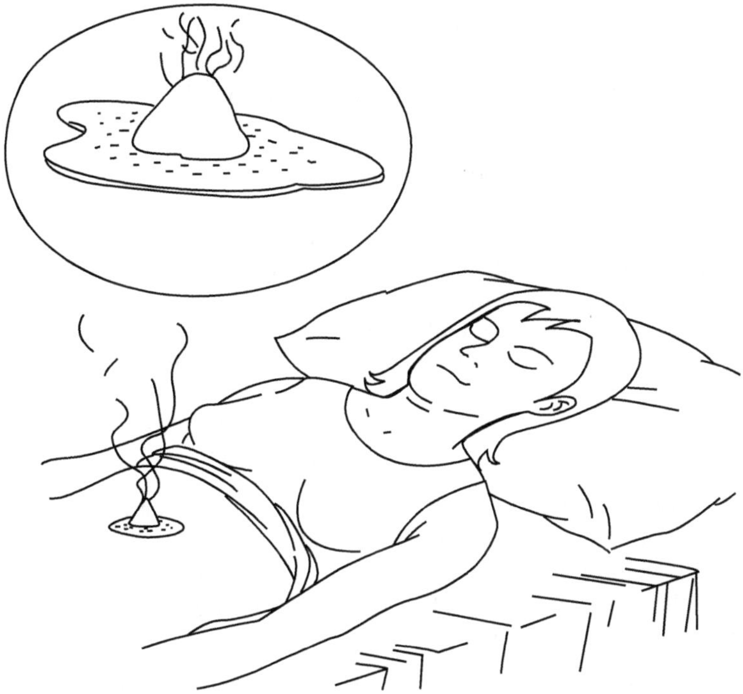

Fig. 4.45 Ginger moxibustion

Indirect Moxibustion: This is a method of moxibustion in which the ignited moxa cone or cylinder is kept from the skin by a pad of medicinal substance. It is classified according to the different medicinal substances used. The following are the most commonly used.

Moxibustion with **Ginger** (Fig. 4.45): Cut a slice of fresh ginger about 0.2–0.3 cm thick. Punch several holes in it with a needle and place it on the acupoint. Place the moxa on the ginger and ignite it. When the moxa is burnt up replace it, and continue until the local skin becomes flushed and wet. In general, each treatment needs 5–10 units of moxa. The treatment may be repeated many times according to the pathological condition. Moxibustion with ginger is used to treat abdominal pain due to Cold, diarrhea due to Cold, and joint pains due to Wind-Cold.

Moxibustion with **Garlic**: Cut a slice of garlic about 0.1–0.3 cm thick (a large single clove of garlic is desirable), punch several holes in it with a needle and place it on the acupoint. Place the moxa on the ginger and ignite it. Use a new slice of garlic for every 3–4 units. Continue until the desired effect is achieved. Moxibustion with garlic is used to relieve swelling, draw out pus and stop pain. It is indicated in surgical diseases such as furuncles, boils and abscesses.

Moxibustion with **Salt**: Fill the umbilicus with salt to a level even with the surrounding skin. Place a large moxa cone on top of the salt and ignite it. If the patient feels a little burning pain, replace the moxa cone with a fresh one. In general, 3–9 units are used; however, for urgent conditions there is no limit. Moxibustion with salt has the capacity to rescue Yang, reverse collapse and astringe. It is used to treat such conditions as acute gastroenteritis, severe abdominal pain, collapse of Yang from excessive sweating, and cold limbs with indistinct pulses.

ii Moxibustion with Moxa Sticks

A moxa stick is moxa rolled into the shape of a long thin cylinder and wrapped with paper, much like the rolling of a cigarette. When being used one end of the stick is ignited and this end applied to the acupoint or diseased part of the body.

Moxa sticks are easy to manipulate, produce good therapeutic results and are readily accepted by patients. This technique has become the most often used in clinical practice.

Moxibustion with moxa sticks is classified into "mild-warm moxibustion," "sparrow-peck moxibustion," and "circling moxibustion."

Mild-Warming Moxibustion (Fig. 4.46): Place the lighted end of the moxa stick near the acupoint. The distance is usually about 3 cm, so that the patient feels the warmth and is comfortable without pain. The treatment lasts 10–20 min, until the skin around the acupoint becomes flushed. Mild-warming moxibustion is suitable for treating a variety of conditions.

Sparrow-Peck Moxibustion (Fig. 4.47): Ignite one end of a moxa stick and use it to peck rapidly and repeatedly at the acupoint without actually touching it. The treatment lasts about 5 min. This technique is most often used to treat diseases in infants or as an emergency measure.

Circling Moxibustion: Ignite one end of a moxa stick and circle it about the acupoint, at a distance of roughly 3 cm, to warm it. Each treatment lasts 10–20 min. This technique is suitable for treating rheumatic pain or nervous paralysis.

iii Moxibustion with Warming-Needle

Moxibustion with warming-needle combines needling with moxibustion. It is used when the most effective treatment requires both needle-retention and moxibustion (see Fig. 4.48).

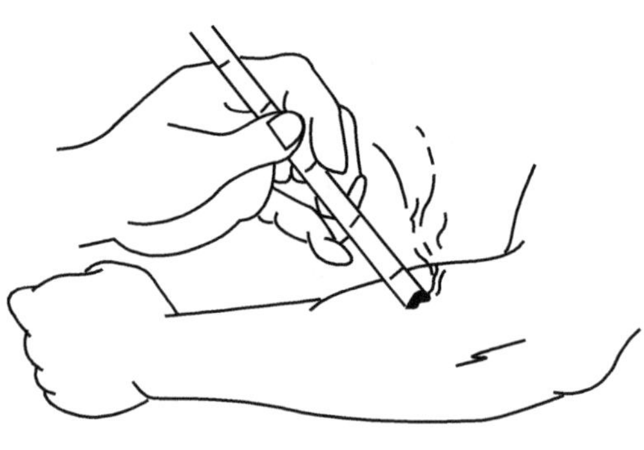

Fig. 4.46 Mild-warming moxibustion

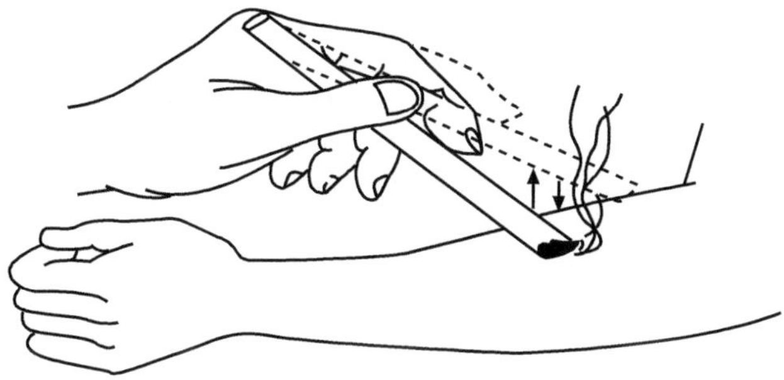

Fig. 4.47 Sparrow-peck moxibustion

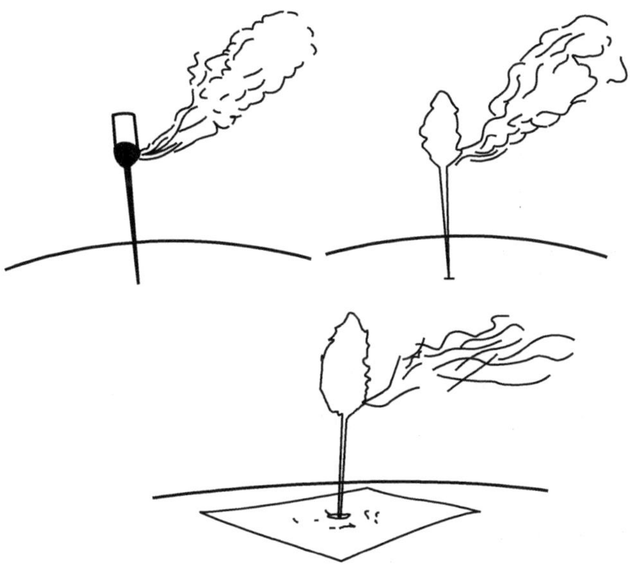

Fig. 4.48 Moxibustion with warming needle

Insert the needle using one of the standard techniques. When meridian Qi has arrived leave the needle in place at the proper depth. Wrap moxa around the handle of the needle or apply a 1–2 cm piece of moxa stick to it. Ignite the moxa and let it burn completely. This technique is suitable for treating many common diseases and for tonification.

2 *Cautions and Precautions of Moxibustion*

1. When several acupoints are treated, the following rules determine the order: the upper body before the lower body; the back before the abdomen; the head before the extremities; and the Yang meridians before the Yin meridians. Fewer units are used at first, more units for subsequent treatment.

2. Adjust the amount of moxibustion – the size of the moxa cones or cylinders and the number of units and duration of treatment – in accordance with the disease, the patient's constitution and age, and the site of moxibustion. As a rule of thumb, use five units of moxa cones or cylinders or treat for 10–20 min with moxa sticks.
3. Contraindications. In general, scarring moxibustion should not be applied to the face, the precordium, the area in the vicinity of any large blood vessel, or over muscles and tendons. In general, do not apply moxibustion in the abdominal or lumbosacral regions of a pregnant woman.
4. For patients in a coma or with numbness or dulled sensation in the extremities, be very careful not to overuse moxibustion to avoid burn injury.
5. Sometimes, a few blisters may result after moxibustion. Small blisters can heal by themselves. Large blisters should be incised with a sterile needle or scalpel and drained, then dressed with sterile gauze.
6. Following scarring moxibustion the patient should not engage in heavy physical labor and must keep the area clean to avoid infection. If the post-moxibustion lesion becomes infected, treat it as appropriate.

II Cupping Therapy

In cupping therapy a jar is applied to the skin to induce local congestion through the removal of air from the jar by heat from ignited material placed in the jar. This therapy warms and promotes the free flow of Qi and blood in the meridians, diminishes swelling and pain, and dispels Cold and Dampness.

1 Types of Jars

The following are the most commonly used jars.

i Bamboo Jar

Cut a section of bamboo 3–5 cm in diameter and 6–8 or 8–10 cm in length, forming a pipe with one closed end. The middle part of the jar should be a little thicker and the rim of the jar should be smoothed. The bamboo jar is light, economical and not easy to break; but it cracks easily from shrinkage if left to dry for long.

ii Pottery Jar

The mouth of the jar is smooth and both ends are smaller than the middle part. The pottery jar can create a strong suction, but is easy to break (see Fig. 4.49).

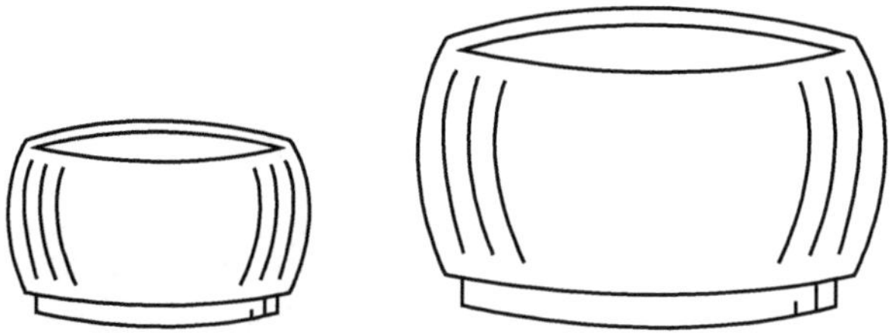

Fig. 4.49 Pottery jars

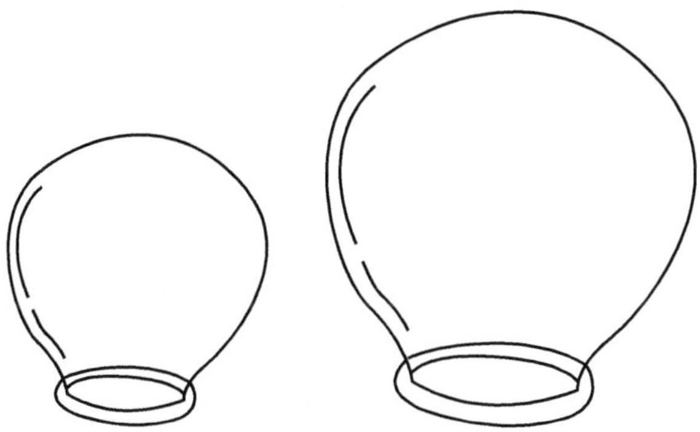

Fig. 4.50 Glass jars

iii Glass Jar

Glass jars have mouths that are smooth and smaller than the bodies. The mouths have lips. The transparency of the glass jar permits easy observation of the congestion in the skin, so that the timing of the treatment can be better controlled. However, glass jars break easily (see Fig. 4.50).

2 *Applications*

Cupping therapy is particularly suitable for rheumatism, acute strains and sprains, facial paralysis, hemiplegia, acute exogenous diseases, cough, stomach pains, and the early stages of abscesses, sores and similar lesions.

3 *Techniques*

i Fire-Flash Technique

Grab a burning alcohol-soaked cotton ball with forceps and move it around the inner wall of the jar. Take it out and immediately place the jar over the selected acupoint (see Fig. 4.51).

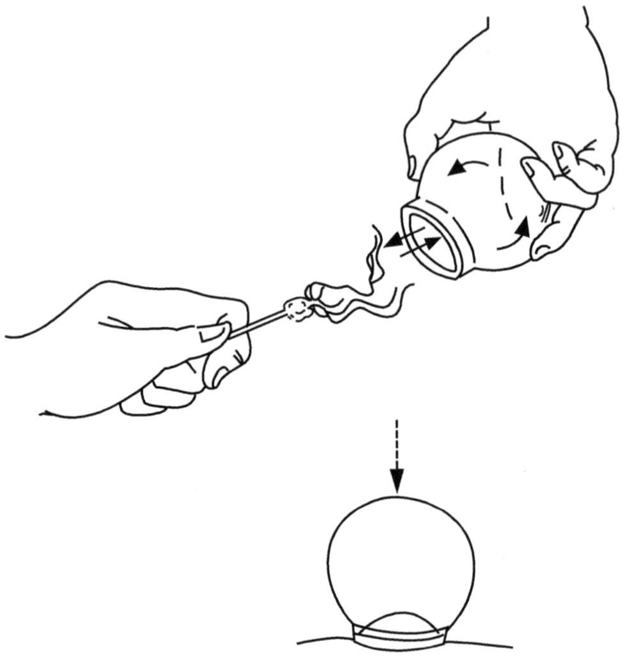

Fig. 4.51 Fire-flash technique

ii Successive Fire-Flash Cupping

In this technique fire-flash cupping is applied in quick succession several times. It is suitable for treating local numbness of the skin or diseases of deficiency with impairment of organ functions.

4 Cup Manipulation

i Retention Cupping

Leave the jar in place for 10–20 min before removing it. Retention cupping may be used to treat most diseases for which cupping therapy is appropriate.

ii Moving Cupping

Also known as walking cupping, this technique is applied in an area with abundant muscle, such as the back, the flank, the buttock and the thigh (see Fig. 4.52).

Smear vaseline over the selected area and apply cupping by one of the techniques described previously. Then slide the jar back and forth several times, until the skin has flushed red or purple. Remove the jar and wipe off the vaseline.

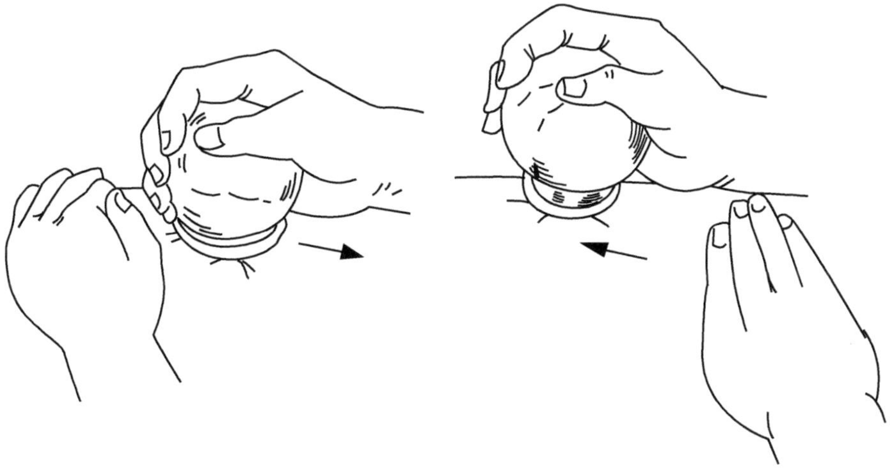

Fig. 4.52 Moving cupping

This technique is mainly useful for treating disorders of obstruction of the meridians or for migratory pain.

iii Cupping With Needle

This technique combines cupping and acupuncture therapy. Insert a filiform needle into the selected acupoint to induce needling sensation. Leave the needle in place. Apply fire-flash to a jar and immediately place the jar over the retained needle. Cupping with needle is mainly used in treating intractable diseases of the deep areas of the body (see Fig. 4.53).

iv Bloodletting Cupping

After pricking the selected acupoint or area with a three-edged needle or the plum-blossom needle, apply cupping immediately to induce more bleeding. In general, leave the jar in place for 10–15 min, then remove the jar and wipe away any remaining blood with sterile gauze. Bloodletting cupping is used to treat various conditions due to stagnation of Qi and blood, such as injuries and snakebites.

5 Removing Jar

To remove the jar following cupping therapy, press the skin by the rim of the jar to break the seal and let air in. The jar can then be removed easily (see Fig. 4.54).

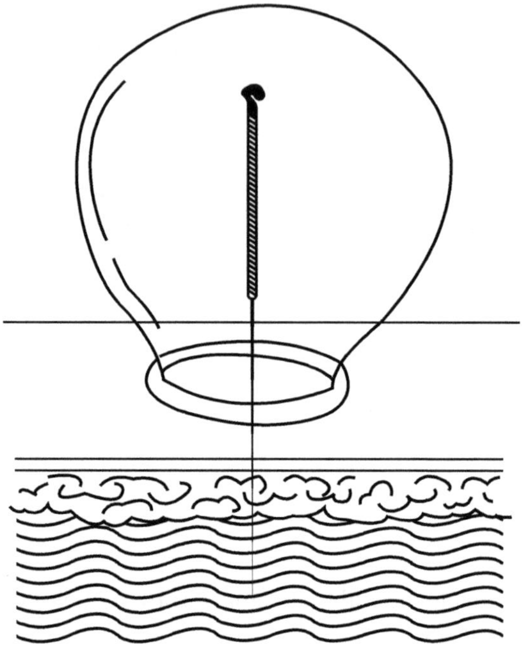

Fig. 4.53 Cupping with needle

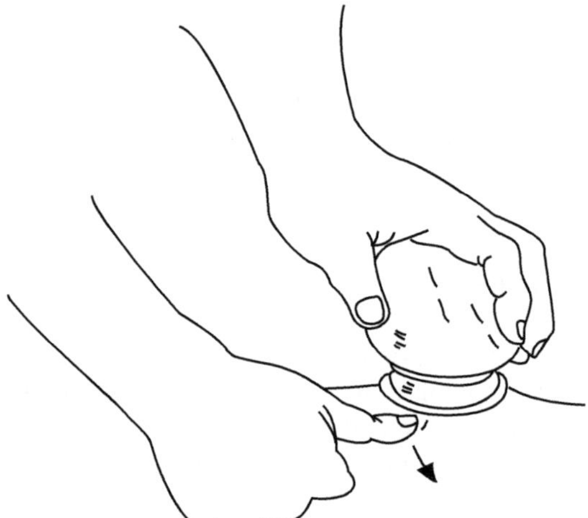

Fig. 4.54 Removing jar

6 *Cautions and Precautions*

1. The mouth of the jar must be round and smooth, without chips or cracks. Otherwise the skin may be injured.
2. Choose sites with abundant muscle mass, and ensure that they are suitable. Sites with hair, joints and depressions are not suitable for cupping therapy since it is difficult to achieve a seal and the jar may fall off.
3. The size of the jar must be chosen to match the site of the acupoint.
4. The duration of jar-retention is usually 15 min. More prolonged retention is likely to cause blisters.
5. Removal of jars should be gentle and slow. Press down on the skin by the rim of the jar to break the seal and allow air to enter the jar, so the jar will come off easily. The physician must not use force to pull or twist the jar off as doing so can injure the skin.
6. It is not advisable to apply cupping therapy to a patient with skin ulcers, high fever and convulsions, skin sensitivity, or edema. It is inappropriate to apply cupping therapy to the abdominal or sacral regions of a pregnant woman.
7. It is normal for the skin to appear flushed or bruised following cupping therapy. If the local blood stasis is severe, it is inadvisable to apply more cupping therapy to the same area. If small blisters appear on the skin it is not necessary to treat them. If the blisters are large, puncture them with a sterile needle, apply gentian violet and cover with sterile dressing to prevent infection.

Guidance for Study

I Aim of Study

This chapter introduces the basic instruments and techniques of acupuncture and moxibustion therapy.

II Objectives of Study

After completing this section learners will

1. Know how to select the appropriate acupuncture needle from the variety that are available;
2. Be familiar the preparations for acupuncture treatment;
3. Be familiar with the techniques of inserting and withdrawing the needles;
4. Be familiar with the angle and depth of needle insertion;
5. Know the fundamental manipulations and the auxiliary manipulations;

6. Be familiar with the reinforcing and reducing methods of acupuncture and the operation of needles;
7. Know the cautions and precautions in the application of acupuncture;
8. Be familiar with the possible accidents during acupuncture and the knowledge for dealing with those problems;
9. Get to know basic skills for using the three-edged needle, the plum blossom needle, electro-acupuncture, scalp acupuncture, ear acupuncture, moxibustion and cupping therapy, and their clinical applications;
10. Be familiar with the techniques of moxibustion therapy, and know the cautions and precautions for their application;
11. Be familiar with the techniques of the commonly used cupping therapy, and know the cautions and precautions for their application.

III Exercises for Review

1. What are the common patient postures used in acupuncture treatment?
2. Describe the standard sterilization procedures used in acupuncture treatment.
3. Describe the standard angles of needle insertion used in acupuncture, and explain their pros and cons.
4. Describe the basic techniques for needle insertion.
5. What are the auxiliary manipulations in acupuncture treatment? Describe them.
6. What is the needling sensation? What are the criteria for the needling sensation?
7. Describe the fundamental manipulations in acupuncture treatment. Explain how they are applied.
8. What are the reinforcing and reducing methods of acupuncture? Explain their techniques and applications.
9. What does the retention of needles mean? Explain its clinical significance.
10. Explain the different techniques for withdrawing an acupuncture needle.
11. Describe the management and prevention of fainting.
12. How does one manage and prevent a stuck needle, a bent needle and a broken needle?
13. Describe the management and prevention of pneumothorax from acupuncture.
14. Describe the management and prevention of hematomas from acupuncture.
15. Describe the techniques for using the three-edged needle. What are the precautions to be observed in its use?
16. How is the plum blossom needle used? What precautions must be observed in its use?
17. Explain the principles and application of electro-acupuncture. What precautions must be observed in its use?
18. Review the stimulation areas for scalp acupuncture. How are they located? What are their clinical applications?
19. Explain how to manipulate the scalp-acupuncture needles. What precautions must be observed in their use?

20. Review the surface anatomic features of the auricular surface. Explain the characteristics of the pattern of distribution of the ear acupoints.
21. Review the locations and applications of the ear acupoints. Give three examples.
22. What are the principles of acupoint selection in ear acupuncture? Describe the techniques of ear acupuncture?
23. Discuss the main types of moxibustion.
24. Describe the techniques of direct moxibustion. What are its main clinical applications?
25. Describe the commonly used techniques of indirect moxibustion. What are its main clinical applications?
26. Explain how the moxa stick is used clinically.
27. What are the contraindications for the clinical application of moxibustion?
28. What is cupping therapy? What are its clinical applications?
29. Describe the techniques of cupping therapy.
30. Discuss the applications and precautions of cupping therapy.

Chapter 5
Principles of Acupuncture Therapeutics

Section 1 Principles of Acupuncture Treatment

The general principles of acupuncture treatment evolved through millennia of acupuncture-moxibustion practice as guided by the theories of CM. In turn, they guide the choice of acupuncture-moxibustion treatment methods and the selection of acupoints and techniques.

I Regulate Yin–Yang

According to CM illness results mainly from a relative imbalance of Yin–Yang, resulting in the excess or deficiency of one or the other. The mechanism of acupuncture is the regulation of Yin–Yang, so that the body is brought back to the physiological state of Yin and Yang in equilibrium.

Regulation of Yin–Yang by acupuncture is achieved through proper needling of the appropriate acupoints. For example, in a patient with dizziness due to hyperactivity of liver-Yang and deficiency of kidney-Yin, treatment is directed at augmenting deficient Yin and suppressing excessive Yang. To augment Yin the acupoints Taixi (KI-3) and Zhaohai (KI-6) of the Kidney Meridian of Foot Shaoyin are selected and a reinforcing technique is applied. To suppress Yang the acupoints Xingjian (LR-2) and Taichong (LR-3) are selected and a reducing technique is applied.

II Strengthen Body Resistance and Eliminate Pathogens

In CM "deficiency" means insufficiency of the body's genuine Qi, whereas "strength" refers to the strength of the disease-causing agents. The goal of acupuncture therapy – "augment the deficient" and "purge the strong" – is mainly achieved by applying needling or moxibustion in order to stimulate the body's auto-regulatory mechanisms.

Z.W. Liu and L. Liu (eds.), *Essentials of Chinese Medicine: Volume 2*,

For example, in a patient with an illness of Heat strength, acupuncture treatment is generally aimed at dispersion of the Heat evil by means of shallow puncturing to induce bleeding. In a patient with an illness of deficiency-Cold, acupuncture treatment is generally aimed at augmenting the deficient while expelling Cold by means of prolonging the retention of the needle and of applying moxibustion. For patients with mixed deficiency and strength, treatment is aimed at simultaneous augmentation of the deficient and purgation of the strong.

III Distinguish Root and Appearance

Briefly, "root" and "appearance" are opposing concepts. The clinical manifestation of an illness is the appearance while the cause and nature of the illness is the root. The body's genuine Qi is the root and the symptoms are the appearance. In a complex illness, the original disease is the root and the complication is the appearance. For a fuller discussion of the root and the appearance, see Volume 1, Part II, Chapter 10, Section 1, Subsection II. In general, if an illness is urgent treat the appearance; if the illness is not urgent treat the root; and if the cause and the symptoms are both urgent treat the root and the appearance simultaneously.

The application of acupuncture therapy depends on the principle of the root and the appearance. The key is to assess what is primary and what is secondary; what takes precedence and what can be delayed; what is serious and what is mild; and what is urgent and what is not. On the basis of this assessment a treatment approach can be selected.

For example, certain illnesses cause constipation or urinary blockage. The first step is to exploit those acupoints that on stimulation can promote defecation or urination – this is "when urgent treat the appearance." When defecation or urination have been re-established, then exploit those acupoints that are suitable for the treatment of the cause of the illness – this is "when not urgent treat the root." In a patient with edema due to deficiency of genuine Qi and strength of evil Qi, stimulate those acupoints that can treat the cause while stimulating those that can promote water mobilization. – This is "when both root and appearance are urgent treat both simultaneously."

Section 2 Acupoint Selection

The selection of acupoints to apply acupuncture is guided by the theory of the meridians and is based on the characteristics and therapeutic properties of the specific acupoints. The most useful principles are listed here.

I Select Acupoints on Diseased Meridian

Select acupoints on the meridian that pertains to the diseased organ. For example, to treat cough due to lung disease it is appropriate to apply acupuncture to the acupoints Zhongfu (LU-1), Chize (LU-5) and others on the Lung Meridian of Hand-Taiyin.

II Combine Interior–Exterior Acupoints

This means that when the illness is in a Yin meridian it is appropriate to select acupoints on the Yang meridian that stands in the exterior–interior relationship to the diseased Yin meridian, in addition to acupoints on this Yin meridian. Similarly, when the disease is in a Yang meridian it is appropriate to select acupoints on the Yin meridian that stands in the interior–exterior relationship to the diseased Yang meridian, in addition to acupoints on this Yang meridian. (For the interior–exterior relationship, see Volume 1, Part I, Chapter 3, Section 4, Subsection II.)

For example, the kidney and the bladder form an interior–exterior dyad. If the Kidney Meridian of Foot-Shaoyin is diseased it is appropriate to apply acupuncture to the acupoints Kunlun (BL-60) and Jinggu (BL-64) on the Bladder Meridian of Foot-Taiyang.

Another application of this principle is the combination of Yuan (Source) and the Luo (Connecting) acupoints (see below).

III Combine Anterior–Posterior Acupoints

Here, anterior refers to the ventral chest and abdomen, which belong to Yin, and posterior refers to the back, which belongs to Yang; hence, this is also known as the combination of abdomen-Yin and the back-Yang acupoints. For example, to treat epigastric pain it is appropriate to select Zhongwan (CV-12) on the abdomen and Weishu (BL-21) on the back.

IV Combine Distant–Local Acupoints

Here, local means in the affected area and distant means away from the affected area but corresponding to it. For example, to treat a disorder of the eye it is appropriate to select Jingming (BL-1), near the inner canthus of the eye, and Xingjian (LR-2), on the dorsal foot.

V Combine Left–Right Acupoints

This principle is based on the fact that the courses of the meridians cross one another. Since the regular meridians are symmetrically distributed, often acupoints on both sides are selected in clinical application to diseases of visceral organs in order to strengthen the coordinated effects.

On the other hand, for many illnesses that mainly affect one side of the body it is appropriate to select acupoints only on the healthy side. For example, left facial paralysis is suitably treated by stimulating the acupoint Hegu (LI-4) on the right hand, and vice versa. Other examples include hemiplegia and rheumatism.

Section 3 Application of Specific Acupoints

The specific acupoints are those on the 14 meridians and have specific clinical significance in acupuncture therapy. These acupoints have been described in Volume 2, Part I, Chapter 3. The student should also review Volume 2, Part I, Chapter 2, Section 3.

I Application of Shu Acupoints

Each of the 12 regular meridians has a set of five Shu acupoints: Jing (Well), Ying (Spring), Shu (Stream), Jing (River) and He (Sea). They are the sites where Qi enters and exits the meridian. Hence, whenever a visceral organ or its meridian is diseased its corresponding Shu acupoints may be selected for the application of acupuncture therapy.

This selection is affected by the season. In spring and summer, because Yang-Qi is ascendant the body's Qi floats to the superficies. Shallow needling is appropriate. Also, the Jing (Well) and Ying (Spring) acupoints are located where the muscles are relatively thin and superficial; and the Jing (River) and He (Sea) acupoints are located where the muscles are relatively thick and deep. Hence, the Jing (Well) and Yin (Spring) acupoints are mostly selected in spring and summer while the Jing (River) and He (Sea) acupoints are mostly selected in autumn and winter.

Selection of the Shu acupoints may be based on their therapeutic properties. Examples include the following. The Jing (Well) acupoints are selected for epigastric distention. The Ying (Spring) acupoints are selected for febrile illnesses. The Shu (Stream) acupoints are selected for heaviness of the body and pain in the joints. The Jing (River) acupoints are selected for cough and labored breathing caused by Cold or Heat. The He (Sea) acupoints are selected for diarrhea due to retrograde flow of Qi.

Like the five principal *zang* organs, the five Shu acupoints of each meridian also have the relationships of the Five Elements. These relationships are tabulated in

Table 5.1 Shu acupoints of Yin meridians

	Jing (Well) (Wood)	Ying (Spring) (Fire)	Shu (Stream) (Earth)	Jing (River) (Metal)	He (Sea) (Water)
Lung Hand-Taiyin	Shaoshang (LU-11)	Yuji (LU-10)	Taiyuan (LU-9)	Jingqu (LU-8)	Chize (LU-5)
Pericardium Hand-Jueyin	Zhongchong (PC-9)	Laogong (PC-8)	Daling (PC-7)	Jianshi (PC-5)	Quze (PC-3)
Heart Hand-Shaoyin	Shaochong (HT-9)	Shaofu (HT-8)	Shenmen (HT-7)	Lingdao (HT-4)	Shaohai (HT-3)
Spleen Foot-Taiyin	Yinbai (SP-1)	Dadu (SP-2)	Taibai (SP-3)	Shangqiu (SP-5)	Yinlingquan (SP-9)
Liver Foot-Jueyin	Dadun (LR-1)	Xingjian (LR-2)	Taichong (LR-3)	Zhongfeng (LR-4)	Ququan (LR-8)
Kidney Foot-Shaoyin	Yongquan (KI-1)	Rangu (KI-2)	Taixi (KI-3)	Fuliu (KI-7)	Yinggu (KI-10)

Table 5.2 Shu acupoints of Yang meridians

	Jing (Well) (Metal)	Ying (Spring) (Water)	Shu (Stream) (Wood)	Jing (River) (Fire)	He (Sea) (Earth)
Large Intestine Hand-Yangming	Shangyang (LI-1)	Erjian (LI-2)	Sanjian (LI-3)	Yangxi (LI-5)	Quchi (LI-11)
Sanjiao Hand-Shaoyang	Guanchong (SJ-1)	Yemen (SJ-2)	Zhongzhu (SJ-3)	Zhigou (SJ-6)	Tianjing (SJ-10)
Small Intestine Hand-Taiyang	Shaoze (SI-1)	Qiangu (SI-2)	Houxi (SI-3)	Yanggu (SI-5)	Xiaohai (SI-8)
Stomach Foot-Yangming	Lidui (ST-45)	Neiting (ST-44)	Xiangu (ST-43)	Jiexi (ST-41)	Zusanli (ST-36)
Gallbladder Foot-Shanyang	Zuqiaoyin (GB-44)	Xiaxi (GB-43)	Zulinqi (GB-41)	Yangfu (GB-38)	Yanglingquan (GB-34)
Bladder Foot-Taiyang	Zhiyin (BL-67)	Zutonggu (BL-66)	Shugu (BL-65)	Kunlun (BL-60)	Weizhong (BL-40)

Tables 5.1 and 5.2. (For the theory of the Five Elements, see Volume 1, Part I, Chapter 1, Section 2, Subsection III.) Selection of the Shu acupoints may also be based on such relationships. For example, the Liver Meridian belongs to the Wood Element. Thus, a strength illness in the Liver Meridian may be treated by applying the reducing technique at the acupoint Xingjian (LR-2) – the Ying (Spring) acupoint of the Liver Meridian – since Xingjian belongs to the Fire Element. This is an example of "if strong purge its son." Liver insufficiency may be treated by applying stimulation to the acupoint Ququan (LR-8) – the He (Sea) acupoint of the Liver Meridian – since Ququan belongs to the Water Element. This is an example of "if deficient strengthen its mother." Other examples include the following. Hyperactivity of the liver may be treated by applying the reducing technique to the acupoint Shaofu (HT-8) – the Ying (Spring) acupoint of the Heart Meridian – since Shaofu belongs to the Fire Element. Deficiency of the liver may be treated by applying the reinforcing technique to the acupoint Yingu (KI-10) – the He (Sea) acupoint of the Kidney Meridian – since Yingu belongs to the Water Element.

II Application of Back-Shu and Front-Mu Acupoints

The Back-Shu and the Front-Mu acupoints are closely related to illnesses of the *zang–fu* organs. When there is abnormality in the *zang–fu* organ a reaction, either tenderness or sensitivity, can be detected in the corresponding Back-Shu or Front-Mu acupoints (see Table 5.3). For this reason, when an internal organ is affected the Back-Shu and the Front-Mu acupoints pertaining to that organ may be selected in combination for treatment. For example, the acupoints Weishu (BL-21) and Zhongwan (CV-12) may be selected for treating gastric disorders.

Sometimes the Back-Shu and the Front-Mu acupoints are used independently. The Back-Shu acupoints are mainly used to treat disorders of the *zang* organs and the Front-Mu acupoints, on the chest and abdomen, are mainly used to treat disorders of *fu* organs. For example, Feishu (BL-13) is selected to treat lung disorders with productive cough and chest fullness. Zhongwan (CV-12) may be needled to treat disorders of the stomach with pain and vomiting.

In addition, the Back-Shu acupoints of the *zang* organs can be used to treat disorders of the sense organs and other parts of the body. For example, Ganshu (BL-18) may be used to treat disorders of the eye and of the tendons and joints. Xinshu (BL-15) may be used to treat disorders of the tongue, pulse and blood vessels. Pishu (BL-20) may be used to treat disorders of the mouth and muscles. Feishu (BL-13) may be used to treat disorders of the nose and skin. Shenshu (BL-23) may be used to treat disorders of the ear and bone marrow.

III Application of Yuan and Luo Acupoints

The Yuan (Source) acupoints of the six Yang meridians are located behind the Shu (Stream) acupoints of those meridians, whereas the Yuan acupoints of the six Yin meridians are the same as the Shu (Stream) acupoints of those meridians. They have

Table 5.3 Back-Shu and Front-Mu acupoints of internal organs

Back-Shu Acupoint	Internal Organ	Front-Mu Acupoint
Feishu (BL-13)	Lung	Zhongfu (LU-1)
Jueyinshu (BL-14)	Pericardium	Tanzhong (CV-17)
Xinshu (BL-15)	Heart	Juque (CV-14)
Ganshu (BL-18)	Liver	Qimen (LR-14)
Pishu (BL-20)	Spleen	Zhangmen (LR-13)
Shenshu (BL-23)	Kidney	Jingmen (GB-25)
Weishu (BL-21)	Stomach	Zhongwan (CV-12)
Danshu (BL-19)	Gallbladder	Riyue (GB-24)
Pangguangshu (BL-28)	Bladder	Zhongji (CV-3)
Dachangshu (BL-25)	Large Intestine	Tianshu (ST-25)
Sanjiaoshu (BL-22)	Sanjiao	Shimen (CV-5)
Xiaochangshu (BL-27)	Small Intestine	Guanyuan (CV-4)

Table 5.4 Yuan and Luo acupoints of regular meridians

Yin Meridians	Yuan Acupoint	Luo Acupoint	Yang Meridians	Yuan Acupoint	Luo Acupoint
Lung Meridian of Hand-Taiying	Taiyuan (LU-9)	Lieque (LU-7)	Large Intestine Meridian of Hand-Yangming	Hegu (LI-4)	Pianli (LI-6)
Pericardium Meridian of Hand-Jueyin	Daling (PC-7)	Neiguan (PC-6)	Sanjiao Meridian of Hand-Shaoyang	Yangchi (SJ-4)	Waiguan (SJ-5)
Heart Meridian of Hand-Shaoyin	Shenmen (HT-7)	Tongli (HT-5)	Small Intestine Meridian of Hand-Taiyang	Wangu (SI-4)	Zhizheng (SI-7)
Spleen Meridian of Foot-Taiyin	Taibai (SP-3)	Gongsun (SP-4)	Stomach Meridian of Foot-Yangming	Chongyang (ST-42)	Fenglong (ST-40)
Liver Meridian of Foot-Jueying	Taichong (LR-3)	Ligou (LR-5)	Gallbladder Meridian of Foot-Shaoyang	Qiuxu (GB-40)	Guangming (GB-37)
Kindey Meridian of Foot-Shaoyin	Taixi (KI-3)	Dazhong (KI-4)	Bladder Meridian of Foot-Taiyang	Jinggu (BL-64)	Feiyang (BL-58)
Du Meridian		Changqiang (GV-1)	Ren Meridian		Jiuwei (CV-15)

an intimate relationship with the *fu*-organ sanjiao, which is the organ through which genuine Qi flows to the Yang meridians. Genuine Qi originates between the kidneys and distributes throughout the body. It coordinates the interior and the exterior, connects the superior and the inferior, and promotes the physiological activities of the *zang–fu* organs. Thus, acupuncture on the Yuan acupoints can facilitate the movement of genuine Qi in the sanjiao and help regulate the functions of the internal organs (see Table 5.4).

There are all together 15 Luo (Connecting) acupoints, one on each of the 12 regular meridians, one on the Ren Meridian, one on the Du Meridian, and one belonging to the spleen.

The Luo acupoints of the regular meridians have an intimate relationship with the collateral meridians, which link the interior and the exterior of the body. Hence, one of the characteristics of the Luo acupoints is their application to disorders involving those meridians in an exterior–interior relationship. For example, Gongsun (SP-4) can be used to treat not only diseases of the Spleen Meridian but also those of the Stomach Meridian (the Spleen and Stomach Meridians forming an interior–exterior dyad).

As for Changqiang (GV-1), Jiuwei (CV-15) and Dabao (SP-21, the extra spleen Luo acupoint), they are used mainly to treat their respective diseased parts and disorders of the internal organs.

IV Application of Confluence Acupoints

The application of these eight Confluence acupoints is based on their being the confluence of the Qi of the irregular meridians with the Qi of the regular meridians. (See Table 5.5). For example, acupoint Neiguan (PC-6) is the Confluence acupoint of the Yinwei Meridian and Gongsun (SP-4) is the Confluence acupoint of the Chong Meridian; and those two meridians are confluent in the heart, chest and stomach. They are suitable for use in treating fullness in the chest and abdomen, epigastric pain and anorexia.

V Application of Influential Acupoints

The Eight Influential Acupoints are where the vital essence and energy of the *zang* organs, *fu* organs, Qi, blood, tendons, vessels, bones and marrow join together. In clinical practice, any disorders affecting any of these tissues may be treated by applying acupuncture therapy to their respective Influential Acupoints. (See Table 5.6). For example, Zhongwan (CV-12) is used to treat disorders of the *fu* organs, and Tanzhong (CV-17) for diseases of Qi.

VI Application of Lower He (Sea) Acupoints

The ***Spiritual Pivot*** states that "disorders of the six *fu*-organs can be treated by the He (Sea) acupoints." According to this theory the Lower He acupoints are

Table 5.5 Confluence acupoints

Irregular Meridian	Confluence Acupoint	Applications
Chong Yinwei	Gongsun (SP-4) Neiguan (PC-6)	Diseases of heart, chest and stomach
DaiYangwei	Zulinqi (GB-41) Waiguan (SJ-5)	Diseases of outer canthus, back of ear, shoulder, neck, cheek
Du Yangqiao	Houxi (SI-3) Shenmai (BL-62)	Diseases of inner canthus, nape, ear and shoulder
Ren Yinqiao	Lieque (LU-7) Zhaohai (KI-6)	Diseases of lung system, throat and chest

Table 5.6 Influential acupoints

Tissue/Organ	Influential Acupoint	Tissue/Organ	Influential Acupoint
Zang organs	Zhangmen (LR-13)	Tendons	Yanglingquan (GB-34)
Fu organs	Zhongwan (CV-12)	Vessels	Taiyuan (LU-9)
Qi	Tanzhong (CV-17)	Bone	Dazhu (BL-11)
Blood	Geshu (BL-17)	Marrow	Juegu (GB-39)

Table 5.7 Lower He (Sea) acupoints

Yang Meridians of Hand	Small Intestine of Taiyang Meridian	Xiajuxu (ST-39)
	Sanjiao of Shaoyang Meridian	Weiyang (BL-39)
	Large Intestine of Yangming Meridian	Shangjuxu (ST-37)
Yang Meridians of Foot	Urinary Bladder of Taiyang Meridian	Weizhong (BL-40)
	Gallbladder of Shaoyang Meridian	Yanglingquan (GB-34)
	Stomach of Yangming meridian	Zusanli (ST-36)

Table 5.8 Xi (Cleft) acupoints

Meridian	Xi (Cleft) Acupoint	Meridian	Xi (Cleft) Acupoint
Lung Meridian of Hand-Taiyin	Kongzui (LU-6)	Kidney Meridian of Foot-Shaoyin	Shuiquan (KI-5)
Pericardium Meridian of Hand-Jueyin	Ximen (PC-4)	Stomach Meridian of Foot-Yangming	Liangqiu (ST-34)
Heart Meridian of Hand-Shaoyin	Yinxi (HT-6)	Gallbladder Meridian of Foot Shaoyang	Waiqiu (GB-36)
Large Intestine Meridian of Hand-Yangming	Wenliu (LI-7)	Bladder Meridian of Foot-Taiyang	Jinmen (BL-63)
Sanjiao Meridian of Hand-Shaoyang	Huizong (SJ-7)	Yinwei Meridian	Zhubin (KI-9)
Small Intestine Meridian of Hand-Taiyang	Yanglao (SI-6)	Yangwei Meridian	Yangjiao (GB-35)
Spleen Meridian of Foot-Taiyin	Diji (SP-8)	Yinqiao Meridian	Jiaoxin (KI-8)
Liver Meridian of Foot-Jueyin	Zhongdu (LR-6)	Yangqiao Meridian	Fuyang (BL-59)

suitable for treating diseases of their respective *fu*-organs. For example, abscess of the large intestine can be treated by applying acupuncture to Shangjuxu (ST-37) because it is the Lower He (Sea) acupoint of the Large Intestine Meridian of Hand-Yangming (see Table 5.7).

VII Application of Xi (Cleft) Acupoints

Each of the 12 regular meridians has one Xi (Cleft) acupoint. In addition, one Xi acupoint can be found on each of the Yinwei, Yangwei, Yinqiao and Yangqiao Meridians. In all there are 16 Xi acupoints. The Xi acupoints are used primarily in treating acute pain and disorders of their respective meridians and organs. For example, Kongzui (LU-6) is used to treat hemoptysis, and Ximen (PC-4) is useful for cardiac pain and chest fullness (Table 5.8).

Guidance for Study

I Aim of Study

This chapter describes the principles of acupuncture therapy and the selection of acupoints.

II Objectives of Study

After completing this chapter the learners will

1. Know the functions and therapeutic principles of acupuncture;
2. Know the general principles for the selection of acupoints for acupuncture therapy;
3. Be familiar with the basics of the clinical application of specific acupoints.

III Exercises for Review

1. Describe the basic principles of acupuncture and moxibustion therapy.
2. Explain the selection of acupoints.
3. Describe the principles of acupoint selection. Give examples.
4. Describe the applications and clinical significance of specific acupoints.

Part II
Chinese *Materia Medica*

Chapter 6
Basic Theory of Chinese *Materia Medica*

From practical clinical experiences spanning a very long time CM has distilled a basic and systemic theory of Chinese herbs. This theory explains the properties and actions of the herbs and guides their selection for use in drugs for clinical application.

Section 1 Properties of Herbs

The properties and actions of herbs are a basic concept of CM. Its principal components are the following: the four natures and five flavors; the ascending, descending, floating and sinking; meridian affinity; and toxicity.

I Nature and Flavor

The nature and flavor of an herb are high-level concepts that summarize its clinical properties. Essentially all herbs have nature and flavor. Herbs with the same nature but different flavors have different actions. Similarly, herbs with the same flavor but different natures have different actions. Both the nature and the flavor of an herb must be taken into account in order to understand its actions and to apply it effectively in clinical practice.

For this reason, in all Chinese medical texts through the ages whenever an herb is discussed its nature and flavor are mentioned first.

1 Nature

The four natures of herbs refer to the properties of "cold," "hot," "warm" and "cool." These four belong to two opposing categories, warm and hot in one and cool and cold in the other. Within each category there are some common aspects and some

Z.W. Liu and L. Liu (eds.), *Essentials of Chinese Medicine: Volume 2*,

different ones. Thus, warm and hot have some common aspects, but the warm nature is weaker than the hot nature. Cool and cold have their common aspects, but the cool nature is weaker than the cold nature. For some herbs, the descriptive terms strongly hot, strongly cold, mildly warm and mildly cool are also used.

The nature of an herb derives from the effects of its actions on the organic body. It corresponds with the coldness or hotness character of the illness it is used to treat. The herb that acts to eliminate or reduce Heat is said to be of cold or cool nature. Conversely, one that acts to eliminate or reduce Cold is said to be of hot or warm nature.

Shennong's Herbal Classic states: "Use herbs of hot nature to cure diseases of Cold. Use herbs of cold nature to cure diseases of Heat." ***Plain Questions*** also advises: "Warm what is cold, and chill what is hot." These aphorisms clarify the fundamental principle in the application of herbal therapeutics.

There are some herbs that have a neutral nature. This means that these herbs are of a nature that is neither significantly warm nor significantly cool. Among them some are mildly warm and some mildly cool. Thus their neutrality still falls within the categorization of the four natures; it is a relative, not an absolute, property.

2 *Flavor*

There are many flavors in CM, but five are regarded as the basic ones. The five basic flavors are the following: acrid, sweet, sour, bitter and salty.

In addition to how the herbs taste their flavors also reflect their actions. Two herbs with different flavors tend to have different actions, whereas two herbs with similar flavors tend to have similar actions. Also, the flavors of acrid, sweet and bland belong in Yang and the flavors of sour, bitter and salty belong in Yin.

The actions of the five flavors are as follows.

i Acrid

Herbs with acrid flavor have the actions of dispersing and promoting the movement of Qi and blood. In general, herbs used to treat illnesses of the exterior (such as mahuang, *Ephedra*, and bohe, *Mentha*) or Qi or blood stagnation (such as muxiang, *Aucklandia*, and honghua, *Carthamus*) have acrid flavor.

ii Sweet

Herbs with sweet flavor have restorative, stomach-regulating or spasm-soothing actions. In general, herbs used to treat deficiencies (such as dangshen, *Codonopsis*, and shudihuang, *Rehmannia*), soothe spasm and pain, or harmonize the actions of other herbs (such as yitang, maltose, and gancao, *Glycyrrhiza*) have sweet flavor.

Most sweet herbs are also moist and are useful for moistening Dryness.

iii Sour

Herbs with sour flavor act to astringe and arrest secretion or discharge. In general, herbs used to treat sweating due to debility or diarrhea have sour flavor. For example, shanzhuyu (*Cornus*) and wuweizi (*Schisandra*) can arrest spermatorrhea and sweating. Wubeizi (*Melaphis*) can astringe the intestines to stop diarrhea.

iv Bitter

Herbs with bitter flavor have the ability to eliminate and to dry.

Elimination has several meanings. It can mean the removal of Heat by catharsis; for example, dahuang, *Rheum*, is used to treat constipation due to Heat accumulation in the intestines and stomach. It can mean suppressing abnormally rising Qi; for example, xingren (*Prunus armeniaca*) is used to control cough or asthma due to abnormally rising lung-Qi. It can mean dispersion of Heat; for example, zhizi (*Gardenia*) is used to sedate from agitation due to strong Heat.

The drying action is exploited to treat illnesses of Dampness. Illnesses of Dampness may be due to Dampness–Cold or Dampness–Heat. Herbs with bitter flavor and warm nature, such as cangzhu (*Atractylodes*), are used to treat Cold–Dampness illnesses. Herbs with bitter flavor and cold nature, such as huanglian (*Coptis*), are used to treat Heat–Dampness illnesses.

In addition, herbs with bitter flavor also augment Yin. Huangbai (*Phellodendron*) and zhimu (*Anemarrhena*) can purge Fire and preserve Yin; they are often used to treat flaccid-paralysis caused by blazing kidney-Fire arising in deficiency of kidney-Yin.

v Salty

Herbs with salty flavor have the ability to soften and dissolve hard masses (such as walengzi, *Arca inflate*) and to induce catharsis (such as mangxiao, sodium sulfate). Such herbs are often used to treat scrofula, subcutaneous nodules, abdominal masses, as well as constipation due to Heat accumulation.

vi Bland and Astringent

In addition to the five basic flavors, some herbs are bland and some have astringent properties. Though these are strictly speaking not flavors, they are usually grouped with the flavors.

Some bland herbs (such as fuling, *Poria*, and zhuling, *Polyporus*) have the ability to promote the excretion of Dampness by inducing diuresis. These herbs are often used to treat edema or difficulty with urination.

Astringent herbs have similar actions to those of sour herbs. Most of them are used to treat such conditions as sweating due to debility, diarrhea, frequent urination, spermatorrhea, or hemorrhage. For example, longgu (*Os Draconis*) and muli (*Ostrea*) can arrest spermatorrhea. Wumei (*Prunus mume*) can astringe the intestines to stop diarrhea.

II Lifting, Lowering, Floating and Sinking

In the clinical manifestations of many illnesses the symptoms often show a tendency for movement upward (such as vomiting and cough), downward (such as diarrhea, metrorrhagia and rectal prolapse), outward (such as spontaneous sweating and night sweats) or inward (such as unresolved exterior symptoms extending to the interior). In treating each patient's illness, therefore, it is necessary to apply herbs that have the ability to reverse or eliminate such tendencies. This is the underlying concept of lifting, lowering, floating and sinking.

Lifting and lowering are opposites; so are floating and sinking. Floating is floating to the surface of the body and means dispersion. Sinking is sinking to the interior and means catharsis. In general, herbs that augment Yang, clear the superficies, expel Wind, dissipate Cold, induce vomiting and open orifices have the ability to lift and float. Conversely, herbs that purge Heat, promote diuresis to reduce Dampness, sedate mental agitation, subdue hyperactive Yang, extinguish endogenous Wind, dissipate accumulations, suppress abnormally rising Qi, astringe and relieve cough and labored breathing have the ability to lower and to sink.

There are also some herbs that do not have prominent lifting, lowering, floating or sinking actions, or that can go one way or the other depending on circumstances. For example, mahuang (*Ephedra*) can induce diaphoresis (floating) as well as relieve asthma and promote diuresis (sinking). Chuanxiong (*Ligusticum*) can go to the head (lifting) as well as the liver (lowering). These herbs are few in number, however.

An herb's ability to lift, lower, float or sink tends to correlate with its nature and flavor. Herbs that lift and float usually have acrid flavor and warm or hot nature. Herbs that lower and sink usually have sour or bitter flavor and cold or cool nature.

In addition, an herb's ability to lift, lower, float or sink is influenced by its processing. For example, frying with wine gives some herbs the ability to lift; cooking with ginger the ability to float; frying with vinegar the ability to astringe; and frying with salt water the ability to lower. Other herbs in a formula also may constrain the actions of any one herb, such as the lifting and floating ability of one herb counteracting the lowering and sinking ability of another. By these manipulations, the ability to lift, lower, float or sink of every kind of herb can be controlled.

III Meridian Affinity

Many herbs act only upon parts, not the whole, of the body. An herb's meridian affinity indicates which meridian, its associated visceral organ and its branches the herb acts upon selectively. For example, though all herbs of cold nature have the ability to clear Heat some are more effective at clearing Heat from the lung, some from the liver, and so on. Similarly, some restoratives are more effective at nourishing the lung, others the spleen, yet others the kidney, and so on. The comprehensive and systematic analysis of how the many herbs affect the many parts of the body has resulted in the principle of meridian affinity.

Meridian affinity is based on the theory of the *zang–fu* viscera and of the meridians as well as empirical clinical experiences. The meridians and their collateral branches link the interior and the exterior. Illness in exterior of the body can affect the internal organs, and similarly illness in an internal organ can be reflected in exterior. Because of this linkage it is possible by analyzing the symptoms expressed in interior to infer which meridian system is diseased. For example, abnormality of the Lung Meridian can manifest labored breathing and coughing. Abnormality of the Liver Meridian can manifest flank pain and tetany or convulsion. Abnormality of the Heart Meridian can manifest disturbances of consciousness and palpitations. By correlating the actions of herbs with the pathology of illnesses and the meridian linkage system it is possible to understand how a specific herb can affect a specific internal organ or meridian and their abnormal changes. In this way, the physician can achieve important therapeutic results. For example, jiegeng (*Platycodon*) and xingren (*Prunus armeniaca*) can cure chest tightness and cough; thus they have affinity for the Lung Meridian. Quanxie (*Buthus martensii*) can stop convulsions; thus it has affinity for the Liver Meridian. Zhusha (cinnabar) can sedate; thus it has affinity for the Heart Meridian.

An illness of any internal organ may be of Cold or of Heat, may be due to strength of pathogenic evil or to deficiency, and may show a tendency to ascend and float or to descend and sink. When prescribing herbs, the physician must take into full consideration and correlate the meridian affinity of herbs with their flavor and nature and their lifting-lowering and floating-sinking properties. For example, a lung illness with cough may be of Cold or Heat, may be due to strength or deficiency, and may be in the exterior or in the interior. Though huangqin (*Scutellaria*), ganjiang (*Zingiber*), baihe (*Lilium*), tinglizi (*Lepidium*) and others all have affinity for the Lung Meridian, huangqin cools lung-Heat, ganjiang warms lung-Cold, baihe strengthens the lung and tinglizi purges pathogenic evil from the lung. The differences between them are great indeed. Thus, it is essential to take into full consideration all of each herb's properties in order to apply the herbs accurately and achieve ideal therapeutic effects.

Furthermore, the pathological changes of an illness of one visceral organ and its meridians affect those of other visceral organs and their meridians. In the clinical application of herbs, therefore, the physician must focus not only on herbs but also on one particular meridian. For example, illnesses of the lung often have associated spleen insufficiency; their treatment requires the incorporation of herbs that strengthen the spleen so that the lung receives nourishment and can heal. The abnormal ascent of liver-Yang is often due to deficiency of kidney-Yin; its treatment requires the incorporation of herbs that nourish kidney-Yin, so that liver-Yin is also nourished and can now subdue liver-Yang. In summary, accurate application of herbs requires thorough understanding of each herb's meridian affinity as well as its other properties while at the same time full consideration of the interrelationship between the *zang–fu* organs and their meridians and branches. (Review the Theory of the Five Elements, Volume 1, Part I, Chapter 1, Section 2, Subsection III, and the Relationship between the *Zang* and *Fu* Organs, Volume 1, Part I, Chapter 3, Section 4.)

IV Toxicity

Toxicity as used in CM has two meanings, a broader and a narrower.

Since ancient times toxicity has been recognized as an intrinsic property of herbs. Indeed, it is because herbs have toxicity that they are able to cure illnesses. The *Internal Classic* states: "When using highly toxic herbs stop when six-tenths of the illness is cured. When using ordinarily toxic herbs stop when seven-tenths of the illness is cured. When using mildly toxic herbs stop when eight-tenths of the illness is cured. When using non-toxic herbs stop when nine-tenths of the illness is cured." ***Shennong's Herbal Classic*** asserts that herbs that attack illness and can effect a cure are toxic whereas those that restore deficiencies and may be taken for prolonged periods are nontoxic. In general, toxic herbs have strong therapeutic actions. More recent CM authorities have stated: "All herbs that can eliminate pathogenic factors and preserve health may be said to be toxic." This is toxicity in the broader sense.

In its narrower sense, toxicity refers to undesirable effects of herbs. When herbs are used improperly there may be harmful consequences. For this reason, in the description of individual herbs in more recent herbals there is the annotation of "poisonous" or "not poisonous" "Poisonous" in this context refers to toxicity in its narrower sense.

Once the concept of the toxicity of herbs is properly understood the physician can exploit the approach of "using toxicity to fight toxicity" For example, appropriately selected toxic herbs are used to lessen the virulence of various skin and other external illnesses, eliminate disease-causing factors and kill parasites. When a particular herb is required but is toxic in the narrower sense, it is often possible to add other herbs with toxic properties that counteract the toxicity of the first herb. By balancing several herbs with different toxic properties but otherwise compatible in the same compound formula it is generally possible to eliminate or significantly reduce the undesirable effects and ensure safety and efficacy in achieving the desired therapeutic effects.

Section 2 Clinical Use of Herbs

In CM herbs may be used singly or in combination. To prescribe properly it is essential for the physician to master the indications and contraindications, the dosage and the administration of herbs, and the principles of drug interaction. Only then can safety be assured and the desired therapeutic result obtained.

I Herb Interactions

The ancient physicians summarized the interactions between herbs as principles. These are sometimes called the "seven facets of herbs."

1 Single

Certain illnesses may be treated with a single herb. In general these are relatively simple illnesses, so that a single herb can achieve a cure. For example, huangqin (*Scutellaria*) by itself is quite effective for hemoptysis caused by Heat in the lung. Many popular remedies contain single herbs. They are convenient, inexpensive and easy to use.

But if an illness is complex a single herb is not likely to take care of all aspects of the illness. For such an illness it becomes necessary to use two or more herbs. When several herbs are involved it becomes necessary to consider their interactions and to ensure that they are compatible.

2 Mutual Reinforcement

Mutual reinforcement is a type of interaction in which herbs with similar properties complement and reinforce one another in such a way that together they achieve a greater therapeutic effect than the herbs can individually. For example, shigao (gypsum) and zhimu (*Anemarrhena*) together are much more effective in cooling Heat and purging Fire. Dahuang (*Rheum*) and mangxiao (*Mirabilite*) together are much more potent in purging Heat through catharsis.

3 Assistance

Assistance means that when two herbs with overlapping properties are used together, one herb enhances the therapeutic effect of the other. For example, huangqi (*Astragalus*) augments Qi and promotes diuresis and fuling (*Poria*) promotes diuresis and strengthens the spleen; used together fuling enhances the diuretic effect of huangqi. Similarly, huangqin (*Scutellaria*) cools Heat and purges Fire and dahuang (*Rheum*) induces catharsis and purges Heat; used together dahuang enhances huangqin's ability to cool Heat and purge Fire.

4 Restraint

Restraint means that when two herbs are used together one may reduce or restrict the actions of the other. For example, raw ginger (*Zingiber*) reduces some of the effects of raw banxia (*Pinellia*), especially its poisonous effects; thus ginger is said to restrain banxia. In addition, physicians of the Jin and Yuan eras compiled the following list:

Puxiao (*Mirabilite*) restrains liuhuang (sulfur)
Arsenic restrains mercury
Mituoseng (lead oxide) restrains langdu (*Stellera*, *Euphorbia*)
Qianniu (*Pharbitis*) restrains badou (*Croton*)
Yujin (*Curcuma*) restrains dingxiang (*Syzygium*)
Xijiao (rhinoceros horn) restrains chuanwu (*Aconitum*)
Sanleng (*Sparganium*) restrains yaxiao (*Mirabilite*)
Shizhi (*Halloysite*) restrains guangui (*Cinnamomum*)
Wulingzhi (*Trogopterus*, *Pleropus*) restrains renshen (*Panax*)

5 Antidote

An antidote is an herb that can significantly reduce or eliminate the poisonous effects of another. For example, fangfeng (*Saposhnikovia*) is antidotal to pishi (arsenolite).

6 Mutual Inhibition

Mutual inhibition is the interaction in which the therapeutic effects of both herbs may be reduced or lost when the herbs are used together. For example, laifuzi (*Raphanus*) lowers Qi and renshen (*Panax*) augments Qi. When used together neither can significantly affect Qi. Other examples readily come to mind, such as using warming herbs together with cooling herbs.

7 Antagonism

In antagonism two or more herbs used together may produce poisonous or undesirable effects that the herbs individually do not have or do not have to any significant degree. Physicians of the Jin and Yuan eras compiled the following list:

Gancao (*Glycyrrhiza*) antagonizes gansui (*Euphorbia kansui*), daji (*Euphorbia pekinensis*), haizao (*Sargassum*) and yuanhua (*Daphne*)

Wutou (*Aconitum*) antagonizes beimu (*Fritillaria*) gualou (*Tricosanthes*), banxia (*Pinellia*), bailian (*Ampelopsis*) and baiji (*Bletilla*)
Lilu (*Veratrum*) antagonizes renshen (*Panax*), shashen (*Glehnia*), danshen (*Salvia*), xuanshen (*Scrophularia*), xixin (*Asarum*) and shaoyao (*Paeonia*)

8 Summary

The complementation of herbs may be summarized in the following hour statements:

1. Some herbs promote curative effects through cooperation. Such cooperation should be exploited fully.
2. Some herbs offset or reduce the curative effects of other herbs. This must be taken into account fully.
3. Some herbs can relieve or diminish the poisonous or undesirable effects of other herbs. This interaction should be exploited when applying herbs that are acrid or are potentially poisonous.
4. Some herbs are harmless when used alone, but may produce poisonous or undesirable effects when used together. Such combinations must be avoided in principle.

II Contraindications

1 Incompatibility of Herbs

Certain combinations of herbs must not be used. These are described in the previous subsection. They are all based on empirical experience. Some have not been studied; nevertheless, the wise course to follow is not to use them.

2 Contraindications in Pregnancy

If used in pregnancy some herbs injure genuine Qi and others harm the fetus or may induce abortion. On the basis of their degree of harmful effect these may be groups in two categories.

i Contraindicated Herbs

These are herbs that must not be used in pregnancy. In general, they are either highly poisonous or act vigorously. Some of the most common of these

contraindicated herbs are badou (*Croton*), qianniu (*Pharbitis*), daji (*Euphorbia pekinensis*), banmao (*Mylabris*), shanglu (*Phytolacca*), shexiang (*Moschus*), sanleng (*Sparganium*), ezhu (*Curcuma*), shuizhi (*Hirudo*, *Whitmania*) and mengchong
(*Tabanus*).

ii Herbs to Use with Caution

Herbs that should be used in pregnancy only with caution mostly act to remove stasis, mobilize Qi or break accumulations, or are acrid in taste and hot in nature. Unless there is a special need they should be avoided in pregnancy. Examples include taoren (*Prunus persica*), honghua (*Carthamus*), dahuang (*Rheum*), zhishi (*Citrus aurantium*), fuzi (*Aconitum*), ganjiang (*Zingiber*) and rougui (*Cinnamomum*).

3 Dietary Avoidance

When prescribing certain herbs the physician must advise the patient to avoid certain food items. In general, the patient should avoid any food that is not easy to digest (raw, cold, glutinous, oily and fishy) and any that is spicy. Examples of specific food items to avoid include the following.

Changshan (*Dichroa fibrifuga*): avoid onion.
Dihuang (*Rehmannia*), heshouwu (*Polygonum*): avoid onion, garlic and radish.
Bohe (*Mentha*): avoid the flesh of the soft-shelled turtle.
Fuling (*Poria*): avoid vinegar.
Biejia (*Amyda*): avoid amaranth.
Fengmi (honey): avoid raw onion.

III Dosage and Administration

1 Dosage

The dosage of an herb is the amount of the herb to be used in preparing the herbal formula to be taken. In Volume 2, Part II, Chapter 7, for each herb described the range of usual dosage is given. Two facts must be borne in mind.

1. This dosage applies when the herb is used by itself.
2. It is the amount to be used by an average adult in one day.

2 Adjustment of Dosage

A number of considerations affect the actual amount of an herb used.

1. When an herb is included in a compound prescription with other herbs, its amount is generally reduced from its single-herb dosage.
2. In a compound formula, the amount of the main herbs is usually larger than that of the auxiliary herbs.
3. The amount of an herb to be prepared as decoction is usually larger than that for preparation as pill or powder.
4. Patient Factors: The physician must take into account the patient's age, body size and the robustness of constitution. In general, an elderly patient has a lower tolerance for herbs, since their Qi and blood tend to be in decline; the amount should be suitably reduced. Because of their smaller size children require smaller amounts. As a rule of thumb, for children under the age of five use one quarter of the usual adult dosage, and for children 6 years of age or older use half of the usual adult dosage. In general, for a patient of weak constitution reduced dosage is appropriate.
5. Illness Factors: In general, smaller dosage is required in a prolonged illness and larger dosage in a recent illness. For restorative herbs, larger dosage is required for those who are old or debilitated by illness; but the amount should be small in the beginning and increased gradually. For serious illnesses the drug should be potent and in relatively large dosage, whereas for mild illnesses the drug should be mild and in relatively small dosage to avoid injuring genuine Qi.
6. Herb Factors: In general, if an herb is of light quality its dosage should be relatively small; and if it is of heavy quality its dosage should be relatively larger. On the other hand, if the herb's flavor and nature are strong its dosage should be relatively smaller; and if they are mild its dosage needs to be relatively larger. In the case of an herb that is toxic, its dosage must be carefully controlled to avoid undesirable effects.

3 Administration

i Preparation of Decoction

Put an appropriate amount of clean water in a suitable-sized pot, a little more than just enough to cover the herbs. In general the herbs are boiled with high heat for several minutes followed by simmering with low heat for a short while. How long an herb should be decocted depends upon its properties. Aromatic herbs are usually decocted for a short time to avoid loss of effectiveness. Restorative herbs, which are often greasy, are decocted for a long time to ensure full potency. Most mineral herbs require even longer decoction.

Because of differences in the duration of cooking, not all herbs are added at once. Mineral herbs are added first and are cooked for about 10 min before aromatic herbs are added. Herbs that are small in size, such as powders or seeds, are wrapped in gauze.

Some herbs are prepared separately. Medicinal herbs not suitable for decoction and gelatinous herbs should be melted separately and mixed with the supernatant decocted from the other herbs. Liquid herbs should be added to the supernatant from the other herbs. Expensive herbs are often made into powders and mixed with the supernatant from the other herbs at the time of administration.

ii Administration

1. Decoctions are usually taken while warm, but herbs that disperse Wind–Cold are best taken hot. Herbs for treating vomiting or drug intoxication are taken in small portions in quick succession. Sometimes herbal prescriptions drugs are taken cold while cooling herbal prescriptions taken warm as appropriate for clinical reasons. Solid herbal preparations, such as pills and powders, are usually swallowed with warm water unless there is a special requirement.
2. Timing: The timing of administration is determined by the clinical requirements and the properties of the herb. Most herbal preparations, including those that strengthen the stomach or stimulate the stomach and the intestines are taken after meals. Restorative or nourishing drugs are taken mostly before meals. Regardless, take the preparation about an hour before or after the meal. Herbs for expelling parasites and cathartics are taken on an empty stomach. Herbal preparations to induce sleep are taken at bedtime.
3. Frequency: The decoction is usually taken in three portions spread evenly through the day. If the illness is not serious or is chronic, it may be taken in two portions a day. If the illness is serious, it is best to divide the decoction into six portions and take one portion every 4 h to ensure continual effect.
4. Duration: Some herbs must not be taken longer than clinically necessary. For example, potent herbal preparations, especially those that induce sweating and catharsis, must be stopped as soon as the desired therapeutic effect has been obtained to avoid injuring vital Qi.

Guidance for Study

I Aim of Study

This chapter introduces the basic properties of herbs, their interactions and the principles governing their dosage and administration.

II Objectives of Study

Upon completion of this chapter, the learners will

1. Know the basic properties of herbs and the principles of their clinical application;
2. Understand the clinical significance of the four natures and the five flavors;
3. Understand the concepts of lifting and lowering, floating and sinking, and meridian affinity, as well as their clinical significance and the factors that affect these properties;
4. Understand the relationship between the nature and flavor of herbs and their ability to lift, lower, float or sink;
5. Understand the concept of toxicity and its clinical significance;
6. Understand the principles of herb interaction, including its "seven facets," and the principles of complementation;
7. Understand the precautions and contraindications when prescribing herbs, especially in pregnancy;
8. Know the basic principles governing dosage and the decoction of herbs.

III Exercises for Review

1. Explain the nature and flavor of Chinese medical herbs. What is the clinical significance of nature and flavor of herbs? What is the relationship between nature and flavor?
2. Explain the concepts of lifting and lowering, floating and sinking, and their clinical significance. Which factors influence lifting, lowering, floating and sinking?
3. What is meridian affinity? How does it affect the clinical application of herbs?
4. Explain the concept of toxicity, in its broader and narrower meaning.
5. What are the seven facets of herb interaction? Explain their clinical significance.
6. Discuss the cautions and contraindications for prescribing herbs.
7. Describe and explain the factors that determine dosage.
8. Describe how a decoction is prepared. Explain the principles of its administration.

Chapter 7
Commonly Used Herbs

In this chapter 154 of the most commonly used medicinal herbs are described. Since there are so many of them, some systems for classifying them are necessary. In this textbook the following scheme is adopted:

Section 1: herbs that release exterior
Section 2: herbs that cool Heat
Section 3: herbs that induce catharsis
Section 4: herbs that dispel Wind–Dampness
Section 5: aromatic herbs that dissipate Dampness
Section 6: herbs that drain water
Section 7: herbs that warm interior
Section 8: herbs that regulate Qi
Section 9: herbs that relieve food retention
Section 10: herbs that stimulate blood circulation and remove blood stasis
Section 11: herbs that dissolve Phlegm or stop cough and relieve asthma
Section 12: herbs that restore
Section 13: herbs that calm the mind
Section 14: herbs that calm liver and extinguish Wind
Section 15: aromatic herbs that open orifices (resuscitate)
Section 16: herbs that stop bleeding
Section 17: herbs that stabilize and astringe
Section 18: herbs that expel worms

In addition, Appendix III provides an alphabetical listing of these herbs, both by their names in *pinyin* and by their Latin names. Appendix IV provides photos of these herbs.

Section 1 Herbs That Release Exterior

Herbs that release the exterior have as their principal action the dispersion of exogenous pathogenic evils from the exterior of the body. Their principal clinical use is to release the exterior by dispelling exogenous Wind–Cold or Wind–Heat,

Z.W. Liu and L. Liu (eds.), *Essentials of Chinese Medicine: Volume 2*,

with such symptoms as Cold-aversion, fever, headache, body aches, with or without sweating, and a floating pulse. Since illnesses of the exterior are of two main kinds, Wind–Cold and Wind–Heat, these herbs are accordingly organized in two groups: warm-acrid herbs and cool-acrid.

Because of their acrid flavor some of these herbs are quite useful for treating edema, cough and asthma. In illnesses with rashes that have not completely erupted, they can be helpful to induce full eruption of the rash so that the patient can recover. In addition, certain exterior-releasing herbs act to remove Dampness and relieve aches. They are used to treat aches in the limbs caused by Wind–Dampness.

When prescribing exterior-releasing herbs, in addition to selecting herbs depending upon whether the illness is one of exogenous Wind–Cold or Wind–Heat, the physician must also take into account the possibility that the patient may have unbalanced deficiency of genuine Qi. In such a situation it is important to add herbs that augment Yang, nourish Qi or enrich Yin. When applying cool-acrid herbs in the early stages of Heat illnesses, it is wise to add appropriate herbs that clear Heat and remove poisons.

When treating with exterior-releasing herbs with a strong diaphoretic action it is important not to induce sweating excessively to avoid damaging Yang-Qi and body fluids. These herbs are contraindicated in those patients who have profuse sweating or are in late stages of fluid depletion. Also, patients who suffer chronically from skin conditions such as abscesses, difficult and painful urination, or persistent blood loss, exterior-releasing herbs must be used with great caution even when they contract an exterior illness.

I Warm-Acrid Herbs That Release Exterior

1 Mahuang (Ephedra sinica)

Chinese name: 麻黄. *Pharmaceutical name*: Herba Ephedrae.

Part Used: stalk.

Flavor/Nature: acrid, slightly bitter; warm.

Meridian Affinity: Lung and Bladder Meridians.

Actions: promotes sweating; relieves wheezing; promotes urination.

Indications: (1) Strength illnesses of the exterior caused by exogenous Wind and Cold. The main chief symptoms are chills, fever, headache, nasal congestion, absence of sweating, and a floating and taut pulse. (2) Cough and asthma due to Wind–Cold invading the lung and disturbing the dispersion of lung-Qi. (3) Edema complicating an illness of the exterior.

Dosage/Administration: 5–10 g. Decocted first before other herbs. Fresh mahuang is used to induce sweating. Prepared mahuang is often used to moisten the lung and relieve asthma.

Cautions/Contraindications: Because this herb is quite potent in inducing sweating, it is contraindicated in a patient with spontaneous sweating, night sweats due to Yin deficiency, or cough and asthma due to kidney failing to receive Qi.

2 *Guizhi (Cinnamomum cassia) (Cinnamon)*

Chinese name: 桂枝. Pharmaceutical name: *Ramulus Cinnamomi*.

Part Used: twig.

Flavor/Nature: acrid, sweet; warm.

Meridian Affinity: Heart, Lung and Bladder Meridians.

Actions: promotes sweating in exterior illnesses; warms meridians and unblocks Yang.

Indications: (1) Headache, fever and chills caused by Wind and Cold. (2) Shoulder, back and limb pain due to rheumatism caused by Wind–Cold–Dampness. (3) Rheum and Phlegm accumulation due to deficiency of heart and spleen Yang, impairing the movement of Yang-Qi and in turn water and Dampness stagnation. (4) Rheumatism of the chest, palpitation of the heart, and a hesitant and intermittent pulse. (5) Amenorrhea or dysmenorrhea due to Cold invading the meridians.

Dosage/Administration: 3–10 g.

Cautions/Contraindications: Because of its acrid flavor and warm nature guizhi can readily injure Yin and move blood. It is contraindicated in illnesses of Heat, Yin deficiency with Yang hyperactivity, and Heat in the blood causing bleeding. It must be used with great caution in pregnancy or during excessive menstrual flow.

3 *Xixin (Asarum heterotropoides, sieboldii) (Manchurian Wild Ginger)*

Chinese name: 细辛. Pharmaceutical name: *Herba Asari*.

Part Used: root.

Flavor/Nature: acrid; warm.

Meridian Affinity: Lung and Kidney Meridians.

Actions: expels Wind, dispels Cold, clears nasal passages, stops pain, warms the lungs and transforms Phlegm.

Indications: (1) Illnesses of the exterior due to exogenous Wind and Cold. (2) Headache, rhinitis, sinusitis, toothache, rheumatism pain. (3) Cold and Phlegm accumulation in the lung causing cough and labored breathing.

Dosage/Administration: In decoction, 1.5–3 g.

Cautions/Contraindications: Xixin is contraindicated in a patient with profuse sweating due to Qi deficiency, headache due to Yang excess and Yin deficiency, or dry cough due to Dryness in the lung damaging Yin. In general, avoid overdose. Xixin is incompatible with lilu (*Veratrum*).

4 Zisu (Perilla frutescens)

Chinese name: 紫苏. Pharmaceutical name: *Perillae*.

Part Used: zisugeng, stalk; zisuye, leaf; zisuzi, ripe seeds.

Flavor/Nature: acrid; warm.

Meridian Affinity: Lung and Spleen Meridians.

Actions: disperses Wind and Cold from the exterior, moves Qi and unblocks the middle-jiao, and counteracts fish and crab toxins.

Indications: (1) Illnesses of exogenous Wind and Cold with fever, Cold-intolerance, headache, nasal congestion, and cough or chest tightness.

Dosage/Administration: 3–10 g. Do not overcook.

5 Jingjie (Schizonepeta tenuifolia)

Chinese name: 荆芥. Pharmaceutical name: *Herba Schizonepetae*.

Part Used: whole herb (above ground portion).

Flavor/Nature: acrid; slightly warm.

Meridian Affinity: Lung and Liver Meridians.

Actions: dispels Wind and relieves the exterior; and stops bleeding.

Indications: (1) Wind and Cold in the exterior, with headache, fever, Cold-intolerance and no sweating. (2) Itchy rashes of the skin and measles prior to full eruption. (3) Early stages of sores and furuncles associated with an exterior illness.

(4) Charred jingjie has the ability to stop bleeding, and is used in hematochezia, epistaxis and metrorrhagia.

Dosage/Administration: 3–10 g. Cook for about 5 min and do not overcook. For stopping bleeding, must be charred.

6 Fangfeng (Saposhnikovia divaricata)

Chinese name: 防风. Pharmaceutical name: *Radix Saposhnikoviae.*

Part Used: root.

Flavor/Nature: acrid, sweet; slightly warm.

Meridian Affinity: Bladder, Liver and Spleen Meridians.

Actions: expels Wind and releases the exterior, dispels Dampness, stops pain, and relieves spasm.

Indications: (1) Exterior illnesses due to Wind and Cold with headache, body aches and Cold-intolerance. (2) Rheumatism due to Wind, Cold and Dampness, joint pains and spasm of the limbs. (3) Opisthotonos, trismus and tetany due to tetanus.

Dosage/Administration: 3–10 g.

Cautions/Contraindications: Fangfeng is principally used for illnesses induced by exogenous Wind. In convulsions of blood insufficiency or blazing Fire in Yin deficiency, it must be used only with great caution.

7 Qianghuo (Notopterygium incisum, franchetti, forbesi)

Chinese name: 羌活. Pharmaceutical name: *Rhizoma et Radix Notopterygii.*

Part Used: root and rhizome.

Flavor/Nature: acrid, bitter; warm.

Meridian Affinity: Bladder and Kidney Meridians.

Actions: releases exterior, disperses Cold, expels Wind, eliminates Dampness, and stops pain.

Indications: (1) Exogenous Cold and Wind, with Cold-intolerance, fever, headache and body aches. (2) Limb joint, shoulder and back aching pain due to Wind–Cold–Dampness – especially in the upper part of body.

Dosage/Administration: 3–10 g.

8 *Baizhi (Angelica dahurica, anomala, taiwaniana)*

Chinese name: 白芷. Pharmaceutical name: *Radix Angelicae Dahuricae*.

Part Used: root.

Flavor/Nature: acrid; warm.

Meridian Affinity: Lung and Stomach Meridians.

Actions: releases the exterior, expels Wind and dries Dampness, reduces swelling and eliminates pus, and stops pain.

Indications: (1) Exogenous Wind and Cold with headache and nasal congestion. (2) Illness in the Yang Ming Meridian with headache, supra-orbital pain, headache and toothache. (3) Boils and furuncles with swelling and pain. (4) Vaginal discharge due to Cold and Dampness.

Dosage/Administration: 3–10 g.

II Cool-Acrid Herbs That Release Exterior

1 *Bohe (Mentha haplocalyx) (Peppermint)*

Chinese name: 薄荷. Pharmaceutical name: *Herba Menthae*.

Part Used: whole herb (above ground portion).

Flavor/Nature: acrid; cold.

Meridian Affinity: Lung and Liver Meridians.

Actions: dispels Wind and Heat, clears the head, eyes and throat, and promotes the eruption of rashes.

Indications: (1) Exterior illnesses due to Wind–Heat and initial stages of seasonal febrile illnesses with headache, fever, and cold-aversion. (2) Headache and eye inflammation caused by Wind–Heat attacking upward. (3) Initial stages of measles or Wind–Heat binding the exterior without eruption of rashes. (4) Stagnation of liver-Qi causing chest tightness and rib and flank pain.

Dosage/Administration: 2–10 g. Cook for about 5 min only. Do not overcook.

Cautions/Contraindications: Contraindicated in spontaneous sweating due to weakness in the exterior.

2 *Niubangzi (Arctium lappa) (Burdock Fruit)*

Chinese name: 牛蒡子. Pharmaceutical name: *Fructus Arctii.*

Part Used: ripe fruit.

Flavor/Nature: acrid, bitter; cold.

Meridian Affinity: Lung and Stomach Meridians.

Actions: disperses Wind–Heat, detoxifies and promotes the eruption of rashes, soothes the throat and relieves swelling.

Indications: (1) Exterior illnesses due to Wind–Heat with cough but difficulty with expectoration, and swollen and painful throat. (2) Initial stages of measles before full eruption or Wind–Heat illnesses with rashes. (3) Boils, abscesses and mumps due to Heat poison.

Dosage/Administration: 3–10 g.

Cautions/Contraindications: Niubangzi can promote defecation. It is contraindicated in Qi deficiency with diarrhea.

3 *Sangye (Morus alba) (Mulberry)*

Chinese name: 桑叶. Pharmaceutical name: *Folium Mori.*

Part Used: leaf.

Flavor/Nature: bitter, sweet; cold.

Meridian Affinity: Lung and Liver Meridians.

Actions: dispels Wind and clears Heat, purifies the liver and brightens the eyes.

Indications: (1) Exogenous illnesses of Wind–Heat with fever, headache, dizziness, cough and sore throat. (2) Heat or Heat–Wind in the Liver Meridian with eye inflammation, irritation and excessive tearing.

Dosage/Administration: 5–10 g as decoction, pill or powder. For external use the supernatant from decoction to wash the eyes.

4 *Juhua (Chrysanthemum morifolium) (Chrysanthemum)*

Chinese name: 菊花. Pharmaceutical name: *Flos Chrysanthemi.*

Part Used: flower (inflorescence).

Flavor/Nature: acrid, sweet, bitter; slightly cold.

Meridian Affinity: Liver and Lung Meridians.

Actions: dispels Wind and clears Heat, eliminates poison and brightens the eyes.

Indications: (1) Exogenous illnesses caused by Wind–Heat and initial stages of febrile illnesses with headache and dizziness. (2) Eye inflammation due to Wind–Heat in the Liver Meridian or abnormal rise of liver-Fire. (3) Headache and vertigo due to stirring of liver-Wind or abnormal rise of liver-Fire.

Dosage/Administration: 10–15 g as decoction or pill.

5 *Chaihu (Bupleurum chinense, scorzonerifolium) (Thoroughwax)*

Chinese name: 柴胡. Pharmaceutical name: *Radix Bupleuri*.

Part Used: root.

Flavor/Nature: bitter, acrid; slightly cold.

Meridian Affinity: Pericardium, Liver, Sanjiao and Gallbladder Meridians.

Actions: releases exterior and relieves fever, mobilizes liver-Qi and raises Yang-Qi.

Indications: (1) Cold evil in Shaoyang causing alternating fever and chills, chest and flank distention, a bitter taste, dry throat and blurred vision. (2) Depression and gelling of liver-Qi causing epigastric and flank pain and distention, or headache, or in females irregular and painful menstruation. (3) Sinking of Qi leading to prolapse of the rectum or the uterus, or shortness of breath and fatigue.

Dosage/Administration: 3–10 g.

Cautions/Contraindications: The nature of Chaihu is to raise and disperse. It is contraindicated in a patient who has deficiency of kidney-Yin and abnormal rise of liver-Yang.

6 *Gegen (Pueraria lobata) (Kudzu Vine)*

Chinese name: 葛根. Pharmaceutical name: *Radix Puerariae*.

Part Used: bulbous root.

Flavor/Nature: sweet, acrid; cool.

Meridian Affinity: Spleen and Stomach Meridians.

Actions: releases exterior and muscles, raises Yang and promotes full eruption of rashes, reduces Heat and generates fluids.

Indications: (1) Exogenous illnesses with fever, headache, neck and back stiffness and pain. (2) Initial stages of measles with fever and cold-intolerance and before the rashes erupt. (3) Dysentery due to Dampness–Heat or diarrhea due to spleen insufficiency. (4) Thirst in febrile illness and diabetes.

Dosage/Administration: 10–30 g as decoction, pill or powder. For stopping diarrhea roast in slow fire.

7 *Chantui (Cryptotympana atrata) (Cicada)*

Chinese name: 蝉蜕. Pharmaceutical name: *Periostracum Cicadae*.

Part Used: molt.

Flavor/Nature: sweet; cold.

Meridian Affinity: Lung and Liver Meridians.

Actions: dispels Wind–Heat, promotes the eruption of rashes, brightens the eyes and clears corneal opacities, suppresses endogenous Wind and relieves spasm.

Indications: (1) Exogenous Wind–Heat illnesses and the initial stages of febrile illnesses with headache. (2) Initial stages of measles before full eruption of the rash. (3) Wind–Heat in the Liver Meridian, eye inflammation, corneal opacities and excessive tearing. (4) Heat–Wind in the Liver Meridian, night terror in infants and tetanus.

Dosage/Administration: 3–10 g as decoction, pill or powder.

Section 2 Herbs That Cool Heat

Heat-cooling herbs have as their principal action the cooling of Heat. These herbs are of cool or cold nature, which enables them to purge Heat, dry Dampness, cool blood, eliminate poison and reduce fever due to deficiencies. This group of herbs is principally used to treat conditions in which the exterior has been cleared of pathogenic evil but Heat is strong in the interior although there is no stagnation in the interior. Examples include exogenous Heat illnesses with high fever, irritability and thirst. Other conditions include dysentery due to Dampness–Heat, illnesses with high fever and macular rashes, furuncles and abscesses, and illnesses of Yin deficiency.

Because of differences in causation, progression and the patients' constitution, there are several varieties of illnesses of interior Heat with varying clinical manifestations. Taking into account these differences, as well as the varying responses to the herbs, Heat-cooling herbs are classified into five main categories. (1) Herbs that cool Heat and purge Fire have the capability to clear Heat from the Qi Level.

They are used to treat illnesses of Heat in the Qi Level showing such symptoms as high fever, irritability and thirst. (For the Qi Level, see Volume 1, Part II, Chapter 9, Section 5.) (2) Herbs that cool Heat and dry Dampness are used to treat dysentery, jaundice and other illnesses of Dampness–Heat. (3) Herbs that cool Heat and detoxify its poisons are used to treat such conditions as furuncles and abscesses that result from the poisons of blazing Heat. (4) Herbs that clear Heat and cool the blood have the capability to expel Heat from the Nutritive and the Blood Levels. They are used to treat illnesses of strong exogenous Heat in the Blood Level manifesting such symptoms as hematemesis, epistaxis and rashes. (5) Herbs that eliminate endogenous Heat arising in deficiency states have the capability to reduce fever arising from deficiency-Heat. They are used to treat such serious conditions as the Heat evil injuring Yin, fever in the night and cold in the morning and fever arising in Yin deficiency and steaming heat from the bones in consumptive diseases.

Although it is convenient to categorize the herbs it must be remembered that many of these herbs can fit in more than one category.

When applying Heat-cooling herbs, the physician must first determine whether the Heat is exogenous or endogenous. Three of these five methods apply to exogenous Heat, and two apply to endogenous Heat. At the same time the physician must pay attention to accompanying conditions. If there is illness in exterior as well, this must be released before attempting to cool interior or exterior and interior must be treated simultaneously. If Heat has gelled in interior then it is necessary to add herbs that induce catharsis.

The herbs in this group are all of cold or cool nature. They can injure the spleen and the stomach easily. Great care must be exercised in their usage whenever spleen or stomach Qi is deficient or there is a poor appetite with diarrhea. Heat illnesses readily damage the body fluids and herbs that are bitter and cold readily transform Dryness and injure Yin. Thus, great care must also be exercised in their usage when there is Yin deficiency. If Yin is grossly excessive and expels Yang to exterior, giving rise to genuine Cole and false Heat, Heat-cooling herbs are contraindicated.

I Herbs That Cool Heat and Purge Fire

1 Shigao (Gypsum)

Chinese name: 石膏. Pharmaceutical name: *Gypsum Fibrosum*. Chemical formula: $CaSO_4$.

Part Used: gypsum (group of sulfate minerals called plaster stone).

Flavor/Nature: acrid, sweet; very cold.

Meridian Affinity: Lung and Stomach Meridians.

Actions: clears Heat, purges Fire, and eliminates irritability and thirst.

Indications: (1) Heat evil in the Qi Level with high fever, irritability, thirst and a large surging pulse. (2) Heat in the lung causing cough, labored breathing, viscous sputum and fever. (3) Stomach-Fire blazing upward and causing headache and gingivitis. (4) Calcined gypsum powder is applied topically to treat skin ulcers, eczema, scalds and burns.

Dosage/Administration: 15–60 g. Use raw gypsum for ingestion. Use cooked powder for decoction. Use the calcined powder to external application.

Cautions/Contraindications: Contraindicated in deficiency-Cold of the spleen and the stomach and in endogenous Heat arising in Yin deficiency.

2 *Zhimu (Anemarrhena asphodeloides)*

Chinese name: 知母. Pharmaceutical name: *Rhizoma Anemarrhenae.*

Part Used: rhizome.

Flavor/Nature: bitter, sweet; cold.

Meridian Affinity: Lung, Stomach and Kidney Meridians.

Actions: clears Heat, purges Fire, nourishes Yin and moistens Dryness.

Indications: (1) Febrile illnesses due to strong Heat evil with high fever, irritability, thirst, and a large surging pulse. (2) Cough due to Heat in the lung or Yin deficiency, either without sputum or with thick viscous sputum. (3) Blazing Fire in Yin deficiency, so that both kidney and lung Yin become deficient resulting in low fever, night sweats and agitation. (4) Diabetes due to diabetes with thirst, polydipsia and polyuria.

Dosage/Administration: 6–12 g.

Cautions/Contraindications: Zhimu is of cold and moistening nature and can lubricate the intestines. It is inappropriate in diarrhea due to spleen insufficiency.

3 *Zhizi (Gardenia jasminoides) (Gardenia)*

Chinese name: 栀子. Pharmaceutical name: *Fructus Gardeniae.*

Part Used: fruit.

Flavor/Nature: bitter; cold.

Meridian Affinity: Heart, Lung, Stomach and Sanjiao Meridians.

Actions: purges Fire and relieves irritability, clears Heat and eliminates Dampness, cools blood and detoxifies.

Indications: (1) Agitation due to Heat illness, mental depression, and restlessness. (2) Gelled Dampness–Heat in the liver and gallbladder causing jaundice, fever and scanty dark urine. (3) Disturbed movement of blood leading to hematemesis, epistaxis and hematuria.

Dosage/Administration: 3–10 g.

Cautions/Contraindications: Contraindicated in diarrhea and anorexia due to spleen insufficiency.

4 Xiakucao (Prunella vulgaris) (Self-Heal)

Chinese name: 夏枯草. Pharmaceutical name: *Spica Prunellae*.

Part Used: fruit spike.

Flavor/Nature: bitter, acrid; cold.

Meridian Affinity: Liver and Gallbladder Meridians.

Actions: cools liver-Fire, dissipates accumulations and lowers blood pressure.

Indications: (1) Upward blazing of liver-Fire causing red and swollen eyes, eye pressure, photophobia, headache and dizziness. (2) Scrofula and goiter due to accumulation and gelling of Phlegm and Fire.

Dosage/Administration: 10–15 g.

II Herbs That Cool Heat and Dry Dampness

1 Huangqin (Scutellaria baicalensis) (Baical Skullcap)

Chinese name: 黄芩. Pharmaceutical name: *Radix Scutellariae*.

Part Used: root.

Flavor/Nature: bitter; cold.

Meridian Affinity: Lung, Gallbladder, Stomach and Large Intestine Meridians.

Actions: cools Heat and dries Dampness, purges Fire and detoxifies, stops bleeding and calms the fetus.

Indications: (1) A variety of illnesses caused by Dampness–Heat, such as jaundice, dysentery with diarrhea, abscesses and boils. (2) Febrile illnesses with high fever, irritability, thirst, a yellow tongue coating and a rapid pulse. (3) Cough and labored breathing due to Heat in the lung. (4) Strong Heat in the interior causing abnormal movement of blood and manifesting as hematemesis, hemoptysis, epistaxis, hematochezia or metrorrhagia. (5) Fetal disturbances by Heat.

Dosage/Administration: 3–10 g. In general, use fresh huangqin for cooling Heat, stirfried huangqin to calm the fetus, huangqin prepared in wine to clear Heat from the upper-jiao, and charred huangqin to stop bleeding.

Cautions/Contraindications: Huangqin is bitter and cold, and is harmful to vital Qi. It is contraindicated in deficiency-Cold of the spleen and the stomach with anorexia and loose feces.

2 *Huanglian (Coptis chinensis) (Golden Thread)*

Chinese name: 黄连. Pharmaceutical name: *Rhizoma Coptidis.*

Part Used: rhizome.

Flavor/Nature: bitter; cold.

Meridian Affinity: Heart, Liver, Stomach and Large Intestine Meridians.

Actions: cools Heat, dries Dampness, purges Fire and detoxifies.

Indications: (1) Diarrhea, dysentery and vomiting caused by Dampness–Heat in the stomach and the intestines. (2) Febrile illnesses with high fever, agitation, restlessness, even delirium or coma. (3) Abscesses, furuncles with internal extensions. (4) Swelling and pain of the eyes and ears.

Dosage/Administration: 2–10 g.

Cautions/Contraindications: Huanglian is very bitter and cold. If too much is used or used for too long a period it can easily injure the stomach. It is contraindicated in vomiting due to Cold in the stomach or diarrhea due to spleen insufficiency.

3 *Huangbai (Phellodendron chinense, amurense) (Amur Cork-Tree)*

Chinese name: 黄柏. Pharmaceutical name: *Cortex Phellodendri.*

Part Used: bark.

Flavor/Nature: bitter; cold.

Meridian Affinity: Kidney, Bladder and Large Intestine Meridians.

Actions: cools Heat, dries Dampness, purges Fire and detoxifies and eliminates endogenous Heat.

Indications: (1) Diarrhea, dysentery and vomiting caused by Dampness–Heat in the stomach and the intestines. (2) Abscesses, cellulitis, eczema and similar skin conditions. (3) Endogenous Heat in Yin deficiency with low fever, night sweats, or spermatorrhea.

Dosage/Administration: 3–10 g.

Cautions/Contraindications: Huangbai is very bitter and cold, and can easily injure stomach-Qi. It is contraindicated in deficiency-Cold in the spleen and the stomach.

4 Longdancao (Gentiana scabra, triflora) (Chinese Gentian)

Chinese name: 龙胆草. Pharmaceutical name: *Radix Gentianae.*

Part Used: root.

Flavor/Nature: bitter; cold.

Meridian Affinity: Liver, Gallbladder and Stomach Meridians.

Actions: cools Heat and dries Dampness, purges liver-Fire.

Indications: (1) Dampness–Heat induced jaundice, swelling and itch of the external genitals, vaginal discharge and eczema. (2) High fever, infantile convulsions and spasm of the hands and feet caused by strong Heat in the Liver Meridian, so that the extreme Heat induces endogenous Wind. (3) Flank pain, headache, a bitter taste, red eyes, deafness and swelling and itch of the external genitals due to strong exogenous Heat in the liver and the gallbladder.

Dosage/Administration: 3–6 g.

Cautions/Contraindications: Contraindicated in deficiency-Cold of the spleen and the stomach.

III Herbs That Cool Heat and Detoxify Poison

1 Jinyinhua (Lonicera japonica) (Honeysuckle)

Chinese name: 金银花. Pharmaceutical name: *Flos Lomicerae.*

Part Used: flower buds.

Flavor/Nature: sweet; cold.

Meridian Affinity: Lung, Stomach and Large Intestine Meridians.

Actions: cools Heat and detoxifies poison.

Indications: (1) Fever and mild wind or cold aversion due to exogenous Wind–Heat or early stages of febrile illnesses. (2) Sores, abscesses, furuncles. (3) Bloody or purulent dysentery due to Heat poisons.

Dosage/Administration: 10–15 g.

2 *Lianqiao (Forsythia suspensa) (Weeping Golden Bell)*

Chinese name: 连翘. Pharmaceutical name: *Fructus Forsythiae*.

Part Used: fruit.

Flavor/Nature: bitter; cool.

Meridian Affinity: Lung, Heart and Gallbladder Meridians.

Actions: cools Heat, detoxifies poison, clears abscesses and dissipates accumulations.

Indications: (1) Fever, headache and thirst caused by exogenous Wind–Heat or in the early stages of febrile illnesses. (2) A variety of abscesses, boils, scrofula and nodules induced by the accumulation of Heat poisons.

Dosage/Administration: 6–15 g.

3 *Pugongying (Taraxacum mongolicum) (Dandelion)*

Chinese name: 蒲公英. Pharmaceutical name: *Herba Taraxaci*.

Part Used: whole herb.

Flavor/Nature: bitter, sweet; cold.

Meridian Affinity: Liver and Stomach Meridians.

Actions: cools Heat, detoxifies poison and dissipates Dampness.

Indications: (1) Sores, boils, furuncles and surface and internal abscesses. (2) Jaundice and difficult and painful urination due to Dampness–Heat.

Dosage/Administration: 10–30 g.

Cautions/Contraindications: Excessive doses can cause persistent diarrhea.

4 *Banlangen (Isatis indigotica, tinctoria)*

Chinese name: 板蓝根. Pharmaceutical name: *Radix Isalidis*.

Part Used: root.

Flavor/Nature: bitter; cold.

Meridian Affinity: Heart and Stomach Meridians.

Actions: cools Heat, detoxifies poison, cools blood and soothes the throat.

Indications: (1) Febrile illnesses with fever, headache and sore throat. (2) Mumps, illnesses with macular rashes, abscesses, furuncles and many other conditions caused by Heat poisons.

Dosage/Administration: 10–15 g.

5 *Yuxingcao (Houttuynia cordata)*

Chinese name: 鱼腥草. Pharmaceutical name: *Herba Houttuyniae*.

Part Used: whole herb.

Flavor/Nature: acrid; slightly cold.

Meridian Affinity: Lung Meridian.

Actions: cools Heat, detoxifies poison, eliminates pus and promotes urination.

Indications: (1) Lung abscess with expectoration of bloody and purulent sputum. (2) Heat in the lung causing cough and viscous sputum. (3) Sores and furuncles due to Heat poison. (4) Heat-induced urethritis with dysuria.

Dosage/Administration: 15–30 g.

6 *Shegan (Belamcanda chinenesis) (Blackberry Lily)*

Chinese name: 射干. Pharmaceutical name: *Rhizoma Belamcandae*.

Part Used: rhizome.

Flavor/Nature: bitter; cold.

Meridian Affinity: Lung Meridian.

Actions: cools Heat, detoxifies poison, dissipates Phlegm and soothes the throat.

Indications: (1) Swollen and painful throat with accumulation of Heat and Phlegm. (2) Cough and labored breathing due to accumulation of Phlegm.

Dosage/Administration: 6–10 g.

Cautions/Contraindications: Contraindicated in pregnancy.

IV Heat-Clearing and Blood-Cooling Herbs

1 Baitouweng (Pulsatilla chinensis and Other Species) (Nodding Anemone)

Chinese name: 白头翁. Pharmaceutical name: *Radix Pulsatillae*.

Part Used: root.

Flavor/Nature: bitter; cold.

Meridian Affinity: Large Intestine Meridian.

Actions: cools Heat, detoxifies poison and cools blood.

Indications: (1) Dysentery due to Dampness–Heat. (2) Bloody and purulent dysentery due to Heat poison with fever, abdominal pain and tenesmus.

Dosage/Administration: 6–15 g.

2 Shengdihuang (Rehmannia glutinosa)

Chinese name: 生地黄. Pharmaceutical name: *Radix Rehmanniae*.

Part Used: (raw) root tuber.

Flavor/Nature: sweet, bitter; cold.

Meridian Affinity: Heart, Liver and Kidney Meridians.

Actions: cools Heat and blood, nourishes Yin and generates body fluids.

Indications: (1) Febrile illnesses in which Heat has entered the Nutritive and Blood Levels, causing fever, dry mouth and a red or crimson tongue. (2) Heat in the Blood Level forcing blood to move erratically, resulting in hematemesis, epistaxis, hematuria, metrorrhagia or other forms of bleeding. (3) Heat illnesses in which Yin has been injured, resulting in a red tongue and a dry mouth or thirst with polydipsia. (4) Diabetes.

Dosage/Administration: 10–30 g.

Cautions/Contraindications: Shengdihuang is of cold and impeding nature. It must not be used to treat patients in whom the spleen is insufficient, producing abdominal distention and loose feces, and Dampness has impeded Qi movement.

3 Chishaoyao (Paeonia lactiflora, veitchii, obovata) (Red Peony)

Chinese name: 赤芍药. Pharmaceutical name: *Radix Paeoniae Rubra.*

Part Used: root.

Flavor/Nature: bitter; slightly cold.

Meridian Affinity: Liver and Spleen Meridians.

Actions: cools Heat and blood, dissolves hematoma and stops pain.

Indications: (1) Febrile illnesses due to Heat in the Blood Level causing fever, macular rashes, erratic blood movement that results in hematemesis, epistaxis and other bleeding. (2) Amenorrhea or dysmenorrhea due to blood stasis. (3) Ecchymosis, swelling and pain caused by trauma. (4) Sores, furuncles and cellulitis; and swelling and pain of the eyes.

Dosage/Administration: 1–15 g.

Cautions/Contraindications: Contraindicated in amenorrhea due to deficiency-Cold. Incompatible with lilu (*Veratrum nigrum*).

4 Mudanpi (Paeonia suffruticosa) (Tree Peony)

Chinese name: 牡丹皮. Pharmaceutical name: *Cortex Moutan Radicis.*

Part Used: root-bark.

Flavor/Nature: bitter, acrid; slightly cold.

Meridian Affinity: Heart, Liver and Kidney Meridians.

Actions: cools Heat and blood, mobilizes blood and dissolves hematoma.

Indications: (1) Febrile illnesses due to Heat in the Blood Level causing fever, macular rashes, erratic blood movement that results in hematemesis, epistaxis and other bleeding. (2) Late stages of Heat illnesses when Heat resides in the Yin Level, or night fever with dawn cold, or endogenous Heat due to Yin deficiency. (3) Amenorrhea or dysmenorrhea, or masses in the abdomen stasis of blood. (4) Sores, furuncles and interior abscesses.

Dosage/Administration: 6–12 g.

Cautions/Contraindications: Contraindicated in pregnancy or excessive menstruation, as well as blood insufficiency inducing endogenous Cold.

V Endogenous Heat-Cooling Herbs

1 Qinghao (Artemisia annua, apiacea) (Wormwood)

Chinese name: 青蒿. Pharmaceutical name: *Herba Artemisiae Chinghao.*

Part Used: whole herb (above ground portion).

Flavor/Nature: bitter, acrid; cold.

Meridian Affinity: Liver, Gallbladder and Kidney Meridians.

Actions: eliminates deficiency-Heat, cools blood, relieves summer heat; anti-malaria.

Indications: (1) Alternating fever and cold in malaria. (2) Late stages of febrile illnesses when the Heat evil has entered the Yin Levels, with night fever and dawn cold, breaking of fever without sweating, or persistent low grade fever following a febrile illness. (3) Febrile illnesses due to Yin deficiency, causing chronic deficiency-fever syndrome with consumption, recurrent fever and a feverish sensation in the palms and soles. (4) Summer heat-stroke with headache, faintness, with or without sweating and a rapid and surging pulse.

Dosage/Administration: 3–10 g. Do not overcook.

2 Digupi (Lycium chinensis) (Wolfberry)

Chinese name: 地骨皮. Pharmaceutical name: *Cortex Lycii Radicis.*

Part Used: root-bark.

Flavor/Nature: sweet, bland; cold.

Meridian Affinity: Lung and Kidney Meridians.

Actions: cools blood and clears deficiency-Heat, and cools lung-Heat.

Indications: (1) Heat in the blood due to Yin deficiency; chronic infantile malnutrition with fever, and deficiency-fever syndrome with recurrent fever and night sweats. (2) Cough and labored breathing due to Heat in the lung. (3) Hematemesis or epistaxis due to Heat in the blood causing erratic blood movement and extravasation.

Dosage/Administration: 6–15 g.

Cautions/Contraindications: Contraindicated in febrile illnesses due to exogenous Wind–Cold, and in loose feces due to spleen insufficiency.

Section 3 Herbs That Induce Catharsis

Herbs that can cause diarrhea or can lubricate the large intestine and promote defecation are grouped as herbs that induce catharsis. Cathartic herbs, or cathartics, can relax the bowels, eliminate accumulations and mobilize excess fluid and other harmful materials for excretion. Some of them can also purge exogenous Heat. These actions make cathartics appropriate for treating such conditions as constipation, impedance of the intestines with accumulations or retained foods, gelling and accumulation of exogenous Heat in interior, retained water and edema.

When prescribing herbal cathartics, the physician should bear in mind certain precautions. If the interior condition targeted for treatment is accompanied by illness in the exterior, the physician should release the exterior prior to treating the interior condition or attack both simultaneously. Doing so will prevent pathogenic evil extending or spreading from the exterior into interior. If interior condition is accompanied by deficiency of genuine Qi, that is, weakened body resistance, include restorative herbs in the treatment, combining reinforcement and elimination, to prevent impairing vital Qi while purging. Always bear in mind that drastic purging readily injures vital Qi. It must be used with great care or not at all in debilitated patients or in women during pregnancy, following delivery or while menstruating.

Because they readily injure stomach-Qi, patients should stop taking herbalcathartics as soon as the desired therapeutic effect has been attained.

1 Dahuang (Rheum palmatum, officinale) (Rhubarb)

Chinese name: 大黃. Pharmaceutical name: *Radix Rehmanniae*.

Part Used: root tuber.

Flavor/Nature: bitter; cold.

Meridian Affinity: Stomach, Large Intestine and Liver Meridians.

Actions: promotes intestinal movement and eliminates retained matter, cools Heat and purges Fire, detoxifies poisons, promotes blood circulation and removes blood stasis.

Indications: (1) Impedance of the intestinal tract and constipation. (2) Heat in the blood causing erratic movement and bleeding, such as hematemesis and epistaxis.

(3) Eye, throat and gingival inflammation caused by upward blazing of Fire. (4) Boils and furuncles due to Heat poison or burn wounds. (5) Conditions of blood stasis.

Dosage/Administration: 3–12 g. Fresh dahuang is somewhat more potent in inducing catharsis than cooked dahuang. When decocted with other herbs it should be added last, since prolonged boiling reduces its cathartic activity. Preparing dahuang with wine further reduces its cathartic activity, but enhances its ability to mobilize blood; thus wine-prepared dahuang is suitable for removing blood stasis but less so for purgation. Charred dahuang is especially commonly used to stop bleeding.

Cautions/Contraindications: Contraindicated in pregnancy, while lactating and during menstruation.

2 Mangxiao (Mirabilite) (Sodium Sulfate)

Chinese name: 芒硝. Pharmaceutical name: *Natrii Sulfas.*

Part Used: crystals (group of sulfate minerals called Glauber's salts).

Flavor/Nature: salty, bitter; cold.

Meridian Affinity: Stomach and Large Intestine Meridians.

Actions: induces catharsis, softens the hard and cools Heat.

Indications: (1) Accumulation of Heat leading to dry constipation. (2) Sore throat, oral ulcers, red eyes, skin boils and furuncles.

Dosage/Administration: 10–15 g. Dissolve in the strained decoction or in boiled water.

Cautions/Contraindications: Contraindicated in pregnancy.

3 Fanxieye (Cassia angustifolia) (Senna)

Chinese name: 番泻叶. Pharmaceutical name: *Folium Sennae.*

Part Used: leaflets.

Flavor/Nature: sweet, bitter; cold.

Meridian Affinity: Large Intestine Meridian.

Actions: induces catharsis and eliminates.

Indications: constipation.

Dosage/Administration: (1) To facilitate defecation: 1.5–3 g. (2) To purge: 5–10 g.

Cautions/Contraindications: Contraindicated in pregnancy, during menstruation and while lactating.

Section 4 Herbs That Dispel Wind–Dampness

These herbs have as their principal action the dispelling of Wind–Dampness and the relieving of the pain of joints. They do so even when Wind and Dampness are lodged in the meridians and their branches in addition to the muscles and skin. Some can also relax the sinews, release obstruction in the meridians, stop pain generally or strengthen the sinews and bones. As a group they are suitable for treating arthritis and rheumatism due to Wind–Dampness, spasm of the sinews and vessels, numbness and weakness, hemiplegia, aching pain in the back and knees and paresis of the lower limbs.

In prescribing Wind–Dampness-dispelling herbs the physician must select them in accordance with the characteristics and location of the rheumatism, and supplement them with other herbs as required by associated symptoms. For example, if the pathogenic evils are in the exterior or the pain is confined to the upper body, add herbs that dispel Wind and release the exterior. If the pathogenic evils have entered the meridian branches and have impeded the movement of Qi and blood, add herbs that promote blood circulation and unblock meridians. If Cold and Dampness are strong, add herbs that warm the meridians. If Wind and Dampness have persisted for a long time and have transformed into Heat, add herbs that cool Heat. If the illness has lasted a long time and the patient's Qi and blood have become deficient, add herbs that augment Qi and nourish blood. If the liver and the kidney have become insufficient, leading to lumbar pain and lower limb weakness, add herbs that strengthen the liver and the kidney. Many other examples will be encountered elsewhere in the book.

Most cases of rheumatism are chronic. For convenience, Wind–Dampness-dispelling herbs can be prepared ahead of time and for long-term use. These are mainly in the forms of medicinal spirits, pills or powders. Preparing these herbs as medicinal spirits enhances their effectiveness in dispelling Wind and Dampness.

Herbs in this group are acrid, warm, sweet and drying. They tend to injure Yin and blood readily. Great care must be taken when using them in Yin and blood deficiency.

1 Duhuo (Angelica pubescens)

Chinese name: 独活. Pharmaceutical name: *Radix Angelicae Pubescentis*.

Part Used: root.

Flavor/Nature: acrid, bitter; warm.

Meridian Affinity: Liver, Kidney and Bladder Meridians.

Actions: dispels Wind–Dampness, stops pain and releases the exterior.

Indications: (1) Rheumatism with pain due to Wind–Dampness, particularly, in the low part of body. (2) Wind and Cold in the exterior, combined with Dampness.

Dosage/Administration: 3–10 g.

Cautions/Contraindications: Use with great care in Yin and blood deficiency.

2 *Mugua (Chaenomeles speciosa, lagenaria) (Chinese Quince)*

Chinese name: 木瓜. Pharmaceutical name: *Fructus Chaenomelis*.

Part Used: fruit.

Flavor/Nature: sour; warm.

Meridian Affinity: Liver and Spleen Meridians.

Actions: relaxes sinews, unblocks meridians, dissolves Dampness and soothes the stomach.

Indications: (1) Wind–Dampness-induced rheumatism with pain, spasm or tightness of the sinews and vessels, and swelling, pain and tinea of the feet. (2) Vomiting and diarrhea accompanied by spasm of the sinews.

Dosage/Administration: 6–12 g.

Cautions/Contraindications: Use with great care in Yin and blood deficiency.

3 *Fangji (Stephania Tetrandra)*

Chinese name: 防己. Pharmaceutical name: *Radix Stephaniae Tetrandrae*.

Part Used: root.

Note. There are two main types of fangji: hanfangji [汉防己] (*Stephania tetrandra*) and guangfangji [广防己] (*Aristolochia fangji*). The latter contains aristolochic acid, which is poisonous, and is not used in CM therapeutics.

Flavor/Nature: bitter, acrid; cold.

Meridian Affinity: Bladder, Kidney and Spleen Meridians.

Actions: dispels Wind–Dampness and stops pain, and promotes urination.

Indications: (1) Rheumatism due to Wind–Dampness. (2) Edema, ascites, and beri-beri.

Dosage/Administration: 5–10 g.

Cautions/Contraindications: Use with great care in Yin and blood deficiency. Because fangji is quite bitter and cold it must not be used in large doses to avoid injuring stomach-Qi. It is contraindicated in anorexia associated with Yin deficiency and without Dampness–Heat.

4 *Qinjiao (Gentiana macrophylla, crassicaulis) (Large-Leaf Gentian)*

Chinese name: 秦艽. Pharmaceutical name: *Radix Gentianae Macrophyllae*.

Part Used: root.

Flavor/Nature: bitter, acrid; slightly cold.

Meridian Affinity: Stomach, Liver and Gallbladder Meridians.

Actions: dispels Wind–Dampness, relaxes the sinews and clears deficiency-Heat.

Indications: (1) Wind–Dampness-induced rheumatism with body aches and spasm of all the joints and impairment of the hands and feet. (2) Deficiency-fever syndrome with recurrent fever.

Dosage/Administration: 5–10 g.

Cautions/Contraindications: Use with care in Yin and blood deficiency.

5 *Sangjisheng (Loranthus parasiticus) (Mulberry Mistletoe)*

Chinese name: 桑寄生. Pharmaceutical name: *Ramulus Loranthi*.

Part Used: leaf-bearing twigs.

Flavor/Nature: bitter; neutral.

Meridian Affinity: Liver and Kidney Meridians.

Actions: dispels Wind–Dampness, nourishes the liver and the kidney, strengthens the sinews and bones and calms the fetus.

Indications: (1) Wind–Dampness-induced rheumatism with pain, especially in the low back and knees. (2) Threatened abortion and fetal distress.

Dosage/Administration: 10–20 g.

6 *Weilingxian (Clematis chinensis)*

Chinese name: 威灵仙. Pharmaceutical name: *Radix Clematidix.*

Part Used: root.

Flavor/Nature: acrid, salty; warm.

Meridian Affinity: Bladder Meridian.

Actions: dispels Wind–Dampness, unblocks meridians and vessels, stops pain and dissolves bones stuck in the throat.

Indications: (1) Wind–Dampness-induced rheumatism with pain. (2) Any kind of bone stuck in the throat.

Dosage/Administration: 5–10 g. For bone stuck in the throat: 30 g.

Cautions/Contraindications: Use with great care in Yin and blood deficiency. In addition, weilingxian has high affinity for orifices and can injure genuine Qi if taken for a long time. Use with caution in a patient with a weak constitution.

Section 5 Aromatic Herbs That Dissipate Dampness

These herbs have as their principal action the dissipation of Dampness and the stimulation of the spleen. They are all fragrant.

The spleen does not function well with Dampness. If turgid Dampness blocks the middle-jiao internally the transformation and transportation functions of the spleen become impaired. Aromatic Dampness-dissipating herbs are warm and dry. They facilitate the movement and functional activities of Qi, dissipate turgid Dampness, strengthen the spleen and stimulate the stomach. They are especially useful when the spleen is blocked by Dampness and its functions impaired, leading to such symptoms as abdominal distention, vomiting, acid regurgitation, diarrhea, anorexia, weariness, a sweet taste in the mouth with much salivation and a white greasy tongue coating. They are also useful for treating illnesses due to Dampness–Heat and heatstroke.

Illnesses of Dampness may be of Cold–Dampness or Heat–Dampness. When treating an illness caused by Dampness it is important to select an appropriate combination of herbs. For Cold–Dampness supplement with herbs that warm the interior. For Heat–Dampness supplement with herbs that cool Heat and dry Dampness.

The nature of Dampness is viscous and impeding. When it invades the meridians, Qi movement becomes impeded. For this reason when treating with Dampness-dissipating herbs it is common to supplement them with herbs that promote Qi movement. Also, weakening of the spleen can generate Dampness. Treatment of Dampness generated when the spleen is weakened should include herbs that nourish the spleen.

Aromatic Dampness-dissipating herbs are fragrant and contain volatile oils, they must not be overcooked during decoction. Doing so will reduce their therapeutic effect.

The herbs in this group are warm and drying. They can readily injure Yin. They should be avoided or used with great care in Yin deficiency.

1 Cangzhu (Atractylodes lancea)

Chinese name: 苍术. Pharmaceutical name: *Rhizoma Atractylodis*.

Part Used: rhizome.

Flavor/Nature: acrid, bitter; warm.

Meridian Affinity: Spleen and Stomach Meridians.

Actions: dissipates Dampness, strengthens the spleen and dispels Wind–Dampness.

Indications: (1) Dampness blocking the middle-jiao. (2) Rheumatism due to Wind–Cold–Dampness, with painful swelling and weakness of the feet and knees.

Dosage/Administration: 5–10 g.

Cautions/Contraindications: Use with care or avoid in Yin deficiency.

2 Houpo (Magnolia officinalis) (Magnolia)

Chinese name: 厚朴. Pharmaceutical name: *Cortex Magnoliae Oiffcinalis*.

Part Used: bark.

Flavor/Nature: bitter, acrid; warm.

Meridian Affinity: Spleen, Stomach, Lung and Large Intestine Meridians.

Actions: facilitates Qi movement, dries Dampness, eliminates food retention and relieves wheezing.

Indications: (1) Disharmony between the spleen and the stomach, with abdominal distention and pain, due to blockage by Dampness, food retention or impedance of Qi movement. (2) Asthma and cough with much sputum.

Dosage/Administration: 3–10 g.

Cautions/Contraindications: Use with care or avoid in Yin deficiency.

3 Huoxiang (Agastache rugosa) (Giant Hyssop)

Chinese name: 藿香. Pharmaceutical name: *Herba Agastachis.*

Part Used: whole herb.

Flavor/Nature: acrid; slightly warm.

Meridian Affinity: Spleen, Stomach and Lung Meridians.

Actions: dissipates Dampness, relieves summer heat and stops vomiting.

Indications: (1) Dampness accumulating and blocking the middle-jiao. (2) Early stages of Heat–Dampness illnesses. (3) Vomiting.

Dosage/Administration: 5–10 g.

Cautions/Contraindications: Use with care in Yin deficiency.

4 Peilan (Eupatorium fortunei) (Mist Flower)

Chinese name: 佩兰. Pharmaceutical name: *Herba Eupatorii.*

Part Used: stalk and leaves.

Flavor/Nature: acrid; neutral.

Meridian Affinity: Spleen and Stomach Meridians.

Actions: dissipates Dampness and relieves summer heat.

Indications: (1) Dampness accumulating and blocking the middle-jiao. (2) Early stages of Heat–Dampness illnesses.

Dosage/Administration: 5–10 g.

Cautions/Contraindications: Use with care in Yin deficiency.

5 Sharen (Amomum villosum, xanthioides)

Chinese name: 砂仁. Pharmaceutical name: *Fructus Amomi.*

Part Used: ripe fruit.

Flavor/Nature: acrid; warm.

Meridian Affinity: Spleen and Stomach Meridians.

Actions: dissipates Dampness, facilitates Qi movement, warms the middle-jiao and calms the fetus.

Indications: (1) Dampness accumulating and blocking the middle-jiao. (2) Dampness impeding spleen and stomach Qi. (3) Fetal distress.

Dosage/Administration: 3–6 g. In decoction put in last cook for 5 min and so not overcook.

Cautions/Contraindications: Use with care or avoid in Yin deficiency.

Section 6 Herbs That Drain Water and Dampness

These are herbs that have their principal actions of unblocking the water pathways and the dissipation of Dampness (diuresis). They can increase the amount of urine, so that retained water and accumulated Dampness can be excreted as urine.

Some of these herbs also act to clear Dampness–Heat, and are especially suitable for such conditions as difficult and painful urination, edema, accumulated Rheum and Phlegm, jaundice and exudative dermatitis.

Water-draining herbs are sweet or bland in flavor and neutral, slightly cold or cold in nature. Bland flavor is associated with ability to drain water and dissipate Dampness. Cold nature is associated with the ability to cool Heat. In addition to increasing the amount of urine water-draining herbs of cold nature are especially effective in cooling Heat and eliminating Dampness from the lower-jiao. They are often prescribed for dysuria.

When prescribing these herbs pay attention to the character of the illness and add herbs as appropriate. For example, for acute edema associated with symptoms of the Exterior add herbs that soothe the lung and induce sweating. For chronic edema due to deficiency of spleen and kidney Yang add herbs that warm and nourish the spleen and the kidney. For illnesses of simultaneous Dampness and Heat add herbs that cool Heat and purge Fire. For Heat injury to blood vessels and hematuria add herbs that cool blood and stop bleeding.

When water-draining herbs are used inappropriately they can easily damage Yin fluids; hence great care must be exercised when treating patients with Yin deficiency or fluid insufficiency.

1 Fuling (Poria cocos) (Tuckahoe)

Chinese name: 茯苓. Pharmaceutical name: *Poria*.

Part Used: sclerotium.

Flavor/Nature: sweet, bland; neutral.

Meridian Affinity: Heart, Spleen and Kidney Meridians.

Actions: drains water, dissipates Dampness, strengthens the spleen and calms the mind.

Indications: (1) Difficulty with urination and edema due to water retention and Dampness accumulation. (2) Spleen insufficiency. (3) Palpitations of the heart and insomnia.

Dosage/Administration: 10–15 g.

Cautions/Contraindications: Caution in Yin deficiency and fluid insufficiency.

2 Yiyiren (Coix lachryma-jobi) (Job's-Tears)

Chinese name: 薏苡仁. Pharmaceutical name: *Semen Coicis.*

Part Used: seed kernel.

Flavor/Nature: sweet, bland; slightly cold.

Meridian Affinity: Spleen, Stomach and Lung Meridians.

Actions: drains water, dissipates Dampness, strengthens the spleen, reduces rheumatic pain, cools Heat and dissolves pus.

Indications: (1) Difficulty with urination, edema and beri-beri. (2) Diarrhea due to spleen insufficiency. (3) Rheumatism, spasticity of sinews. (4) Lung abscess and intestinal ulcers.

Dosage/Administration: 10–30 g.

3 Zexie (Alisma plantago-aquatica, orientale) (Water Plantain)

Chinese name: 泽泻. Pharmaceutical name: *Rhizoma Alismatis.*

Part Used: stalk tuber.

Flavor/Nature: sweet, bland; cold.

Meridian Affinity: Kidney and Bladder Meridians.

Actions: drains water, dissipates Dampness and purges Fire.

Indications: (1) Difficulty with urination and edema. (2) Diarrhea. (3) Urethritis. (4) Vaginal discharge. (5) Accumulation of Rheum and Dampness.

Dosage/Administration: 5–10 g.

Cautions/Contraindications: Caution in Yin deficiency and fluid insufficiency.

4 *Cheqianzi (Plantago asiatica) (Plantain)*

Chinese name: 车前子. Pharmaceutical name: *Semen Plantaginis*.

Part Used: ripe seed.

Flavor/Nature: sweet; cold.

Meridian Affinity: Kidney, Liver and Lung Meridians.

Actions: drains water, alleviates urethritis, stops diarrhea, clears the liver, brightens the eyes, clears the lung and dissolves Phlegm.

Indications: (1) Difficulty with urination and edema. (2) Urethritis. (3) Diarrhea due to summer heat and Dampness. (4) Inflammation of the eyes and cataract with dimming and blurring of vision. (5) Heat in the lung with cough and much sputum.

Dosage/Administration: 5–10 g. Wrap in cloth to decoct.

Cautions/Contraindications: Caution in Yin deficiency and fluid insufficiency.

5 *Yinchenhao (Artemisia capillaris) (Oriental Wormwood)*

Chinese name: 茵陈蒿. Pharmaceutical name: *Herba Artemisiae capillaris*.

Part Used: tender stalk with leaves.

Flavor/Nature: bitter; slightly cold.

Meridian Affinity: Spleen, Stomach, Liver and Gallbladder Meridians.

Actions: cools Heat and dissipates Dampness, and reduces jaundice.

Indications: Jaundice and accumulation of the Heat–Dampness in the Interior.

Dosage/Administration: 10–30 g.

6 *Jinqiancao (Lysimachia christinae, Glochoma longituba) (Christina Loosestrife)*

Chinese name: 金钱草. Pharmaceutical name: *Herba Lysimachiae*.

Part Used: whole herb.

Flavor/Nature: sweet, bland; neutral.

Meridian Affinity: Liver, Gallbladder, Kidney and Bladder Meridians.

Actions: drains water, relieves urethritis, dissipates Dampness, reduces jaundice, removes poison and reduces swelling.

Indications: (1) Urethritis due to Heat, sand or stones. (2) Jaundice due to Dampness–Heat.

Dosage/Administration: 30–60 g.

7 *Zhuling (Polyporus umbellatus)*

Chinese name: 猪苓. Pharmaceutical name: *Polyporus umbellatus.*

Part Used: dried fungal body.

Flavor/Nature: sweet, bland; neutral.

Meridian Affinity: Liver and Gallbladder Meridians.

Actions: drains water and dissipates Dampness.

Indications: (1) Difficulty with urination. (2) Edema. (3) Diarrhea. (4) Urethritis. (5) Vaginal discharge.

Dosage/Administration: 5–10 g.

8 *Huzhang (Polygonum cuspidatum) (Giant Knotgrass)*

Chinese name: 虎杖. Pharmaceutical name: *Rhizoma Polygoni Cuspidati.*

Part Used: root and rhizome.

Flavor/Nature: bitter; cold.

Meridian Affinity: Liver, Gallbladder and Lung Meridians.

Actions: normalizes the gallbladder and reduces jaundice, cools Heat and removes its poisons, mobilizes blood and removes stasis, stops cough and removes sputum.

Indications: (1) Jaundice due to Dampness–Heat. (2) Urethritis and vaginal discharge. (3) Burns and scalds. (4) Abscesses and furuncles. (5) Bites by venomous snakes or other animals. (6) Blood stasis and ecchymosis. (7) Amenorrhea. (8) Traumatic injuries. (9) Cough due to Heat in the lung.

Dosage/Administration: 10–30 g.

Cautions/Contraindications: Contraindicated in pregnancy. Caution in Yin deficiency and fluid insufficiency.

Section 7 Herbs That Warm Interior

These are herbs that have as their principal action the warming of and dispelling Cold from interior. They are of acrid flavor and hot nature; these are the properties that make them so suitable for treating illnesses of interior Cold.

There are two types of interior Cold illnesses: those of exogenous Cold invading the interior and suppressing Yang-Qi of the spleen and the stomach, and those of endogenous Cold arising out of deficiency of Yang-Qi or injury of Yang-Qi by excessive sweating. In either case, interior-warming herbs are appropriate treatment.

When prescribing interior-warming herbs it is appropriate to modify the combination of herbs depending on the clinical condition. For exogenous Cold invading interior but associated with symptoms of exterior, add herbs that release the exterior. For Qi stagnation due to congealing by Cold, add herbs that mobilize Qi. For accumulation of Cold and Dampness in interior, add herbs that strengthen the spleen and dissolve Dampness. For Yang deficiency in the spleen and the kidney, add warming herbs that strengthen the spleen and the kidney. For Yang collapse and Qi depletion, add herbs that can vigorously augment and support genuine Qi.

The herbs in this group are acrid and hot, and they are drying. If applied improperly they can easily injure body fluids. In illnesses of Heat or Yin deficiency and in pregnancy they must be used with great care or are contraindicated.

1 Fuzi (Aconitum carmichaeli) (Monkshood)

Chinese name: 附子. Pharmaceutical name: *Radix Aconiti Lateralis Praeparata.*

Part Used: lateral (secondary) root.

Flavor/Nature: acrid; hot. This herb is toxic.

Meridian Affinity: Heart, Kidney and Spleen Meridians.

Actions: rescues Yang and reverses collapse, augments Fire and Yang, and dispels Cold and stops pain.

Indications: (1) Yang exhaustion. (2) Deficiency of Yang-Qi. (3) Rheumatism with pain caused by Wind–Cold–Dampness.

Dosage/Administration: 3–15 g. Only the processed roots can be used. To reduce toxic properties, cook for 30–60 min before adding the other herbs to decoct.

Cautions/Contraindications: Contraindicated in pregnancy. Caution in illnesses of Heat or Yin deficiency.

1a Chuanwu (Aconitum carmichaeli) (Monkshood)

Chinese name: 川烏. Pharmaceutical name: *Radix Aconiti.*

Part Used: axial or main root.

Flavor/Nature: acrid; bitter, hot. This herb is extremely toxic.

Meridian Affinity: Heart, Kidney, Liver and Spleen Meridians.

Actions: dispels Wind and Dampness, disperses Cold and stops pain.

Indications: (1) Rheumatism due to Wind–Cold–Dampness. (2) Pain due to Cold or trauma.

Dosage/Administration: 3–9 g. Pre-boil for 30–60 min before adding the other herbs to decoct. Can be used externally. Only can the processed herb be used for oral taking.

Cautions/Contraindications: Contraindicated in pregnancy. Unprepared Chuanwu is for external used only.

2 Rougui (Cinnamomum cassia) (Cinnamon)

Chinese name: 肉桂. Pharmaceutical name: *Cortex Cinnamomi.*

Part Used: bark.

Flavor/Nature: acrid, sweet; hot.

Meridian Affinity: Kidney, Spleen, Heart and Liver Meridians.

Actions: augments Fire and Yang, dispels Cold and stops pain, and warms and unblocks meridians and vessels.

Indications: (1) Kidney-Yang deficiency, fading of Gate-of-Life Fire. (2) Pain associated with Cold in the abdomen, Cold–Dampness induced rheumatism or blood stasis due to Cold causing amenorrhea or dysmenorrhea. (3) Lumbar pain. (4) Deficiency of Qi and blood with endogenous Cold leading to deep purulent boils or abscesses that fail to drain or having drained fail to heal.

Dosage/Administration: 2–5 g as decoction, pill or powder. Mix with freshly prepared decoction.

Cautions/Contraindications: Contraindicated in blazing Fire in Yin deficiency, exogenous Heat in the interior, erratic blood flow due to Heat in the blood and in pregnancy.

3 *Ganjiang (Zingiber officinale) (Ginger)*

Chinese name: 干姜. Pharmaceutical name: *Rhizoma Zingiberis*.

Part Used: dried rhizome.

Flavor/Nature: acrid; hot.

Meridian Affinity: Spleen, Stomach, Heart and Lung Meridians.

Actions: warms the middle-jiao, rescues Yang, warms the lung and dissipates Rheum.

Indications: (1) Illnesses of Cold in the spleen and the stomach. (2) Yang exhaustion. (3) Cold and Rheum residing in the lung.

Dosage/Administration: 3–10 g.

Cautions/Contraindications: Use with great caution in pregnancy.

4 *Wuzhuyu (Evodia rutaecarpa)*

Chinese name: 吴茱萸. Pharmaceutical name: *Fructus Evodiae*.

Part Used: unripe fruit.

Flavor/Nature: acrid, bitter; hot. This herb is somewhat toxic.

Meridian Affinity: Liver, Spleen and Stomach Meridians.

Actions: dispels Cold and stops pain, regulates the liver and suppresses Qi, dries Dampness.

Indications: (1) Epigastric and abdominal pain due to Cold or hernia. (2) Headache. (3) Diarrhea due to deficiency Cold. (4) Beri-beri due to Cold–Dampness causing pain, or the abnormal Qi of beri-beri rising into the abdomen. (5) Vomiting with acid regurgitation. (6) Aphthous sores on the tongue and in the mouth. In this case, wuzhuyu is ground into a powder and applied in vinegar to the sole, drawing Fire downward.

Dosage/Administration: 1.5–5 g.

Cautions/Contraindications: Wuzhuyu is acrid and hot. It is highly potent in its drying effect and can easily damage Qi and stir up Fire. It must not be used in excess or for too long. It is contraindicated in any patient with endogenous Heat in Yin deficiency.

5 Dingxiang (Syzygium caryophyllata, aromaticum) (Clove)

Chinese name: 丁香. Pharmaceutical name: *Flos Caryophylli.*

Part Used: flower bud.

Flavor/Nature: acrid; warm.

Meridian Affinity: Spleen, Stomach and Kidney Meridians.

Actions: warms the middle-jiao and suppresses abnormal Qi ascent; and warms the kidney and assists Yang.

Indications: (1) Vomiting, hiccup, anorexia and diarrhea due to Cold in the stomach. (2) Impotence due to deficiency of kidney-Yang.

Dosage/Administration: 2–5 g.

Cautions/Contraindications: Incompatible with Yujin (Curcuma wenjujin).

Section 8 Herbs That Regulate Qi

These are herbs that have their principal actions of promoting the functional activities of Qi and of facilitating Qi movement. Qi-regulating herbs are generally aromatic, and have acrid and bitter flavor and warm nature. They are efficacious in normalizing Qi activities and movement, strengthening the spleen, unblocking the liver and releasing stagnation, and are particularly suitable for treating Qi stagnation or suppressing abnormally ascending Qi caused by impedance of Qi movement.

Impedance of Qi movement is manifested mainly through effects on the functions of the lung, the liver, the spleen and the stomach. Qi stagnation generally shows tightness or an oppressed sensation, distention and pain. Abnormal Qi ascent generally shows hiccups, vomiting or labored breathing.

Because of differences in location, progression and severity, the actual symptoms may also differ. Hence, when prescribing Qi-regulating herbs the physician must choose them to suit the actual illness and supplement them appropriately. For example, for obstruction of Qi caused by exogenous pathogenic evils, add herbs that ventilate the lung, dissolve sputum and stop cough. For cough and dyspnea due to Phlegm and Heat in the lung, add herbs that cool Heat and dissolve Phlegm. For stagnation of spleen and stomach Qi with associated Dampness and Heat, add herbs that cool Heat and dissipate Dampness. For Cold and Dampness blocking the spleen, add herbs that warm the middle-jiao and dry Dampness. For food retention and indigestion, add herbs that promote digestion and relieve retention. For insufficiency of the spleen and the stomach, add herbs that augment Qi and strengthen the spleen.

Many symptoms can accompany the stagnation of liver-Qi. Depending on the specific associated symptoms, it may be necessary to add herbs that nourish the liver, soften the liver, promote blood circulation, regulate the Nutritive Level, stop pain or strengthen the spleen.

Most Qi-regulating herbs are acrid and drying, and can easily consume Qi and injure Yin. They must be used with great care in deficiency of both Qi and Yin.

1 *Chenpi (Citrus tangerina, reticulata) (Tangerine)*

Chinese name: 陈皮. Pharmaceutical name: *Exocarpium Citri Crandis*.

Part Used: mature pericarp (mature fruit peel).

Flavor/Nature: acrid, bitter; warm.

Meridian Affinity: Spleen and Lung Meridians.

Actions: regulates Qi, harmonizes the middle-jiao, dries Dampness and dissolves Phlegm.

Indications: (1) Epigastric or abdominal distention, eructation, hiccup and vomiting due to stagnation of spleen and stomach Qi. (2) Chest tightness, abdominal distention, anorexia, lassitude, loose feces and a thick greasy tongue coating caused by accumulated Dampness blocking the middle-jiao. (3) Blockage of the lung and loss of its normal descent due to Phlegm and Dampness blocking the lung, leading to much coughing with copious sputum.

Dosage/Administration: 3–10 g.

Cautions/Contraindications: Use with great caution in conditions of strong exogenous Heat with a red tongue and decreased body fluids.

2 *Zhishi (Citrus aurantium) (Immature Orange)*

Chinese name: 枳实. Pharmaceutical name: *Fructus Aurantii Immaturus*. (Some authorities identify zhishi as the tiny fruit of *Poncirus trifoliata*, the trifoliate orange.)

Part Used: immature fruit.

Flavor/Nature: bitter, acrid; slightly cold.

Meridian Affinity: Spleen, Stomach and Large Intestine Meridians.

Actions: breaks Qi blockage, moves retained food, dissolves Phlegm and eliminates accumulations.

Indications: (1) Food retention with abdominal pain and constipation. (2) Dysentery with diarrhea and tenesmus. (3) Turbid Phlegm impeding Qi movement.

Dosage/Administration: 3–10 g.

Cautions/Contraindications: Use with great caution in insufficiency of the spleen and the stomach and in pregnancy.

3 Muxiang (Aucklandia lappa)

Chinese name: 木香. Pharmaceutical name: *Radix Aucklandiae*. (Some authorities identify muxiang as the root of *Saussurea lappa*, costus.)

Part Used: root.

Flavor/Nature: acrid, bitter; warm.

Meridian Affinity: Spleen, Stomach, Large Intestine and Gallbladder Meridians.

Actions: mobilizes Qi, harmonizes the middle-jiao and stops pain.

Indications: (1) Impedance of spleen and stomach Qi causing anorexia, indigestion with food retention, epigastric and abdominal distention and pain, borborygmus, diarrhea, dysentery and tenesmus. (2) Impairment of spleen functions leading to liver dysfunction. (3) Deficiency of spleen and stomach Qi causing loss of transportation, epigastric and abdominal distention and anorexia or vomiting, diarrhea, preference for pressure and warmth and a white greasy tongue coating.

Dosage/Administration: 3–10 g. Use fresh muxiang to mobilize Qi and baked muxiang to stop diarrhea.

Cautions/Contraindications: Use with caution in Yin deficiency with blazing Fire.

4 Xiangfu (Cyperus rotundus) (Nutgrass)

Chinese name: 香附. Pharmaceutical name: *Rhizoma Cyperi*.

Part Used: rhizome.

Flavor/Nature: acrid, slightly bitter and sweet; neutral.

Meridian Affinity: Liver and Sanjiao Meridians.

Actions: unblocks the liver and regulates Qi, regulates menstruation and stops pain.

Indications: (1) Distending flank, abdominal and epigastric pain due to stagnation of liver-Qi. (2) Irregular menstruation, dysmenorrhea and mastitis.

Dosage/Administration: 6–12 g.

5 Chuanlianzi (Melia toosendan) (Chinaberry)

Chinese name: 川楝子. Pharmaceutical name: *Fructus Toosendan.*

Part Used: mature fruit.

Flavor/Nature: bitter; cold. Chuanlianzi is mildly poisonous.

Meridian Affinity: Liver, Stomach, Small Intestine and Bladder Meridians.

Actions: mobilizes Qi, stops pain, kills parasites and cures tinea.

Indications: (1) Flank, epigastric, abdominal and hernia pain caused by stagnation of liver-Qi or disharmony between the liver and the stomach. (2) Abdominal pain due to parasite infestation.

Dosage/Administration: 3–10 g.

Cautions/Contraindications: Chuanlianzi is bitter and cold. It is not used in endogenous Cold in the spleen and the stomach. In some cases, it happened in vomiting after taking decoction of the herb.

6 Xiebai (Allium macrostemon) (Long Stem Onion)

Chinese name: 薤白. Pharmaceutical name: *Bulbus Allii Macrostemi.*

Part Used: bulb.

Flavor/Nature: acrid, bitter; warm.

Meridian Affinity: Lung, Stomach and Large Intestine Meridians.

Actions: unblocks Yang-Qi, dissipates masses, mobilizes Qi and disperses accumulation.

Indications: (1) Cold–Phlegm–Dampness accumulation in the chest causing stagnation of Yang-Qi in the chest, which in turn causes chest tightness and pain or thoracic rheumatism with dyspnea and productive cough. (2) Stagnation of stomach-Qi causing dysentery with diarrhea and tenesmus.

Dosage/Administration: 5–10 g.

Cautions/Contraindications: Contraindicated in Qi deficiency without stagnation, poor appetite due to weak stomach and onion-intolerance.

Section 9 Herbs That Relieve Food Retention

These are herbs that have their principal action of promoting of digestion and relief of food retention. In addition, most of these herbs also induce appetite and settle the stomach. Several individual herbs also strengthen spleen function.

Food-retention-relieving herbs are appropriate for treating insufficiency of the spleen and the stomach with resultant indigestion, as well as epigastric and abdominal distention, eructation, vomiting and irregular defecation due to food retention.

When prescribing these herbs add appropriate supplemental herbs in accordance with the varying symptoms manifested by the patients. Under ordinary circumstances, retained food in the middle-jiao often blocks Qi movement so that the spleen and the stomach show symptoms of blockage. In such situations it is appropriate to add Qi-regulating herbs to unblock Qi movement. Doing so in turn facilitates digestion and food movement. If there are symptoms of Cold, add interior-warming herbs to dispel Cold and eliminate sluggishness. Chronic food retention can sometimes transform into endogenous Heat. In this situation add bitter-cold cathartics to purge Heat and stimulate bowel movement. If turgid Dampness blocks the middle-jiao then it is important to use as the main treatment method spleen-strengthening and stomach-harmonizing rather than rely only on herbs that relieve food retention.

1 Maiya (Hordeum vulgare) (Barley)

Chinese name: 麦芽. Pharmaceutical name: *Fructus Hordei Germinatus*.

Part Used: sprout.

Flavor/Nature: sweet; neutral.

Meridian Affinity: Spleen, Stomach and Liver Meridians.

Actions: enhances digestion, harmonizes the middle-jiao and stops lactation.

Indications: (1) Food retention, indigestion, anorexia, epigastric and abdominal distention. (2) Persistent lactation or retained milk. (3) Liver-Qi stagnation.

Dosage/Administration: 10–15 g. For stopping persistent lactation: 30–60 g.

Cautions/Contraindications: Contraindicated for women in lactation.

2 Shenqu (Massa medicata fermentata) (Medicated Leaven)

Chinese name: 神曲. Pharmaceutical name: Leaven.

Flavor/Nature: sweet, acrid; warm.

Meridian Affinity: Spleen and Stomach Meridians.

Actions: promotes digestion and harmonizes the stomach.

Indications: Food retention with epigastric and abdominal distention, anorexia, borborygmus and diarrhea.

Dosage/Administration: 6–15 g.

Cautions/Contraindications: Use with caution in Yin deficiency or stomach Fire. Shenqu may induce abortion.

3 Shanzha (Crataegus pinnatifida) (Chinese Hill Haw)

Chinese name: 山楂. Pharmaceutical name: *Fructus Crataegi*.

Part Used: mature fruit.

Flavor/Nature: sour, sweet; slightly warm.

Meridian Affinity: Spleen, Stomach and Liver Meridians.

Actions: enhances digestion, relieves food retention, mobilizes blood and dissolves hematoma.

Indications: (1) Indigestion with food (especially meat) retention, epigastric and abdominal distention and pain, and diarrhea. (2) Post-partum blood stasis and abdominal pain, and persistent lochia.

Dosage/Administration: 10–15 g. May increase to 30 g.

4 Laifuzi (Raphanus sativus) (Radish)

Chinese name: 莱菔子. Pharmaceutical name: *Semen Raphani*.

Part Used: ripe seed.

Flavor/Nature: acrid, sweet; neutral.

Meridian Affinity: Spleen, Stomach and Lung Meridians.

Actions: enhances digestion, relieves food retention, lowers Qi and dissolves sputum.

Indications: (1) Indigestion, food retention and impeded movement of spleen and stomach Qi causing epigastric and abdominal distention, eructation and acid regurgitation or abdominal pain, diarrhea yet incomplete evacuation. (2) Cough and asthma due to exogenous pathogenic evil, with much viscous sputum.

Dosage/Administration: 6–10 g.

Cautions/Contraindications: Laifuzi is very wearing on Qi. Contraindicated in Qi deficiency without food retention or viscous sputum.

Section 10 Herbs That Stimulate Blood Circulation and Remove Blood Stasis

These are herbs that have their principal action of stimulating blood circulation and of removing blood stasis. They are especially efficacious at dispersion, including reversing stasis, dissolving hematomas, stimulating blood circulation, restoring menstrual flow, ameliorating rheumatism, reducing swelling and stopping pain.

The main application of these herbs is the condition of blood stasis. This is a commonly seen condition with four major presentations: (1) aches, pain or numbness, (2) masses in the interior or the exterior, or traumatic hematomas, (3) internal hemorrhage with dark purple blood clots, and (4) ecchymosis on the skin, mucous membranes or the tongue. Blood stasis develops in the course of many illnesses, and it is itself also the cause of further disease.

Since there are many causes of blood stasis, when prescribing herbs that stimulate blood circulation and remove blood stasis the physician must form a firm diagnosis and select and add herbs appropriate to the clinical requirements. For example, if the blood stasis is due to Cold gelling Qi and impeding blood flow, add herbs that warm the interior and dispel Cold. If it is due to Heat consuming Yin and blood, add herbs that cool Heat and blood. For rheumatism with pain due to Wind–Dampness, add herbs that dispel Wind and dissipate Dampness. For blood stasis associated with deficiency of genuine Qi, add herbs that restore the deficient.

In the human body Qi and blood are intimately interrelated. When Qi moves so does blood, and when Qi becomes impeded then blood becomes static. Hence, when prescribing herbs that stimulate blood circulation and relieve stasis it is appropriate to include herbs that stimulate Qi movement. Doing so enhances the ability of the herbs to stimulate blood circulation and relieve stasis.

1 Chuanxiong (Ligusticum chuanxiong, wallichii) (Sichuan Lovage)

Chinese name: 川芎. Pharmaceutical name: *Rhizoma Chuanxiong*.

Part Used: rhizome.

Flavor/Nature: acrid; warm.

Meridian Affinity: Liver, Gallbladder and Pericardium Meridians.

Actions: mobilizes blood and Qi, dispels Wind and stops pain.

Indications: (1) Irregular menstruation, dysmenorrhea, amenorrhea, difficult labor and post-partum abdominal, subcostal pain and limb numbness. (2) Traumatic injuries, boils and abscesses. (3) Headache and rheumatism due to Wind–Dampness.

Dosage/Administration: 3–10 g.

Cautions/Contraindications: Chuanxiong is acrid and warm, and it raises and disperses. It is contraindicated whenever there is Yin deficiency with blazing of Fire, with a red and dry tongue. In women it is also contraindicated when there is excessive menstruation or a bleeding condition.

2 Yujin (Curcuma wenyujin, aromatica) (Tumeric)

Chinese name: 郁金. Pharmaceutical name: *Radix Curcumae*.

Part Used: root tuber.

Flavor/Nature: acrid, bitter; cold.

Meridian Affinity: Heart, Liver and Gallbladder Meridians.

Actions: mobilizes blood, stops pain, mobilizes Qi and relieves Qi stagnation, cools blood and clear the heart, stimulates gallbladder function and reduces jaundice.

Indications: (1) Stagnation of liver-Qi and stasis of blood in the interior resulting in pain and distention in the chest, the subcostal region and the abdomen, in irregular or painful menstruation, and in abdominal masses. (2) Blockage of the orifices by Dampness–Heat causing chest and epigastric tightness and mental confusion. (3) Phlegm accumulation causing blockage of heart-Qi causing convulsions or dementia.

Dosage/Administration: 6–12 g.

Cautions/Contraindications: Incompatible with dingxiang (*Syzygium*).

3 Yanhusuo (Corydalis yanhusuo)

Chinese name: 延胡索. Pharmaceutical name: *Rhizoma corydalis*.

Part Used: tuber.

Flavor/Nature: acrid, bitter; warm.

Meridian Affinity: Heart, Liver and Spleen Meridians.

Actions: mobilizes blood and Qi and stops pain.

Indications: pain in the chest, epigastrium, abdomen and limbs due to Qi stagnation and blood stasis.

Dosage/Administration: 5–10 g. Powder: 1.5–3 g.

4 *Danshen (Salvia miltiorrhiza) (Red Sage)*

Chinese name: 丹参. Pharmaceutical name: *Radix Salveae Miltiorrhizae*.

Part Used: root, rhizome.

Flavor/Nature: acrid; slightly cold.

Meridian Affinity: Heart, Pericardium and Liver Meridians.

Actions: mobilizes blood circulation and remove blood stasis, cools blood, shrinks abscesses, nourishes blood and calms the mind.

Indications: (1) Irregular menstruation, amenorrhea, and post-partum abdominal pain. (2) Heart and abdominal pain, abdominal masses and limb pains. (3) Swelling and pain of boils and abscesses. (4) Exogenous Heat evil in the Nutritive and Blood Levels, with high fever, agitation, delirium or faint rashes, a red or crimson tongue, palpitations of the heart and insomnia.

Dosage/Administration: 5–15 g.

Cautions/Contraindications: Incompatible with lilu (*Veratrum*).

5 *Yimucao (Leonurus heterophyllus, japonicus) (Mother-Wort)*

Chinese name: 益母草. Pharmaceutical name: *Herba Leonuri*.

Part Used: whole herb (above ground portion).

Flavor/Nature: acrid, bitter; slightly cold.

Meridian Affinity: Heart, Liver and Bladder Meridians.

Actions: mobilizes blood circulation, removes blood stasis, promotes diuresis and reduces swelling.

Indications: (1) Blood-stasis-induced irregular menstruation, amenorrhea, low abdominal pain and distention, post-partum abdominal pain and persistent lochia. (2) Traumatic hematoma and ecchymosis. (3) Oliguria and edema.

Dosage/Administration: 10–15 g.

6 Taoren (Prunus persica) (Peach)

Chinese name: 桃仁. Pharmaceutical name: *Semen Persicae.*

Part Used: nut kernel.

Flavor/Nature: bitter; neutral.

Meridian Affinity: Heart, Liver, Lung and Large Intestine Meridians.

Actions: mobilizes blood circulation, removes blood stasis, moistens the intestines and facilitates defecation.

Indications: (1) Dysmenorrhea, amenorrhea and post-partum abdominal pain. (2) Traumatic injuries and pain from stasis. (3) Lung or intestinal abscesses. (4) Intestinal dehydration with constipation.

Dosage/Administration: 6–10 g.

Cautions/Contraindications: Contraindicated in pregnancy and diarrhea.

7 Honghua (Carthamus tinctorius) (Safflower)

Chinese name: 红花. Pharmaceutical name: *Flos carthami.*

Part Used: flower.

Flavor/Nature: acrid; warm.

Meridian Affinity: Heart and Liver Meridians.

Actions: mobilizes blood circulation, removes blood stasis and unblocks channels.

Indications: (1) Dysmenorrhea, amenorrhea, abdominal masses and post-partum abdominal pain. (2) Traumatic injuries. (3) Ecchymosis due to impedance of blood flow by Heat.

Dosage/Administration: 3–10 g.

Cautions/Contraindications: Contraindicated in pregnancy.

8 Niuxi (Achyranthes bidentata)

Chinese name: 牛膝. Pharmaceutical name: *Radix Achyranthis Bidentatae.*

Part Used: root.

Flavor/Nature: bitter, sour; neutral.

Meridian Affinity: Liver and Kidney Meridians.

Actions: mobilizes blood, removes stasis, nourishes the liver and the kidney, strengthens the sinews, promotes diuresis and relieves urethritis, and conducts blood downward.

Indications: (1) Dysmenorrhea, amenorrhea and post-partum abdominal pain due to blood stasis. (2) Traumatic injuries. (3) Aching pain in the waist and the knees, and weakness in the lower limbs. (4) Hematuria, difficulty with urination and urethritis. (5) Hematemesis, epistaxis, toothace, mouth sores, headaches and vertigo.

Dosage/Administration: 6–15 g.

Cautions/Contraindications: Contraindicated in pregnancy and excessive menses.

9 Sanleng (Sparganium stoloniferum) (Bur Reed)

Chinese name: 三棱. Pharmaceutical name: *Tuber Sparganii.*

Part Used: tuber (bark removed).

Flavor/Nature: acrid; neutral.

Meridian Affinity: Liver and Spleen Meridians.

Actions: breaks up and removes blood stasis, mobilizes Qi and stops pain.

Indications: (1) Qi stagnation and blood stasis causing amenorrhea, abdominal pain or abdominal masses. (2) Food retention and Qi stagnation leading to epigastric and abdominal distention and pain.

Dosage/Administration: 3–10 g.

Cautions/Contraindications: Contraindicated in pregnancy and excessive menses.

10 Ezhu (Curcuma aeruginosa, zedoaria) (Zedoary)

Chinese name: 莪术. Pharmaceutical name: *Rhizoma Zedoariae.*

Part Used: rhizome.

Flavor/Nature: acrid, bitter; warm.

Meridian Affinity: Liver and Spleen Meridians.

Actions: breaks up and relieves blood stasis, mobilizes Qi and stops pain.

Indications: (1) Qi stagnation and blood stasis causing amenorrhea, abdominal pain or abdominal masses. (2) Dietary indiscretion resulting in abnormal spleen functions, food retention and epigastric and abdominal distention and pain.

Dosage/Administration: 3–10 g.

Cautions/Contraindications: Contraindicated in pregnancy and excessive menses.

Section 11 Herbs That Dissolve Phlegm or Stop Cough and Relieve Asthma

This group actually comprises two subgroups of herbs. The Phlegm-dissolving herbs act principally to dissolve Phlegm and eliminate sputum. The cough-stopping and asthma-relieving herbs act principally to stop cough and to relieve wheezing and labored breathing. Cough is usually accompanied by sputum and Phlegm usually causes cough. In general, Phlegm-dissolving herbs also can stop cough and relieve asthma and cough-stopping and asthma-relieving herbs also can dissolve Phlegm. The two groups are therefore usually discussed together.

Phlegm-dissolving herbs are mainly used to treat illnesses of Phlegm causing much sputum and cough, cough with labored breathing or sputum that is difficult to expectorate. Cough-stopping and asthma-relieving herbs are mainly used to treat cough and asthma due to either internal injury or exogenous pathogenic agent. Since both internal injury and exogenous illness can produce cough, asthma or much sputum, it is important to select these herbs on the basis of the cause and properties of the clinical condition being treated and to add appropriate supplemental herbs.

For cough with associated hemoptysis it is not appropriate to prescribe Phlegm-dissolving herbs that are harsh and irritating, as these may aggravate the hemoptysis. For cough in the early stages of measles, the main herbs to use are in general those that clear and ventilate the lung rather than cough-stopping herbs. Cough-stopping herbs that are warm or astringent are especially inappropriate as they may aggravate Heat or affect the proper eruption of the measles rash.

1 Banxia (Pinellia ternata)

Chinese name: 半夏. Pharmaceutical name: *Rhizoma Pinelliae.*

Part Used: stalk tuber.

Flavor/Nature: acrid; warm. Banxia is poisonous and it must be processed before use.

Meridian Affinity: Spleen, Stomach and Lung Meridians.

Actions: dries Dampness, dissolves Phlegm, suppresses abnormal Qi ascent, stops vomiting, relieves distention and dissipates accumulations.

Indications: (1) Cough with much sputum and dyspnea due to failure of the spleen to dissolve Dampness, thereby allowing it to accumulate and cause blockage. (2) Abnormal ascent of stomach-Qi causing nausea and vomiting. (3) Chest and epigastric tightness. (4) Globus hystericus, goiter, subcutaneous nodules, abscesses and cellulitis.

Dosage/Administration: 5–10 g.

Cautions/Contraindications: Incompatible with fuzi (*Aconitum*). Because of its warm and dry nature, banxia is contraindicated or used with great caution in dry cough due to Yin deficiency, bleeding conditions, and illnesses of Heat–Phlegm.

2 *Jiegeng (Platycodon grandiflorum)*

Chinese name: 桔梗. Pharmaceutical name: *Radix Platycodonis*.

Part Used: root.

Flavor/Nature: bitter, acrid; neutral.

Meridian Affinity: Lung Meridian.

Actions: removes inhibition on lung-Qi, clears sputum and drains pus.

Indications: (1) Cough with much sputum or sputum that is difficult to expectorate, chest tightness, and sore throat with loss of voice. (2) Lung abscess with chest pain, cough productive of pus and blood, or yellow and foul-smelling sputum.

Dosage/Administration: 3–10 g.

3 *Beimu (Fritillaria cirrhosa, verticillata)*

Chinese name: 贝母. Pharmaceutical name: *Bulbus Fritillaria Cirrhosae*. There are two main varieties of beimu: chuanbeimu (*F. cirrhosa*) and zhebeimu (*F. verticillata, thunbergii*).

Part Used: bulb.

Flavor/Nature: Chuanbeimu: bitter, sweet; cool. Zhebeimu: bitter; cold.

Meridian Affinity: Chuanbeimu: Lung Meridian. Zhebeimu: Lung and Stomach Meridians.

Actions: Chuanbeimu: dissolves sputum, stops cough and moistens the lung. Zhebeimu: dissolves sputum, stops cough, clears Heat and dissipates accumulation.

Indications: (1) Cough due to several causes: lung insufficiency with chronic cough, little sputum and dry throat; exogenous Wind–Heat; and accumulation of Phlegm–Fire with viscous yellow sputum. (2) Scrofula, boils, abscesses, cellulitis and lung abscess. (3) Mastitis.

Dosage/Administration: 3–10 g.

Cautions/Contraindications: Incompatible with fuzi (*Aconitum*).

4 *Gualou (Trichosanthes kirilowii) (Snake-Gourd)*

Chinese name: 瓜蒌. Pharmaceutical name: *Fructus Trichosanthis.*

Part Used: ripe fruit; gualouzi, ripe seed.

Flavor/Nature: sweet; cold.

Meridian Affinity: Lung, Stomach and Large Intestine Meridians.

Actions: Peel: clears the lung and dissolves Phlegm, facilitates Qi and loosens the chest. Seed: moistens the lung and dissolves Phlegm, moistens the intestines and facilitates defecation. Fruit: all the above.

Indications: (1) Heat in the lung causing cough with viscous sputum that is difficult to expectorate. (2) Rheumatism of the chest, accumulation of exogenous disease-causing agent in the chest or chest pain. (3) Dehydrated intestines with constipation. (4) Mastitis (whole herb).

Dosage/Administration: Whole fruit: 10–20 g. Peel: 6–12 g. Seed: 10–15 g.

Cautions/Contraindications: Incompatible with fuzi (*Aconitum*).

5 *Xingren (Prunus armeniaca) (Apricot) (Also Known as Kuxingren)*

Chinese name: 杏仁. Pharmaceutical name: *Semen Armeniacae Amarum.*

Part Used: ripe seed.

Flavor/Nature: bitter; slightly warm. Xingren is mildly poisonous.

Meridian Affinity: Lung and Large Intestine Meridians.

Actions: stops cough, relieves asthma, moistens the intestines and facilitates defecation.

Indications: (1) Any kind of cough and asthma. (2) Constipation due to dehydrated intestines.

Dosage/Administration: 3–10 g.

Cautions/Contraindications: Because it is mildly poisonous do not overdose. Use with great caution in infants.

6 *Baibu (Stemona sessilifolia)*

Chinese name: 百部. Pharmaceutical name: *Radix stemonae*.

Part Used: tuberous root.

Flavor/Nature: sweet, bitter; neutral.

Meridian Affinity: Lung Meridian.

Actions: moistens the lungs, stops cough, and kills lice and parasites.

Indications: (1) Acute or chronic cough, pertussis (whooping cough), and tuberculosis. (2) Pinworm or louse infestation.

Dosage/Administration: 5–10 g.

7 *Zisuzi (Perilla frutescens)*

Chinese name: 紫苏子. Pharmaceutical name: *Fructus perillae*.

Part Used: ripe seeds.

Flavor/Nature: acrid; warm.

Meridian Affinity: Lung and Large Intestine Meridians.

Actions: stops cough, relieves asthma, moistens the intestines and facilitates defecation.

Indications: (1) Accumulated Phlegm blocking normal Qi movement and causing cough and asthma. (2) Intestinal dehydration with constipation.

Dosage/Administration: 5–10 g.

8 *Sangbaipi (Morus alba) (White Mulberry)*

Chinese name: 桑白皮. Pharmaceutical name: *Cortex Mori Radicis*.

Part Used: root bark

Flavor/Nature: sweet; cold.

Meridian Affinity: Lung Meridian.

Actions: purges lung-Heat, relieves asthma, promotes water movement and reduces swelling.

Indications: (1) Lung-Heat with cough productive of much sputum. (2) Edema and difficulty with urination.

Dosage/Administration: 10–15 g.

9 Tinglizi (Lepidium apetalum) (Pepper Weed)

Chinese name: 葶苈子. Pharmaceutical name: *Semen Lepidii seu Descurainiae.*

Part Used: ripe seed.

Flavor/Nature: bitter, acrid; very cold.

Meridian Affinity: Lung and Bladder Meridians.

Actions: lowers Qi, relieves asthma and moves water.

Indications: (1) Cough and asthma due to accumulated Phlegm blocking the lung. (2) Edema and difficulty in urination.

Dosage/Administration: 3–10 g.

Section 12 Herbs That Restore (Tonics)

These herbs have their principal actions of replenishing the vital substances of the body and of strengthening its visceral organs. By doing so they enhance the body's resistance to illness and eliminate the deficiencies.

There are four types of deficiency – of Qi, blood, Yin and Yang. By their actions and applications restorative herbs fall into four categories: those that augment Qi, those that generate blood, those that restore Yin and those that restore Yang. Which herb to prescribe will depend upon the type of deficiency. Moreover, in conditions of deficiency or damage of Qi, blood, Yin and Yang often interact and affect one another. Hence, herbs from the different categories must often be prescribed together – restorative herbs for Qi and Yang together and restorative herbs for blood and Yin together.

Restorative herbs are inappropriate in strength illnesses due to exogenous pathogenic evils. Also, if they are used incorrectly, restoratives can do more harm than good. When prescribing them the physician must take proper care of the spleen and the stomach. To avoid impairing digestion and absorption, as well as to obtain the desired therapeutic effects, the physician must include appropriate herbs that strengthen these organs.

1 *Renshen (Panax ginseng) (Ginseng)*

Chinese name: 人参. Pharmaceutical name: *Radix Ginseng*.

Part Used: root.

Flavor/Nature: sweet, slightly bitter; slightly warm.

Meridian Affinity: Spleen and Lung Meridians.

Actions: powerfully augments genuine Qi, strengthens the spleen and the lung, generates fluids and quenches thirst, calms the mind and improves mental function.

Indications: (1) Qi deficiency on the verge of collapse. (2) Insufficiency of spleen-Qi. (3) Injury to lung-Qi. (4) Injury to fluids with thirst. (5) Agitation and restlessness, insomnia with excessive dreaming, fearfulness and forgetfulness. (6) Weakness of general physical condition.

Dosage/Administration: Decoction: 5–10 g decocted over a slow fire and the ginseng juice added to decoction prepared from the other herbs. Powder: 1–2 g per dose, 2–3 doses per day.

Cautions/Contraindications: Contraindicated in strength illnesses due to exogenous disease evils, and in Heat illnesses in which genuine Qi is not deficient. Incompatible with lilu (*Veratrum*), wulingzhi (*Trogopterus*) or zaojia (*Gleditsia*).

2 *Dangshen (Codonopsis pilosula) (Asia Bell)*

Chinese name: 党参. Pharmaceutical name: *Radix Codonopsis Pilosulae*.

Part Used: root.

Flavor/Nature: sweet; neutral.

Meridian Affinity: Spleen and Lung Meridians.

Actions: tonifies the middle-jiao, augments Qi and generates fluids and blood.

Indications: (1) Deficiency of spleen-Qi. (2) Deficiency of lung-Qi. (3) Illness of Heat injuring fluids, with shortness of breath and thirst. (4) Insufficiency of blood with chlorosis, dizziness and palpitations of the heart.

Dosage/Administration: 10–30 g.

Cautions/Contraindications: Incompatible with lilu (*Veratrum*).

3 Huangqi (Astragalus membranaceus, monaholicus) (Milkvetch)

Chinese name: 黄芪. Pharmaceutical name: *Radix Astragaliseu Hedysari.*

Part Used: root.

Flavor/Nature: sweet; slightly warm.

Meridian Affinity: Spleen and Lung Meridians.

Actions: augments Qi and raises Yang, augments defensive-Qi, consolidates the superficies, promotes drainage of pus and healing, facilitates water movement and reduces swelling.

Indications: (1) Deficiency of spleen and lung Qi or sinking of middle-jiao-Qi. (2) Defensive–Qi deficiency causing weakness of the superficies and spontaneous sweating. (3) Abscesses that are refractory to treatment because of deficiency of Qi and blood. (4) Edema with oliguria.

Dosage/Administration: 10–15 g. May increase to 30–50 g.

Cautions/Contraindications: Because of its ability to augment Qi and raise Yang, huangqi can intensify Fire and can stop sweating. It is therefore inappropriate for use in such conditions as strong exogenous pathogen in the exterior, impedance of Qi by Dampness, food retention, hyperactive Yang in Yin deficiency, and early stages of abscesses or Heat poison still present following drainage.

4 Baizhu (Atractylodes macrocephala)

Chinese name: 白术. Pharmaceutical name: *Rhizoma Atractylodis Macrocephalae.*

Part Used: rhizome.

Flavor/Nature: better, sweet; warm.

Meridian Affinity: Spleen and Stomach Meridians.

Actions: augments Qi, strengthens the spleen, dries Dampness, promotes diuresis, stops sweating and calms the fetus.

Indications: A variety of conditions of spleen-Qi deficiency: (1) Impairment of its transportation and transformation functions causing anorexia, loose feces, epigastric and abdominal distention, lassitude and weakness. (2) Loss of transportation and transformation of water and Dampness causing edema and accumulation of Phlegm and Rheum. (3) Insecure superficies with spontaneous sweating. (4) Fetal distress.

Dosage/Administration: 5–15 g.

Cautions/Contraindications: Baizhu dries Dampness and damages Yin, and is appropriate only for illnesses with Dampness in the middle-jiao. It is contraindicated in all conditions of Yin-deficiency with interior-Heat or exhaustion of body fluids with dehydration.

5 Gancao (Glycyrrhiza uralensis) (Chinese Liquorice)

Chinese name: 甘草. Pharmaceutical name: *Radix Glycyrrhiza*.

Part Used: root and rhizome.

Flavor/Nature: sweet; neutral.

Meridian Affinity: Heart, Spleen, Lung and Stomach Meridians.

Actions: strengthens the spleen and augments Qi, moistens the lung and stops cough, soothes spasm and stops pain, and moderates the properties of other herbs.

Indications: (1) Insufficiency of the spleen and the stomach leading to deficiency of middle-jiao-Qi and causing shortness of breath, lassitude, anorexia and loose feces. (2) Cough and asthma. (3) Abscesses, cellulitis and poisoning from food and herbs. (4) Painful spasms of the epigastrium, abdomen and limbs. (5) To moderate or harmonize the properties and actions of the various herbs.

Dosage/Administration: 2–10 g. Use raw gancao for cooling Heat and eliminating toxin. Use fried Gancao for tonifying the middle-jiao and soothing spasm and pain.

Cautions/Contraindications: Gancao is sweet in flavor and can aid Dampness in blocking Qi. It is contraindicated when Dampness causes chest and abdominal distention and vomiting. Incompatible with daji (*Euphorbia*), yuanhua (*Daphne*), haizao (*Sargassum*).

6 Shanyao (Dioscorea opposita) (Chinese Yam)

Chinese name: 山药. Pharmaceutical name: *Rhizoma Dioscoreae*.

Part Used: rhizome.

Flavor/Nature: sweet; neutral.

Meridian Affinity: Spleen, Lung and Kidney Meridians.

Actions: augments Qi, nourishes Yin, strengthens the spleen, lung and kidney.

Indications: (1) Deficiency of spleen-Qi causing anorexia, loose feces or diarrhea. (2) Lung insufficiency causing cough and labored breathing. (3) Kidney insufficiency leading to spermatorrhea, polyuria and in women vaginal discharge.

Dosage/Administration: Decoction: 10–30 g; may increase to 60–250 g. Powder: 6–10 g.

Cautions/Contraindications: Shanyao nourishes Yin and can aid Dampness. It is contraindicated whenever Dampness is strong or has gelled.

7 *Shudihuang (Rehmannia glutinosa)*

Chinese name: 熟地黄. Pharmaceutical name: *Radix Rehmannia Libosch.*

Part Used: cooked root tuber.

Flavor/Nature: sweet; slightly warm.

Meridian Affinity: Liver and Kidney Meridians.

Actions: nourishes Yin, generates blood, augments essence and enriches the marrow.

Indications: (1) Blood insufficiency with chlorosis, dizziness, palpitations of the heart, insomnia, irregular menstruation or metrorrhagia. (2) Deficiency of kidney-Yin causing recurrent fever, night sweat, spermatorrhea or diabetes.

Dosage/Administration: 10–30 g.

Cautions/Contraindications: Shudihuang is glutinous, more so than shendihuang, and can impair digestion. It is contraindicated whenever there is Qi stagnation with production of much sputum, epigastric and abdominal distention and pain, or anorexia with watery diarrhea.

8 *Heshouwu (Polygonum multiflorum) (Fleece-Flower)*

Chinese name: 何首乌. Pharmaceutical name: *Radix Polygoni Multiflori.*

Part Used: root tuber.

Flavor/Nature: bitter, sweet; warm.

Meridian Affinity: Liver and Kidney Meridians.

Actions: replenishes essence and blood, moistens the intestines and facilitates defecation; detoxifies poisons; and halts malaria.

Indications: (1) Insufficiency of both essence and blood leading to dizziness, blurred vision, premature graying of hair, aches and weakness of the waist and the legs, and spermatorrhea or metrorrhagia and vaginal discharge. (2) Chronic malaria, abscesses, scrofula, and dehydrated intestines with constipation.

Dosage/Administration: 10–30 g.

Cautions/Contraindications: Inadvisable in diarrhea or severe Dampness–Phlegm.

9 Danggui (Angelica sinensis)

Chinese name: 当归. Pharmaceutical name: *Radix Angelicae Sinensis*.

Part Used: root.

Flavor/Nature: sweet, acrid; warm.

Meridian Affinity: Liver, Heart and Spleen Meridians.

Actions: replenishes and mobilizes blood, stops pain and moistens the intestines.

Indications: (1) All varieties of blood insufficiency. (2) Irregular menstruation, amenorrhea and dysmenorrhea. (3) Abdominal pain due to deficiency-Cold, pain due to blood stasis, trauma injuries, pain and numbness of rheumatism. (4) Abscesses and furuncles. (5) Dehydrated intestines with constipation due to blood insufficiency.

Dosage/Administration: 5–15 g.

Cautions/Contraindications: Contraindicated in diarrhea and abdominal distention due to Dampness accumulated in the interior.

10 Baishaoyao (Paeonia lactiflora) (White Peony)

Chinese name: 白芍药. Pharmaceutical name: *Radix Paeoniae Alba*.

Part Used: root.

Flavor/Nature: bitter, sour; slightly cold.

Meridian Affinity: Liver and Spleen Meridians.

Actions: generates blood and astringes Yin, softens the liver and stops pain, and suppresses excessive liver-Yang.

Indications: (1) Irregular menstruation, dysmenorrhea, metrorrhagia, spontaneous sweating, night sweat. (2) Erratic liver-Qi with flank, epigastric and abdominal pain or spasm and pain of the limbs.

Dosage/Administration: 5–10 g. May increase to 15–30 g.

Cautions/Contraindications: Should not be used by itself in deficiency-Cold; incompatible with lilu (*Veratrum*).

11 Ejiao (Equus asinus) (Donkey-Hide Gelatin)

Chinese name: 阿胶. Pharmaceutical name: *Colla Corii Asini.*

Part Used: gelatin from the skin, dried.

Flavor/Nature: sweet; neutral.

Meridian Affinity: Lung, Liver and Kidney Meridians.

Actions: generates blood, stops bleeding, nourishes Yin and moistens the lung.

Indications: (1) Blood insufficiency causing dizziness or palpitations of the heart. (2) Bleeding conditions such as hematemesis, epistaxis, hematochezia and metrorrhagia. (3) Restlessness and insomnia of Yin deficiency. (4) Deficiency-induced fatigue, cough and labored breathing, or dry cough due to Yin deficiency.

Dosage/Administration: 5–10 g dissolved in boiling water or yellow wine.

Cautions/Contraindications: Ejiao is glutinous and can impair digestion. It is contraindicated in spleen-stomach insufficiency, anorexia or vomiting and diarrhea.

12 Beishashen (Glehnia littoralis)

Chinese name: 北沙参. Pharmaceutical name: *Radix Glehniae.*

Part Used: root.

Flavor/Nature: sweet; slightly cold.

Meridian Affinity: Lung and Stomach Meridians.

Actions: clears the lungs, nourishes Yin, tonifies the stomach and generates body fluids.

Indications: (1) Yin deficiency with lung Heat causing dry or consumptive cough and hemoptysis. (2) Febrile illness impairing body fluids and causing dry mouth, thirst and poor appetite.

Dosage/Administration: 10–15 g.

Cautions/Contraindications: Contraindicated in deficiency Cold; incompatible with lilu (*Veratrum*)

13 Yuzhu (Polygonatum odoratum) (Fragrant Solomon's Seal)

Chinese name: 玉竹. Pharmaceutical name: *Rhizoma Polygonati Odorati.*

Part Used: rhizome.

Flavor/Nature: sweet; neutral.

Meridian Affinity: Lung and Stomach Meridians.

Actions: nourishes Yin, moistens the lung, generates fluids and strengthens the stomach.

Indications: Injury to lung and stomach Yin producing dry coughing, fever, and a dry mouth with thirst.

Dosage/Administration: 10–15 g.

Cautions/Contraindications: Yuzhu nourishes Yin and moistens Dryness. It is inappropriate in spleen insufficiency with Dampness–Phlegm.

14 Maimendong (Ophiopogon japonicus) (Lily-Turf)

Chinese name: 麦门冬. Pharmaceutical name: *Radix Ophiopogonis.*

Part Used: root tuber.

Flavor/Nature: sweet, slightly bitter; cool.

Meridian Affinity: Lung, Heart and Stomach Meridians.

Actions: moistens the lung, nourishes Yin, strengthens the stomach and generates fluid.

Indications: (1) Dry cough with viscous sputum. (2) Cough with hemoptysis in consumption. (3) Deficiency of stomach-Yin with a dry tongue and thirst. (4) Agitation and insomnia.

Dosage/Administration: 10–15 g.

Cautions/Contraindications: Contraindicated in cough due to Wind–Cold or accumulation of Phlegm–Rheum and in deficiency-Cold in the spleen and the lung with diarrhea.

15 Gouqizi (Lycium barbarum) (Wolfberry)

Chinese name: 枸杞子. Pharmaceutical name: *Fructus Lycii.*

Part Used: ripe fruit.

Flavor/Nature: sweet; neutral.

Meridian Affinity: Liver, Kidney and Lung Meridians.

Actions: nourishes the liver and the kidney, clears the eyes and moistens the lung.

Indications: (1) Deficiency of liver and kidney Yin causing dizziness, blurred vision, weakness of the waist and knees, spermatorrhea or diabetes. (2) Consumption with cough due to Yin deficiency.

Dosage/Administration: 5–10 g.

Cautions/Contraindications: Because of its ability to nourish Yin and moisten Dryness gouqizi is inappropriate in spleen insufficiency with diarrhea.

16 Baihe (Lilium brownii) (Lily)

Chinese name: 百合. Pharmaceutical name: *Bulbus Lilii.*

Part Used: bulb petals.

Flavor/Nature: sweet; cool.

Meridian Affinity: Lung and Heart Meridians.

Actions: moistens the lung, stops cough, clears the heart and calms the mind.

Indications: (1) Heat in the lung with cough. (2) Consumption with cough and hemoptysis. (3) Restlessness, fearfulness, insomnia and excessive dreaming.

Dosage/Administration: 10–30 g.

Cautions/Contraindications: Contraindicated in cough due to Wind–Cold or diarrhea due to Cold in the middle-jiao.

17 Nuzhenzi (Ligustrum lucidum) (Wax Privet)

Chinese name: 女贞子. Pharmaceutical name: *Fructus Ligustri Lucidi.*

Part Used: ripe fruit.

Flavor/Nature: sweet, bitter; cool.

Meridian Affinity: Liver and Kidney Meridians.

Actions: tonifies the liver and the kidney, cools Heat and clears the eye.

Indications: (1) Deficiency of liver and kidney Yin causing dizziness, blurred vision, weakness in the waist and knees and premature graying of hair. (2) Endogenous Heat in Yin deficiency. (3) Deficiency of liver and kidney Yin causing reduced visual acuity and clouding of vision.

Dosage/Administration: 10–15 g.

Cautions/Contraindications: Contraindicated in Yang deficiency or deficiency-Cold in the spleen and the stomach with diarrhea.

18 Mohanlian (Eclipta prostrata)

Chinese name: 墨旱莲. Pharmaceutical name: *Herba Ecliptae*.

Part Used: whole herb.

Flavor/Nature: sweet, sour; cold.

Meridian Affinity: Liver and Kidney Meridians.

Actions: nourishes Yin, strengthens the kidney, cools blood and stops bleeding.

Indications: (1) Deficiency of liver and kidney Yin with dizziness, blurred vision and premature graying of hair. (2) Yin deficiency and Heat in blood causing hematemesis, epistaxis, hematuria and metrorrhagia.

Dosage/Administration: 10–15 g.

Cautions/Contraindications: Contraindicated in deficiency-Cold in the spleen and the stomach with diarrhea.

19 Guiban (Chinemys reevesii) (Tortoise)

Chinese name: 龟板. Pharmaceutical name: *Plastrum Testudinis*.

Part Used: ventral exoskeleton (plastron).

Flavor/Nature: sweet, salty; cold.

Meridian Affinity: Liver, Kidney and Heart Meridians.

Actions: nourishes Yin, suppresses Yang, strengthens the kidney and bones, generates blood and stimulates the heart.

Indications: (1) Yin deficiency with hyperactive Yang or exogenous Heat damaging Yin allowing the stirring of endogenous Wind in Yin deficiency. (2) Endogenous Heat in Yin deficiency. (3) Kidney insufficiency causing lumbar and lower limb flaccidity in adults or non-closure of the fontanel in infants. (4) Insufficiency of the heart with fearfulness, insomnia and forgetfulness.

Dosage/Administration: 10–30 g. Decocted first.

Cautions/Contraindications: Contraindicated in deficiency-Cold in the spleen and the stomach. Also, according to ancient texts this is contraindicated in pregnancy.

20 Biejia (Amyda sinensis) (Turtle)

Chinese name: 鳖甲. Pharmaceutical name: *Carapax Trionycis*.

Part Used: dorsal exoskeleton (carapace).

Flavor/Nature: salty; cold.

Meridian Affinity: Liver and Spleen Meridians.

Actions: nourishes Yin, suppresses Yang, softens the hard and dissolves masses.

Indications: (1) Endogenous Wind arising in Yin deficiency and causing convulsions or tremors of the fingers. (2) Fever in Yin deficiency. (3) Chronic malaria, amenorrhea and abdominal masses.

Dosage/Administration: 10–30 g. Decocted first.

Cautions/Contraindications: Use with caution in deficiency-Cold of the spleen and stomach, anorexia, diarrhea, or during pregnancy.

21 Yinyanghuo (Epimedium brevicornum, grandiflorum) (Barren-wort)

Chinese name: 淫羊藿. Pharmaceutical name: *Herba Epimedii.*

Part Used: stalk leaves.

Flavor/Nature: acrid, sweet; warm.

Meridian Affinity: Liver and Kidney Meridians.

Actions: tonifies the kidney, augments Yang, dispels Wind and removes Dampness.

Indications: (1) Impotence, frequent urination and lumbar and knee weakness. (2) Rheumatism or numbness of the limbs due to Wind–Cold–Dampness.

Dosage/Administration: 9–12 g.

Cautions/Contraindications: Contraindicated in blazing Fire arising in Yin deficiency.

22 Duzhong (Eucommia ulmoides)

Chinese name: 杜仲. Pharmaceutical name: *Cortex Eucommia.*

Part Used: bark.

Flavor/Nature: sweet; warm.

Meridian Affinity: Liver and Kidney Meridians.

Actions: strengthens the liver, the kidney and the sinews, and calms the fetus.

Indications: (1) Insufficiency of the liver and the kidney causing aching pain in the waist and knees or flaccidity. (2) Fetal distress or habitual abortion.

Dosage/Administration: 10–15 g.

Cautions/Contraindications: Contraindicated in blazing Fire in Yin deficiency.

23 Xuduan (Dipsacus asperoides) (Himalayan Teasel)

Chinese name: 续断. Pharmaceutical name: *Radix Dipsaci.*

Part Used: root.

Flavor/Nature: bitter, sweet, acrid; slightly warm.

Meridian Affinity: Liver and Kidney Meridians.

Actions: strengthens the liver and the kidney, stimulates blood circulation and repairs sinews and bones.

Indications: (1) Lumbar pain, weakness of the feet, spermatorrhea and metrorrhagia. (2) Threatened abortion. (3) Traumatic injuries, poison in wounds, abscesses and furuncles.

Dosage/Administration: 10–20 g.

24 Bajitian (Morinda officinalis)

Chinese name: 巴戟天. Pharmaceutical name: *Radix Morindae Officinalis.*

Part Used: root.

Flavor/Nature: acrid, sweet; slightly warm.

Meridian Affinity: Kidney Meridian.

Actions: strengthens the kidney, augments Yang, dispels Wind and removes Dampness.

Indications: (1) Impotence with polyuria or infertility with irregular menstruation and cold pain in the pelvis. (2) Aching pain in the waist and knees or flaccidity.

Dosage/Administration: 10–15 g.

Cautions/Contraindications: Contraindicated in blazing Fire in Yin deficiency or in Dampness–Heat.

25 Buguzhi (Psoralea corylifolia)

Chinese name: 补骨脂. Pharmaceutical name: *Fructus Psoraleae*.

Part Used: ripe fruit.

Flavor/Nature: bitter, acrid; hot.

Meridian Affinity: Kidney and Spleen Meridians.

Actions: strengthens the kidney, augments Yang, consolidates genitive essence, reduces urine, warms the spleen and stops diarrhea.

Indications: (1) Impotence with cold pain in the waist and knees. (2) Spermatorrhea, urinary incontinence and polyuria. (3) Diarrhea due to Yang deficiency in the spleen and the kidney.

Dosage/Administration: 5–10 g.

Cautions/Contraindications: Buguzhi warms and dries, and can injure Yin and intensify Fire. It is contraindicated in blazing Fire in Yin deficiency and in constipation.

26 Hutaoren (Juglans regia) (Walnut)

Chinese name: 胡桃仁. Pharmaceutical name: *Semen Juglandis Regiae*.

Part Used: kernel.

Flavor/Nature: sweet; warm.

Meridian Affinity: Kidney, Lung and Large Intestine Meridians.

Actions: strengthens the kidney, warms the lung and moistens the intestines.

Indications: (1) Lumbar pain and foot weakness. (2) Asthma and cough due to deficiency-Cold.

Dosage/Administration: 10–30 g.

Cautions/Contraindications: Contraindicated in Yin deficiency with blazing Fire, cough due to Phlegm–Heat or diarrhea.

27 Roucongrong (Cistanche deserticola)

Chinese name: 肉苁蓉. Pharmaceutical name: *Herba Cistanchis*.

Part Used: (scale/leaf-bearing) stalk.

Flavor/Nature: sweet, salty; warm.

Meridian Affinity: Kidney and Large Intestine Meridians.
Actions: strengthens the kidney, aids Yang, moistens the intestines and facilitates defecation.

Indications: (1) Impotence or infertility with cold pain in the waist and knees or weakness of the sinews. (2) Constipation due to dehydration.

Dosage/Administration: 10–15 g.

Cautions/Contraindications: Contraindicated in Yin deficiency with blzaing Fire and diarrhea. Inappropriate in constipation due to strength Heat.

28 Dongchongxiacao (Cordyceps sinensis) (Chinese Caterpillar Fungus)

Chinese name: 冬虫夏草. Pharmaceutical name: *Cordyceps.*

Part Used: stroma of the fungus that parasitizes the larva of insects of the Hepialidae family, together with the larva corpse.

Flavor/Nature: sweet; warm.

Meridian Affinity: Kidney and Lung Meridians.

Actions: strengthens the kidney and lung, stops bleeding and dissolves Phlegm.

Indications: (1) Impotence with spermatorrhea and aching pain in the waist and knees. (2) Chronic cough, labored breathing due to deficiency, and consumption with cough productive of sputum and blood.

Dosage/Administration: 5–10 g.

Cautions/Contraindications: Contraindicated when there is exogenous pathogenic evil in the exterior.

Section 13 Herbs That Calm Mind

These are herbs that have their principal action of calming the mind. They are sometimes also known as tranquilizers or sedatives. Their principal application is the treatment of restlessness, agitation, palpitations of the heart, insomnia, excessive dreaming, as well as infantile convulsions, epilepsy and dementia.

Most herbs in this category derive from minerals or the seeds of plants. In general mineral herbs are heavy and lowering in nature; hence many of them are sedating or tranquilizing. The seed herbs are moistening and restorative in nature; hence many of them strengthen the heart and calm the mind.

When prescribing mind-calming herbs the physician must take full stock of the patient's illness – not only select an appropriate herb, but also supplement and complement it with appropriate other herbs. For example, for Yin deficiency and blood insufficiency, complement the mind-calming herb with herbs that generate blood and augment Yin. For abnormal ascent of liver-Yang, complement with herbs that calm the liver and suppress Yang. For the blazing of heart-Fire, complement with herbs that cool the heart and clear Fire. In such conditions as epilepsy and infantile convulsion, the approach is usually to use herbs that dissolve Phlegm and open orifices or those that calm the liver and extinguish Wind as the main treatment; mind-calming herbs are used only as supplement.

Mineral herbs when taken as pills or powders can easily injure the stomach and impair stomach-Qi. They must be complemented with herbs that nourish the stomach and strengthen the spleen. Some of them are quite toxic and must be used only with great care.

1 Suanzaoren (Ziziphus jujuba Mill. var. spinosa) (Chinese Jujube)

Chinese name: 酸枣仁. Pharmaceutical name: *Semen Ziziphi Spinosae*.

Part Used: ripe seed.

Flavor/Nature: sweet; neutral.

Meridian Affinity: Heart and Liver Meridians.

Actions: nourishes the heart, calms the mind and astringes sweat.

Indications: (1) Insomnia and palpitations. (2) Spontaneous sweating and night sweat in deficiency.

Dosage/Administration: 10–18 g.

2 Baiziren (Biota orientalis) (Chinese Tree of Life)

Chinese name: 柏子仁. Pharmaceutical name: *Semen Biotae*.

Part Used: kernel of ripe seed.

Flavor/Nature: sweet; neutral.

Meridian Affinity: Heart, Kidney and Large Intestine Meridians.

Actions: nourishes the heart, calms the mind, moistens the intestine and facilitates defecation.

Indications: (1) Deficiency of heart-blood causing restlessness, insomnia and palpitations. (2) Dehydration of the intestines with constipation.

Dosage/Administration: 10–18 g.

Cautions/Contraindications: Use cautiously in diarrhea or excessive sputum.

3 *Yuanzhi (Polygala tenuifolia) (Milk Wort)*

Chinese name: 远志. Pharmaceutical name: *Radix Polygalae*.

Part Used: root.

Flavor/Nature: acrid, bitter; slightly warm.

Meridian Affinity: Lung and Heart Meridians.

Actions: stabilizes the heart and calms the mind, dissolves Phlegm and opens orifices, and reduces abscesses and swelling.

Indications: (1) Agitation, palpitations, insomnia and forgetfulness. (2) Phlegm blocking the orifices causing mental confusion, absent-mindedness or infantile convulsion. (3) Abscesses and furuncles.

Dosage/Administration: 6–10 g.

Cautions/Contraindications: Use cautiously in ulcers and gastritis.

4 *Muli (Ostrea gigas, rivularis) (Oyster)*

Chinese name: 牡蛎. Pharmaceutical name: *Concha Ostreae*.

Part Used: shell.

Flavor/Nature: salty; cool.

Meridian Affinity: Liver and Kidney Meridians.

Actions: calms the liver, suppresses Yang, softens the hard, disperses accumulations and astringes.

Indications: (1) Restlessness, agitation, palpitations, insomnia, dizziness, blurred vision and tinnitus due to Yin deficiency and Yang hyperactivity. (2) Scrofula and similar conditions due to accumulation of Phlegm and Fire. (3) Sweating duet to debility, spermatorrhea, vaginal discharge and metrorrhagia.

Dosage/Administration: 15–30 g. Decocted first for 30 to 60 min.

5 *Longgu (Os Draconis) (Fossil Bone)*

Chinese name: 龙骨. Pharmaceutical name: *Fossilia Ossis Mastodi*.

Flavor/Nature: sweet; cold.

Meridian Affinity: Heart and Liver Meridians.

Actions: regulates the liver, suppresses Yang, tranquilizes and calms the mind, astringes.

Indications: (1) Yin deficiency with hyperactive Yang causing agitation, irascibility, dizziness and blurred vision. (2) Restlessness, palpitations, insomnia, infantile convulsions, epilepsy and dementia. (3) Spermatorrhea, vaginal discharge, sweating due to debility and metrorrhagia. (4) In addition, the powder of toasted longgu may be applied topically and has drying and astringent properties. It may be used to treat wet skin lesions such as eczema or newly drained abscesses.

Dosage/Administration: 15–30 g. Decocted first for 30 to 60 min.

6 *Cishi (Magnetitium) (Magnetite)*

Chinese name: 磁石. Pharmaceutical name: *Magnetitum*.

Flavor/Nature: acrid, salty; cold.

Meridian Affinity: Liver, Heart and Kidney Meridians.

Actions: suppresses Yang, tranquilizes, improves visual and auditory acuity, improves respiratory air exchange and relieves asthma.

Indications: (1) Yin deficiency and Yang hyperactivity causing agitation, palpitations, insomnia, dizziness, headache and epilepsy. (2) Deficiency of liver and kidney Yin causing tinnitus, deafness and clouded vision. (3) Kidney insufficiency causing labored breathing.

Dosage/Administration: 10–30g.

Cautions/Contraindications: Use cautiously in spleen and stomach insufficiency.

Section 14 Herbs That Calm Liver and Extinguish Wind

These herbs have their principal actions of extinguishing liver-Wind and of restraining the hyperactive Yang. With these dual actions herbs in this group are used mainly in two kinds of illnesses with hyperactive liver: stirring of liver-Wind in interior with tetany or convulsions, and abnormal ascent of liver-Yang with dizziness and blurring of vision.

When prescribing these herbs the physician must take into account the different causes and associated conditions and symptoms of these two illnesses and supplement or complement them with appropriate additional herbs. The stirring of liver-Wind in interior mostly occurs when Fire or Heat is extreme, known as "extreme Heat generates Wind." The abnormal ascent of liver-Yang is also usually associated with Heat in the liver, and requires treatment by simultaneous purging of Fire and clearing of the liver. When "the Water Element fails to nourish the Wood Element," Yin becomes deficient, blood becomes insufficient and the liver loses its nourishment (see Volume 1, Part I, Chapter 1, Section 2, Subsection III, and Volume 1, Part I, Chapter 3, Section 2). In this situation liver-Wind stirs in the Interior and liver-Yang ascends abnormally. Treatment then requires strengthening of the kidney to augment Yin or generating blood in concert with calming of the liver and extinguishing of Wind. "The liver stores the soul." Hence, when the liver is hyperactive the mental state is often disturbed; and supplemental herbs to calm the mind must be included.

Herbs in this group come mainly from animals. Most of them are of cold or cool nature, but some are of warm or drying nature. These two groups are used differently. In general, cold or cool herbs are not appropriate for spleen insufficiency with chronic infantile convulsion; and warming and drying herbs are not appropriate for Yin deficiency and blood insufficiency.

1 Tianma (Gastrodia elata)

Chinese name: 天麻. Pharmaceutical name: *Rhizoma Gastrodiae*.

Part Used: tuber.

Flavor/Nature: sweet; neutral.

Meridian Affinity: Liver Meridian.

Actions: extinguishes endogenous Wind, stops convulsions, calms the liver and restrains abnormally rising Yang.

Indications: (1) Internal stirring of liver-Wind with spasm or infantile convulsion. (2) Abnormal rise of liver-Yang with dizziness and headache. (3) Additional applications: because of tianma's ability to dispel Wind and Dampness and to stop pain it is also used for Wind–Dampness induced rheumatism with pain, numbness and compromised function of the hands and feet.

Dosage/Administration: 3–10 g.

2 *Gouteng (Uncaria rhynchophylla)*

Chinese name: 钩藤. Pharmaceutical name: *Ramulus Uncariae cum Uncis*.

Part Used: thorn-bearing twig.

Flavor/Nature: sweet; cool.

Meridian Affinity: Liver and Pericardium Meridians.

Actions: extinguishes endogenous Wind, stops convulsions, clears Heat and calms the liver.

Indications: (1) Infantile convulsions. (2) Heat in the liver channels with distending headache or abnormal rise of liver-Yang with dizziness and blurred vision. (3) Additional applications: gouteng is effective in lowering blood pressure and is especially effective for high blood pressure with Heat in the liver or abnormal rise of liver-Yang.

Dosage/Administration: 10–15 g.

3 *Shijueming (Haliotis diversicolor) (Abalone)*

Chinese name: 石决明. Pharmaceutical name: *Concha Haliotidis*.

Part Used: shell.

Flavor/Nature: salty; cold.

Meridian Affinity: Liver Meridian.

Actions: calms the liver, suppresses Yang, and clears the liver and the eyes.

Indications: (1) Dizziness and blurring of vision. (2) Inflammation of the eyes or membranous clouding of vision.

Dosage/Administration: 15–30 g. Decocted first for 30 to 60 min.

4 *Dilong (Pheretima aspergillum) (Earthworm)*

Chinese name: 地龙. Pharmaceutical name: *Pheretima*.

Part Used: whole worm.

Flavor/Nature: salty; cold.

Meridian Affinity: Liver, Spleen and Bladder Meridians.

Actions: clears Heat, extinguishes endogenous Wind, relieves asthma, unblocks channels and promotes diuresis.

Indications: (1) High fever with convulsions. (2) Labored breathing with rattling sputum in the throat. (3) Inflammatory arthritis due to Heat with impaired joint movement. (4) Heat in the bladder with dysuria or anuria. (5) Additional application: dilong also has the ability to lower pressure and can be used to treat high blood pressure due to abnormal rise of liver-Yang.

Dosage/Administration: 5–15 g.

5 Baijiangcan (Bombyx mori) (Silkworm)

Chinese name: 白僵蚕. Pharmaceutical name: *Bombyx Batryticatus.*

Part Used: body of the 4th or 5th stage larva of the silkworm that has died from infection by the fungus *Beauveria bassiana.*

Flavor/Nature: salty, acrid; neutral.

Meridian Affinity: Liver and Lung Meridians.

Actions: extinguishes endogenous Wind, stops convulsions, dispels Wind, stops pain, detoxifies poisons and dissipates accumulations.

Indications: (1) Convulsions due to liver-Wind and strong Phlegm–Heat. (2) Wind–Heat or liver-Heat with headache, inflamed eyes, swollen and painful throat and toothache. (3) Scrofula, subcutaneous nodules, abscesses and erysipelas. (4) Additional application: baijiangcan also dispels Wind and stops itch, and may be used for various rashes.

Dosage/Administration: 3–10 g.

6 Quanxie (Buthus martensii) (Scorpion)

Chinese name: 全蝎. Pharmaceutical name: *Scorpio.*

Part Used: dried body.

Flavor/Nature: acrid; neutral. Poisonous.

Meridian Affinity: Liver Meridian.

Actions: extinguishes endogenous Wind, stops convulsions, detoxifies poisons, dissipates accumulations, unblocks channels and stops pain.

Indications: (1) Acute or chronic infantile convulsions, Wind-induced stroke with facial palsy and tetanus. (2) Abscesses, scrofula and subcutaneous nodules. (3) Refractory migraine or headache. (4) Pain of Wind–Dampness induced rheumatism.

Dosage/Administration: 2–5 g.

Cautions/Contraindications: This herb is poisonous and must not be overdosed. Use with great caution in endogenous Wind due to blood insufficiency.

7 Wugong (Scolopendra subspinipes) (Centipede)

Chinese name: 蜈蚣. Pharmaceutical name: *Scolopendra.*

Part Used: dried body.

Flavor/Nature: acrid; warm. Poisonous.

Meridian Affinity: Liver Meridian.

Actions: extinguishes endogenous Wind, stops convulsions, detoxifies poisons, dissipates accumulations, unblocks channels and stops pain.
Indications: (1) Acute or chronic infantile convulsions and tetanus. (2) Abscesses, scrofula and subcutaneous nodules. (3) Refractory migraine or headache. (4) Pain of Wind–Dampness induced rheumatism.

Dosage/Administration: 1–3 g.

Cautions/Contraindications: Contraindicated in pregnancy. This herb is poisonous and must not be overdosed.

Section 15 Aromatic Herbs That Open Orifices (Resuscitate)

These aromatic and acrid herbs have their principal actions of opening orifices and of reviving consciousness. Most orifice-opening herbs have affinity for the Heart Meridian. They are mainly used to treat two types of illnesses: coma or delirium due to Heat occupying the pericardium or turbid Phlegm blocking the orifices, and acute coma due to a convulsion or Wind invasion (stroke).

Coma may be caused by an illness of deficiency or of strength. Coma caused by a deficiency is said to be "prostrate." Its typical manifestation is a pattern of symptoms that includes cold sweat, cold limbs and an indistinct pulse on the verge of collapse. Coma caused by strong exogenous pathogenic evil is said to be "closed." It mainly manifests such symptoms as a tight jaw, clenched fists and a forceful pulse. "Closed" coma may further be classified as Cold-closure or Heat-closure. The typical pattern of symptoms of Cold-closure coma includes a green face, a cold body, a white tongue coating and a slow pulse. The typical pattern of symptoms of

Heat-closure coma includes a red face, a feverish body, a yellow tongue coating and a rapid pulse.

"Prostrate" coma is best treated by the method of reviving Yang, rescuing from prostration, augmenting Qi and stopping Qi escape. It should not be treated with herbs that open orifices.

"Closed" coma, on the other hand, is appropriately treated with orifice-opening herbs. Coma due to Cold-closure should be treated by orifice opening and warming. Coma due to Heat-closure should be treated by orifice opening and cooling. In addition, the physician must supplement or complement the treatment with herbs in accordance with the specific cause and the associated symptoms of the illness.

Orifice-opening herbs are acrid and aromatic, and are volatile. They are intended for urgent use and aim at treating the appearance (see Volume 1, Part I, Chapter 5, Section 1, Subsection II). They are to be used only briefly in order to avoid damaging genuine Qi. They are also contraindicated in "prostrate" coma. For oral administration they should in general be prepared as pills. Only a few can be appropriately administered as decoction.

1 Shichangpu (Acorus gramineus, tatarinowii) (Sweet Flag)

Chinese name: 石菖蒲. Pharmaceutical name: *Rhizoma Acori Graminei*.

Part Used: rhizome.

Flavor/Nature: acrid; warm.

Meridian Affinity: Heart and Stomach Meridians.

Actions: opens orifices and calms the mind, dissolves Dampness and harmonizes the stomach.

Indications: (1) Turbid Dampness blocking the orifices causing mental confusion or forgetfulness and tinnitus. (2) Accumulation of Dampness and obstruction of Qi causing chest and abdominal distention or pain. (3) Additional application: shichangpu may also be used to treat Wind–Cold rheumatism, traumatic injuries, abscesses and various skin lesions.

Dosage/Administration: 5–8 g.

2 Shexiang (Moschus moschiferus) (Musk)

Chinese name: 麝香. Pharmaceutical name: *Moschus*.

Part Used: dried secretion from the glands of the prepuce.

Flavor/Nature: acrid; warm.

Meridian Affinity: Heart and Spleen Meridians.
Actions: opens orifices, restores consciousness, mobilizes blood, dissipates accumulations, stops pain and stimulates labor and delivery.

Indications: (1) In Heat illnesses where Heat has entered the pericardium, causing coma, convulsions or delirium, and similar "closed" coma. (2) Abscesses and furuncles. (3) Tearing pain in the heart and abdomen, traumatic injuries and pains of rheumatism. (4) Fetal death or retention of the placenta.

Dosage/Administration: 0.06–0.1 g as pills or powders only.

Cautions/Contraindications: Contraindicated in pregnancy. (Nowadays, natural shexiang is replaced by laboratory-produced shexiang.)

3 Suhexiang (Liquidambar orientalis) (Storax)

Chinese name: 苏合香. Pharmaceutical name: *Styrax*.

Part Used: balsam (resin) from the tree.

Flavor/Nature: acrid; warm.

Meridian Affinity: Heart and Spleen Meridians.

Actions: opens orifices, eliminates turbidity and stops pain.

Indications: (1) Sudden Cold-closure coma, such as stroke or blockage by Phlegm. (2) Cold pain and distention in the chest and abdomen.

Dosage/Administration: 0.3–1 g in pills only.

4 Bingpian (Dryobalanops aromatica) (Borneol)

Chinese name: 冰片. Pharmaceutical name: *Borneolum Syntheticum*.

Part Used: crystals formed from the resin of the tree.

Flavor/Nature: acrid, bitter; cool.

Meridian Affinity: Heart, Spleen and Lung Meridians.

Actions: opens orifices, restores consciousness, cools Heat and stops pain.

Indications: (1) Coma and convulsions. (2) Abscesses, pain and swelling in the throat, aphthous sores in the mouth and eye disorders.

Dosage/Administration: 0.03–0.1 g, in pill and power only.

Cautions/Contraindications: Use very cautiously in pregnancy.

Section 16 Herbs That Stop Bleeding

These are herbs that have their principal action of stopping bleeding. They are used mainly to treat bleeding conditions such as hemoptysis, epistaxis, hematemesis, hematuria, metrorrhagia, ecchymosis and traumatic bleeding.

Herbs that stop bleeding come with a variety of associated properties, such as blood cooling, astringent, clot dissolving and channel warming. When prescribing, the physician must select the most suitable herbs for the whole patient and combine it with appropriate supplementary herbs to enhance the therapeutic effect. For example, if the bleeding is due to Heat in the blood driving it to flow erratically, add herbs that cool Heat and blood. If it is due to Yin deficiency with hyperactive Yang, add herbs that nourish Yin and suppress Yang. If it is due to blood stasis, add herbs that mobilize Qi and blood. If it is due to deficiency Cold, add herbs that warm Yang, augment Qi or strengthen the spleen as appropriate for the clinical condition. If excessive bleeding has depleted Qi and brought it to the verge of collapse, herbs that stop bleeding used alone are too slow in action for such an urgent situation; it is necessary to add herbs that augment genuine Qi vigorously to avoid prostration.

When applying herbs that stop bleeding and cool blood or that stop bleeding and astringe, the physician must take note whether there is blood stasis as well. If the clots that resulted from the stasis have not been completely reabsorbed, the physician must add herbs that mobilize blood and eliminate clots to avoid leaving residual clots.

1 Xiaoji (Cephalanoplos segetum) (Field Thistle)

Chinese name: 小蓟. Pharmaceutical name: *Herba Cephalanoploris.*

Part Used: whole herb or root.

Flavor/Nature: sweet; cold.

Meridian Affinity: Heart and Liver Meridians.

Actions: cools blood, stops bleeding, detoxifies poison and shrinks abscesses.

Indications: (1) Hemoptysis, epistaxis, hematemesis, hematuria or metrorrhagia due to Heat in the blood causing erratic blood movement. (2) Abscesses and furuncles due to Heat poisoning.

Dosage/Administration: 10–15 g. May use 30–60 g if fresh.

2 Diyu (Sanguisorba officinalis) (Garden Burnet)

Chinese name: 地榆. Pharmaceutical name: *Herba Cephalanoploris.*

Part Used: root.

Flavor/Nature: bitter, sour; cool.

Meridian Affinity: Liver, Stomach and Large Intestine Meridians.

Actions: cools blood, stops bleeding, detoxifies poison and shrinks abscesses.

Indications: (1) Hemoptysis, epistaxis, hematemesis, hematuria or metrorrhagia due to Heat in the blood causing erratic blood movement. (2) Burns, eczema and skin breakdowns.

Dosage/Administration: 10–15 g.
Cautions/Contraindications: Contraindicated in extensive burns.

3 *Baiji (Bletilla striata)*

Chinese name: 白及. Pharmaceutical name: *Rhizoma Bletillae*.

Part Used: tuber.

Flavor/Nature: bitter, sweet, astringent; cool.

Meridian Affinity: Lung, Liver and Stomach Meridians.

Actions: astringes, stops bleeding, reduces swelling and generates new flesh.

Indications: (1) Hemoptysis, hematemesis and traumatic bleeding. (2) Abscesses, furuncles and skin fissures on the hands and feet. (3) Lung abscess.

Dosage/Administration: 3–10 g.

Cautions/Contraindications: Incompatible with fuzi (*Aconitum*).

4 *Sanqi (Panax pseudoginseng, var. notojinseng)*

Chinese name: 三七. Pharmaceutical name: *Radix Pseudogiseng*.

Part Used: root.

Flavor/Nature: sweet, slightly bitter; warm.

Meridian Affinity: Liver and Stomach Meridians.

Actions: dissolves clots, stops bleeding, mobilizes blood and relieves pain.

Indications: (1) Various types of bleeding. (2) Traumatic injuries. (3) Swelling and pain due to blood stasis.

Dosage/Administration: 3–10 g.

Cautions/Contraindications: Sanqi is warm in nature. If the bleeding is accompanied by symptoms of Yin deficiency, such as a dry mouth, add herbs that nourish Yin and cool blood.

5 *Qiancao (Rubia cordifolia) (India Madder)*

Chinese name: 茜草. Pharmaceutical name: *Radix Rubiae*.

Part Used: root.

Flavor/Nature: bitter; cold.

Meridian Affinity: Liver Meridian.

Actions: cools blood, stops bleeding, mobilizes blood and removes stasis.

Indications: (1) Bleeding conditions due to Heat in the blood. (2) Amenorrhea due to blood stasis. (3) Traumatic injuries, pain due to blood stasis and joint pains of rheumatism.

Dosage/Administration: 10–15 g.

6 *Aiye (Artemisia argyi) (Argy Wormwood)*

Chinese name: 艾叶. Pharmaceutical name: *Folium Artemisiae Argyi*.

Part Used: leaf.

Flavor/Nature: bitter, acrid; warm.

Meridian Affinity: Liver, Spleen and Kidney Meridians.

Actions: warms channels, stops bleeding, dispels Cold and relieves pain.

Indications: (1) Various types of bleeding. (2) Deficiency-Cold in the lower-jiao with cold pain in the abdomen, irregular menstruation, dysmenorrhea and vaginal discharge.

Dosage/Administration: 3–10 g.

Section 17 Herbs That Stabilize and Astringe

These are herbs that have their principal actions of astringing and stabilizing. Most of them are sour and astringent. Individual herbs have the ability to hold back sweat, stop diarrhea, hold back semen, reduce diuresis, curtail vaginal discharge, stop bleeding or stop cough. Hence they are suitable for use in a patient in whom the constitution has been weakened by chronic illness or genuine Qi is infirm. Such a patient may show symptoms of unrestrained flow, such as spontaneous sweating, night sweat, chronic diarrhea, dysentery, spermatorrhea, premature ejaculation, enuresis, polyuria, chronic cough with labored breathing, persistent metrorrhagia and persistent vaginal discharge.

Stabilizing-astringing herbs treat only the appearance, not the root. They can prevent exhaustion of genuine Qi from the unrestrained and continual loss and avoid other complications. However, the fundamental cause of illnesses with such unrestrained loss is deficiency of genuine Qi. Hence complete treatment of both root and appearance requires the use of complementary restorative herbs. For example, for spontaneous sweating due to Qi deficiency or night sweat due to Yin deficiency, add respectively herbs that augment Qi or nourish Yin. For chronic diarrhea, dysentery and persistent vaginal discharge due to insufficiency of the spleen and the kidney, add herbs that nourish and strengthen the spleen and the kidney. For premature ejaculation, spermatorrhea, enuresis and polyuria due to kidney insufficiency, add herbs that nourish and strengthen the kidney. For infirmity of the Ren and Chong Meridians causing metrorrhagia, add herbs that nourish the liver and the kidney and those that reinforce the Ren and Chong Meridians. For chronic cough and labored breathing due to insufficiency of the lung and the kidney, add herbs that nourish the lung and enhance the kidney's capacity to receive Qi.

Stabilizing-astringing herbs have the disadvantage of potentially retaining disease-causing evils. In general, if the exogenous pathogenic evil is still present in the exterior, if Dampness has accumulated in the interior, or if interior Heat has not been cleared, then it is inappropriate to prescribe these herbs.

1 Fuxiaomai (Triticum aestivum) (Wheat)

Chinese name: 浮小麦. Pharmaceutical name: *Fructus Tritici Leves*.

Part Used: shriveled wheat grains (that float on water).

Flavor/Nature: sweet; cool.

Meridian Affinity: Heart Meridian.

Actions: augments Qi, eliminates Heat and stops sweating.

Indications: (1) Spontaneous sweating or night sweat. (2) Deficiency-fever syndrome.

Dosage/Administration: 15–30 g.

2 Wuweizi (Schisandra chinensis)

Chinese name: 五味子. Pharmaceutical name: *Fructus Schisandrae.*

Part Used: ripe fruit.

Flavor/Nature: sour; warm.

Meridian Affinity: Lung, Kidney and Heart Meridians.

Actions: astringes the lung, nourishes the kidney, generates fluids, reduces sweating, holds back semen, stops diarrhea and calms the heart and the mind.

Indications: (1) Chronic cough and labored breathing due to deficiency. (2) Fluid depletion with thirst, spontaneous sweating or night sweat. (3) Spermatorrhea, premature ejaculation, or persistent diarrhea. (4) Palpitations, insomnia and excessive dreams.

Dosage/Administration: 3–9 g.

Cautions/Contraindications: Contraindicated when there is exogenous illness in the exterior still, when there is exogenous Heat in the interior, when cough has just started or in the early stages of measles.

3 Wumei (Prunus mume) (Plum)

Chinese name: 乌梅. Pharmaceutical name: *Fructus Pruni Mume.*

Part Used: not quite ripe fruit, heat or sun dried.

Flavor/Nature: sour; neutral.

Meridian Affinity: Liver, Spleen, Lung and Large Intestine Meridians.

Actions: astringes the lung and intestines, generates fluid and subdues roundworms.

Indications: (1) Persistent cough due to lung insufficiency. (2) Persistent diarrhea or dysentery. (3) Diabetes due to deficiency-Heat. (4) Vomiting and abdominal pain due to roundworms.

Dosage/Administration: 3–10 g.

Cautions/Contraindications: Contraindicated when there is exogenous illness in the exterior still or when there is exogenous Heat in the interior.

4 Lianzi (Nelumbo nucifera) (Lotus)

Chinese name: 莲子. Pharmaceutical name: *Semen Nelumbinis.*

Part Used: ripe seed.

Flavor/Nature: sweet, astringent; neutral.

Meridian Affinity: Spleen, Kidney and Heart Meridians.

Actions: strengthens the spleen and stops diarrhea, strengthens the kidney and astringes semen, and nourishes the heart and calms the mind.

Indications: (1) Spleen insufficiency with persistent diarrhea and anorexia. (2) Kidney insufficiency with spermatorrhea or premature ejaculation. (3) Restlessness, palpitations and insomnia.

Dosage/Administration: 6–15 g.

Cautions/Contraindications: Contraindicated in dry constipation.

5 Shanzhuyu (Cornus officinalis) (Bunchberry)

Chinese name: 山茱萸. Pharmaceutical name: *Fructus Corni*.

Part Used: fruit (sarcocarp).

Flavor/Nature: sour; slightly warm.

Meridian Affinity: Liver and Kidney Meridians.

Actions: nourishes the liver and the kidney and astringes.

Indications: (1) Liver and kidney insufficiency with dizziness, blurred vision, aching and weakness of the waist and the knees and impotence. (2) Spermatorrhea, premature ejaculation, urine incontinence and persistent sweating of debility.

Dosage/Administration: 6–12 g.

Cautions/Contraindications: Contraindicated in blazing of kidney-Fire, chronic accumulation of Dampness–Heat or difficulty with urination.

6 Sangpiaoxiao (Paratenodera sinensis) (Praying Mantis)

Chinese name: 桑螵蛸. Pharmaceutical name: *Ootheca Mantidis*.

Part Used: egg case.

Flavor/Nature: sweet, salty; neutral.

Meridian Affinity: Liver and Kidney Meridians.

Actions: tonifies the kidney, augments Yang, holds back semen and astringes urine.

Indications: (1) Kidney insufficiency and Yang exhaustion causing spermatorrhea, premature ejaculation, urinary incontinence, polyuria and profuse vaginal discharge. (2) Male impotence.

Dosage/Administration: 3–10 g.
Cautions/Contraindications: Contraindicated in Yin deficiency with much Fire causing excessive Heat in the bladder and polyuria.

Section 18 Herbs That Expel Parasites

These are herbs that have their principal actions of killing or expulsion of parasites. They are mainly used to treat infestations by such parasites as the roundworm, pinworm, tapeworm and hookworm.

Patients infested with such parasitic worms often show peri-umbilical pain, vomiting, excessive salivation, anorexia or polyphagia, pica and itch in the anus, nose or ear. If the infestation is massive and persistent the patient may develop a sallow complexion and emaciation with potbelly, or edema and weakness. On the other hand, when the infestation is relatively mild or short in duration, many patients do not show any symptoms. In such cases the infestation can be diagnosed only by examining the feces.

In clinical practice, the specific herbs to be selected must accord with the type of parasite and the condition of the patient. In addition, supplementary or complementary herbs must be included as appropriate. For example, if there is retention or stagnation, add herbs that relieve retention or dissipate stagnation. If there is constipation, add cathartic herbs to facilitate expulsion of the worms. If the spleen and the stomach are weakened, so that digestion and transportation are impaired, add herbs that strengthen the spleen and the stomach. If the patient's constitution is weak, treat with restorative herbs simultaneously or prior to treatment with worm-expelling herbs.

Among these herbs there are several that are quite toxic. When prescribing them pay careful attention to their dosage to avoid injuring genuine Qi. When fever is high or abdominal pain is severe, it is best to postpone temporarily the administration of these herbs. Use with great caution in the pregnant or elderly patients.

1 Shijunzi (Quisquslis indica) (Rangoon Creeper)

Chinese name: 使君子. Pharmaceutical name: *Fructus Quisqualis*.

Part Used: ripe fruit.

Flavor/Nature: sweet; warm.

Meridian Affinity: Spleen and Stomach Meridians.

Actions: kills parasites and relieves accumulation.

Indications: Roundworm infestation and infantile malnutrition.
Dosage/Administration: 6–10 g.

Cautions/Contraindications: Overdosing can cause hiccup, dizziness and vomiting. These symptoms generally resolve when the herb is discontinued.

2 *Kuliangenpi (Melia azedarach, toosendan) (Chinaberry)*

Chinese name: 苦楝根皮. Pharmaceutical name: *Cortex Meliae*.

Part Used: root bark. (Kulianpi is the bark of the tree.)

Flavor/Nature: bitter; cold. Poisonous.

Meridian Affinity: Spleen, Stomach and Liver Meridians.

Actions: kills parasites and cures tinea.

Indications: (1) Roundworm, hookworm and pinworm infestation. (2) Tinea capitis and scabies (applied topically).

Dosage/Administration: 6–10 g.

Cautions/Contraindications: Do not overdose or prolong treatment. Contraindicated in weak constitution or liver diseases. It can induce vomiting in some cases.

3 *Binglang (Areca catechu) (Betel Palm)*

Chinese name: 槟榔. Pharmaceutical name: *Semen Arecae*.

Part Used: ripe seed.

Flavor/Nature: acrid, bitter; warm.

Meridian Affinity: Stomach and Large Intestine Meridians.

Actions: kills parasites, relieves accumulation and mobilizes Qi and water.

Indications: (1) Intestinal parasites. (2) Food retention and Qi stagnation causing abdominal distention, constipation, diarrhea or dysentery with tenesmus. (3) Edema and the swelling and pain of beri-beri. (4) In addition, may be effective in malaria.

Dosage/Administration: 6–15 g. May increase to 30–60 g when used alone for tapeworm and intestinal fluke infestation.

Cautions/Contraindications: Contraindicated in diarrhea due to spleen insufficiency.

4 Nanguazi (Cucurbita moschata) (Pumpkin)

Chinese name: 南瓜子. Pharmaceutical name: *Semen Cucurbitae Moschatae*.

Part Used: seed.

Flavor/Nature: sweet; neutral.

Meridian Affinity: Stomach and Large Intestine Meridians.

Actions: kills parasites.

Indications: Tapeworm or roundworm infestation.

Dosage/Administration: 60–120 g.

Guidance for Study

I Aim of Study

This chapter presents the most commonly used herbs in CM in 18 basic categories. For each herb it provides essential information on its properties, meridian affinity, actions and indications, dosages and cautions and contraindications.

II Objectives of Study

Upon completion of this chapter, the learners will

1. Be familiar with the 18 basic categories of herbs;
2. Be familiar with the essential information on the properties, meridian affinity, actions and indications, dosages and cautions and contraindications in the use of each herb.

III Exercises for Review

1. What are herbs that release exterior? Compare and contrast the actions and indications of warm-acrid and cool-acrid herbs for releasing exterior.
2. What are the actions and indications of mahuang (*Ephedra*)? What considerations should be taken into account when prescribing it?
3. What are the actions and indications of guizhi (*Cinnamomum*)?
4. What are the actions and indications of zisu (*Perilla*)?

5. Compare and contrast the actions and indications of jingjie (*Schizonepeta*) and fangfeng (*Saposhnikovia*).
6. Describe the actions and indications of bohe (*Mentha*), chantui (*Cryptotympana*), chaihu (*Bupleurum*), gegen (*Pueraria*), qianghuo (*Notopterygium*), xixin (*Asarum*).
7. Characterize herbs that cool heat. Compare and contrast the actions and indications of the main subcategories.
8. Describe the actions and indications of shigao (Gypsum) and zhimu (*Anemarrhena*).
9. Describe the actions and indications of zhizi (*Gardenia*) and baitouweng (*Pulsatilla*).
10. Huangqin (*Scutellaria*), huanglian (*Coptis*) and huangbai (*Phellodendron*) all cool Heat and dry Dampness. What are the differences between them?
11. Describe the actions and indications of longdancao (*Gentian*)?
12. Which kind of fetal distress is huangqin (*Scutellaria*) available to treat?
13. Compare and contrast the actions and indications of qinghao (*Artemisia*) and digupi (*Lycium*).
14. Compare and contrast the actions and indications of longdancao (*Gentian*) and xiagucao (*Prunella*)?
15. Describe the actions and indications of shengdihuang (*Rehmannia*)?
16. Compare and contrast the actions and indications of mudanpi (*Paeonia suffruticosa*) and chishaoyao (*Paeonia lactiflora*)?
17. Compare and contrast the actions and indications of pugongying (*Taraxacum*) and banlangen (*Isatis*)?
18. Describe the actions and indications of herbs that induce catharsis.
19. What precautions should be taken when prescribing cathartic herbs?
20. Dahuang (*Rheum*) is often prepared differently for different purposes. Describe the differences.
21. What are the actions and indications of mangxiao (*Mirabilite*) and fanxieye (*Cassia*) respectively?
22. Describe the actions and indications of herbs that dispel Wind–Dampness?
23. Duhuo (*Angelica pubescens*), fangji (*Stephania*), qinjiao (*Gentiana*), sangjisheng (*Loranthus*) and weilingxian (*Clematis*) are all used to dispel Wind–Dampness. Describe their differences.
24. Compare and contrast the actions and indications of mugua (*Chaenomeles*) and sangjisheng (*Loranthus*).
25. Compare and contrast the actions and indications of fangji (*Stephania*) and qinjiao (*Gentiana*).
26. Compare and contrast the actions and indications of duhuo (*Angelica pubescens*) and qianghuo (*Notopterygium*).
27. Give a brief description of the aromatic herbs that dissipate Dampness? What are their actions and indications?
28. Cangzhu (*Atractylodes*) and houpo (*Magnolia*) both dry Dampness. Describe the differences in their application.

29. Compare and contrast the actions and indications of peilan (*Eupatorium*) and huoxiang (*Agastaches*) respectively?
30. Give a brief description of herbs that drain water. How do they differ from herbs that dissipate Dampness?
31. What are the precautions to be considered when prescribing herbs that dissipate Dampness?
32. Which herbs should be used to treat difficult and painful urination due to stones? Briefly describe their properties and actions.
33. Which herbs should be used to treat jaundice? Briefly describe their properties and actions.
34. Jinqiancao (*Glechoma*), cheqianzi (*Plantago*), zexie (*Alisma*) and zhuling (*Polyporus*) can all be used to treat difficult and painful urination. Compare their suitability and usage.
35. What are the actions and indications of yiyiren (*Coix*)?
36. Briefly describe herbs that warm the interior. What are their actions and indications?
37. Rougui and guizhi are both derived from Cinnamomum cassia. What are their differences? Compare and contrast their actions and indications.
38. What are the actions and indications of ganjiang (*Zingiber*)?
39. Compare and contrast the actions and indications of wuzhuyu (*Evodia*) and dingxiang (*Syzygium*)?
40. Briefly describe the herbs that regulate Qi. What are their actions and indications?
41. Compare and contrast the actions and indications of chenpi (*Citrus tangerina*) and zhishi (*Citrus aurantium*)? Compare and contrast the actions and indications of muxiang (*Aucklandia*) and xiebai (*Allium*).
42. Xiangfu (*Cyperus*) and chuanlianzi (*Melia*) both have affinity for the Liver Meridian. How are they used clinically?
43. Compare and contrast the actions and indications of zhishi (*Citrus aurantium*) and houpo (*Magnolia*).
44. Briefly describe the herbs that relieve food retention. What are their actions and indications?
45. Discuss the combined use of herbs that relieve food retention and herbs that mobilize Qi.
46. Discuss the combined use of herbs that mobilize Qi and herbs that strengthen spleen?
47. Compare and contrast the properties, actions and indications of shanzha (*Crataegus*) and laifuzi (*Raphanus*).
48. Briefly describe herbs that stimulate blood circulation and relieve blood stasis. What are their actions and indications? Which of them are useful for treating traumatic injuries?
49. What are the actions and indications of yimucao (*Leonurus*)? In what ways is it important for gynecology?
50. Compare and contrast the actions and indications of chuanxiong (*Ligusticum*) and danshen (*Salvia*).

51. Compare and contrast the actions and indications of taoren (*Prunus persica*) and honghua (*Carthamus*)?
52. Compare and contrast the actions and indications of sanleng (*Sparganium*) and ezhu (*Curcuma*)?
53. Briefly describe the herbs that dissolve Phlegm, stop cough and relieve asthma. What are their actions and indications?
54. Compare and contrast the actions and indications of banxia (*Pinellia*), gualou (*Trichosanthes*), and jiegeng (*Platycodon*).
55. Mahuang (*Ephedra*), shigao (gypsum), chenpi (*Citrus tangerina*), beimu (*Fritillaria*), gualou (*Trichosanthes*) and xingren (*Prunus armeniaca*) can be all used to treat cough and asthma. Compare and contrast their clinical application.
56. Which illnesses of Phlegm are banxia (*Pinellia*) and gualou (*Trichosanthes*) suitable for treating?
57. Compare and contrast the actions and indications of baibu (*Stemona*), xingren (*Prunus armeniaca*), zisuzi (*Perilla*), sangbaipi (*Morus*), tinglizi (*Lepidium*).
58. Compare and contrast the use of banxia (*Pinellia*) and wuzhuyu (*Evodia*) to treat vomiting.
59. Briefly describe herbs that restore. What are their actions and indications?
60. Compare and contrast the properties, actions and indications of danggui (*Angelica sinensis*) and baishaoyao (*Paeonia*).
61. What are the actions and indications of huangqi (*Astragalus*)? Renshen (*Panax*) and huangqi are both important herbs that restore. Compare and contrast their actions and clinical applications.
62. Compare and contrast the actions and clinical applications of baizhu (*Atractylodes*) and shanyao (*Dioscorea*)?
63. Compare and contrast the actions and indications of dangshen (*Codonopsis*) and gancao (Glycyrrhiza).
64. Compare and contrast the actions and indications of baizhu (*Atractylodes macrocephala*) and cangzhu (*Atractylodes lancea*).
65. Compare and contrast the actions and indications of maimendong (*Ophiopogon*), yuzhu (*Polygonatum*) and shashen (*Glehnia*).
66. Hutaoren (*Juglans*) and dongchongxiacao (Cordyceps) are both used to treat cough and asthma. What are their differences?
67. Shoudihuang (*Rehmannia*) and gouqizi (*Lycium*) both nourish the liver and the kidney. Compare and contrast their actions and clinical applications.
68. Compare and contrast the actions and clinical applications of yinyanghuo (*Epimedium*) and bajitian (*Morinda*)?
69. Compare and contrast the actions and indications of duzhong (*Eucommia*) and xuduan (*Dipsacus*)?
70. Compare and contrast the actions and clinical applications of nuzhenzi (Ligustrum) and mohanlian (*Eclipta*).
71. Compare and contrast the actions and clinical applications of ejiao (*Equus*) and heshouwu (*Polygonum*).

72. Compare and contrast the actions and indications of shengdihuang and shoudihuang (*Rehmannia*).
73. Compare and contrast the actions and indications of baihe (*Lilium*) and guiban (*Chinemys*).
74. Briefly describe the herbs that calm the mind. What are their actions and clinical applications?
75. Compare and contrast the actions and indications of suanzaoren (*Ziziphus*) and baiziren (*Biota*).
76. How is yuanzhi (*Polygala*) used in clinical practice?
77. Compare and contrast the actions and indications of longgu (fossil bone) and muli (*Ostrea*)?
78. Briefly describe herbs that calm the liver and extinguish Wind. What are their actions and clinical applications?
79. Compare and contrast the actions and indications of tianma (*Gastrodia*) and gouteng (*Uncaria*).
80. Compare and contrast the actions and indications of baijiangcan (*Bombyx*), quanxie (*Buthus*) and wugong (*Scolopendra*).
81. Compare and contrast the actions and indications of dilong (*Pheretima*) and shijueming (*Haliotis*).
82. Briefly describe the aromatic herbs that open orifices. What are their actions and clinical applications?
83. Compare and contrast the actions and indications of bingpian (*Dryobalanops*) and shexiang (*Moschus*).
84. Compare and contrast the actions and indications of shichangpu (*Acorus*) and suhexiang (*Liquidambar*).
85. Briefly describe the herbs that stop bleeding. What are their actions and clinical applications?
86. Compare and contrast the actions and indications of xiaoji (*Cephalanoplos*) and diyu (*Sanguisorba*).
87. How are baiji (*Bletilla*) and sanqi (*Panax pseudoginseng*) used clinically?
88. Compare and contrast the actions and indications of qiancao (*Rubia*) and aiye (*Artemisia*).
89. Briefly describe the herbs that stabilize and astringe. What are their actions and clinical applications?
90. Compare and contrast the actions and indications of fuxiaomai (*Triticum*), wuweizi (*Schisandra*), shanzhuyu (*Cornus*), wumei (*Mume*), lianzi (*Nelumbo*) and sangpiaoxiao (*Paratenodera*).
91. Briefly describe the herbs that expel parasites. What are their actions and clinical applications? How should be they supplemented or complemented with other herbs?
92. Describe the precautions to be taken when prescribing shijunzi (*Quisqualis*)?
93. Compare and contrast the actions and indications of kuliangenpi (*Melia*), binglang (*Areca*) and nanguazi (*Cucurbita*).

Part III
Chinese Medicinal Formulas

Chapter 8
Basic Principles of CM Herbal Formulation

Theory, treatment strategy, formulas and herbs together form the fundamentals of traditional Chinese herbal medicine. The physician must diagnose the patient's illness, devise a strategy for treating it and select the herbs to apply. The herbs selected must be compatible with one another and must fully address the root and appearance of the patient's illness.

This chapter introduces the basic principles that govern the construction of medicinal formulas, their preparations and administration.

Section 1 Construction of Herbal Formulas

Illnesses may be simple or complex. Some simple illnesses may be effectively treated with a single herb. More complex illnesses may require a complex prescription containing several herbs, sometimes as many as dozens. A complex prescription must be carefully constructed so that the desired therapeutic efficacy is enhanced and all the causes and symptoms the patient manifests can be addressed.

I Composition of Formulas

The formula is devised on the basis of the causes and symptoms of an illness. These determine the organizing principle for constructing the formula and the organizing principle guides the selection of the specific herbs and the amount of each.

The organizing principle in CM organizes the herbs in a formula in four categories: chief, deputy, assistant and envoy herbs – but not all formulas contain all four categories. The chief herbs are directed against, and have the greatest effect on, the main cause or symptoms. The deputyherbs enhance the effectiveness of the chief herbs; they may also be directed against other important symptoms of the illness or a co-existing illness. The assistant herbs are selected for three functions: to enhance the effects of the chief or deputy herbs; to treat the non-dominant symptoms; and

Z.W. Liu and L. Liu (eds.), *Essentials of Chinese Medicine: Volume 2*,

to moderate or eliminate potentially poisonous or harsh effects of the chief, deputy or another assistant herb. The envoy herbs direct the other herbs in the formula to a certain meridian or region of the body or harmonize their actions. There are no strict requirements for the amounts of the chief, deputy, assistant or envoy herbs in the construction of formulas. In general, the number of chief herbs is smaller than the number of deputy or assistant herbs.

An example of a complex prescription is ***Mahuang Tang***, which is designed to treat exogenous illnesses of Cold in exterior. In this illnesses the main symptoms are fever, cold-intolerance, headache, joint aches, absence of sweating, labored breathing, and a floating and tight pulse. ***Mahuang Tang*** is designed to expel exogenous Wind and Cold from exterior, mobilize stagnant lung-Qi and relieve the labored breathing. Its formulation is as follows.

Chief herb: mahuang (*Ephedra*), which is acrid and warm, induces sweating and releases exterior, mobilizes lung-Qi and eases labored breathing.

Deputy herb: guizhi (*Cinnamomum*), which is acrid, sweet and warm, warms the channels, releases the superficies and aids mahuang in inducing sweating and releasing the exterior.

Assistant herb: xingren (*Prunus*), which is bitter and warm, assists mahuang to mobilize lung-Qi and ease labored breathing.

Envoy herb: *gancao* (*Glycyrrhiza*), which is sweet and warm, harmonizes the actions of the other herbs. Since both mahuang and xingren have affinity for the Lung Meridian, there is no need in this formula for an herb to direct them to that meridian.

Analysis of the formula of Mahuang Tang shows that its construction emphasizes synergism between the ingredient herbs in order to obtain greater efficacy and to cover a broader range of symptoms.

II Modification of Formulas

A complex prescription is composed of a number of herbs, and modification of its ingredients may change its effects, efficacy and range of application. Just as a patient's illness and the herbs' properties determine the organizing principles in constructing the herbal formula, so do changes in the patient's clinical condition guide the modification of the formula. This ability to modify the formula gives the physician considerable flexibility to tailor the treatment to the patient's needs and circumstances.

Modification of formulas may involve adding or subtracting of ingredients, changing the amounts of some or all of the ingredients or changing the formulation (physical form) of the formula.

1 Modification of Ingredients

Modification by adding or subtracting ingredients is of two types. In one type, the assistant and envoy herbs are changed. In general, the role of these herbs in the complex prescription is relatively minor, so that changing them does not fundamentally change the applicability of the prescription. This approach is appropriate when the main illness is unchanged. In the other type, the deputy herbs are changed. As the deputy herbs assist the chief herbs and focus on the main symptoms, this type of modification may well change the basic actions and applicability of the formula.

Consider **Mahuang Tang**. The following two examples clearly demonstrate the consequences of modifying the deputy herbs.

In one, the deputy herb, guizhi, is removed. The resulting formula – which has the formula: mahuang, xingren and gancao – is called **San Ao Tang**. Mahuang still serves as the chief herb, but without the cooperation of guizhi its efficacy in inducing sweating is weaker than that of **Mahuang Tang**. Since xingren is now the deputy and its main effect is to stop cough and relieve labored breathing, **San Ao Tang** is more suitable for treating cough and wheezing due to accumulation of Wind–Cold in the lung.

In the other, baizhu (*Atractylodes*) is added as an additional deputy herb. The modified drug is called **Mahuang Jia Zhu Tang**, and is devised for treating the early stages of numbness due to Wind–Cold–Dampness accumulation.

These two formulas both use mahuang as the chief herb. They differ from **Mahuang Tang** only in the subtraction and addition, respectively, of a deputy herb; yet as a result they have different actions and are used to treat different disorders.

2 Modification of Amounts

The actions of an herbal formula depend not only upon the composition of its formulation but also upon the amounts of the individual ingredients. Modification of the amount of even one herb may alter the balance of the interaction of all the ingredient herbs, and may affect the efficacy and application of the formula.

Consider **Xiao Cheng Qi Tang** and **Houpo San Wu Tang**. The formulas of these two complex prescriptions include the same three ingredient herbs, yet because of the different amounts of the individual herbs the roles of the herbs change (reversal of chief and assistant herbs).

Ingredient Herbs	**Xiao Cheng Qi Tang**	**Houpo San Wu Tang**
Houpo (*Magnolia*)	6 g (assistant)	24 g (chief)
Zhishi (*Citrus aurantium*)	6 g (deputy)	12 g (deputy)
Dahuang (*Rheum*)	12 g (chief)	12 g (assistant/envoy)

Xiao Cheng Qi Tang acts mainly to purge accumulated Heat and is used mainly to treat illnesses of Heat accumulation in the Yangming Meridian. **Houpo San Wu Tang** acts mainly to mobilize Qi and relieve abdominal fullness and is used to mainly to treat Qi stagnation with abdominal distention and constipation.

3 *Modification of Formulation*

How an herbal complex prescription is formulated, its physical form, is potentially of consequence. The same formula, with the same ingredient herbs in the same relative amounts, can have different actions and applications when formulated differently. For example, **Li Zhong Wan** (pill) and **Renshen Tang** (decoction) are composed of the same ingredients at the same amounts, yet **Li Zhong Wan** is used to treat deficiency-Cold in the middle-jiao whereas **Renshen Tang** is used to treat deficiency-Cold in the upper and middle-jiao. The effect of **Renshen Tang** is also stronger and more immediate. In general, decoctions are used for acute disorders and pills are often selected for chronic and non-urgent disorders.

Section 2 Classification of Herbal Formulas

Many classification systems for herbal formulas have been devised in traditional CM. There are systems based on the nature or pattern of illnesses or their causes or organ involvement, the composition of the formulas of the herbs and their treatment strategy, as well as various combinations of these systems. This textbook will use a classification system based on the action of the herbs. In this system, the formulas are classified as follows:

Section 1: formulas that release the Exterior
Section 2: formulas that drain downward
Section 3: formulas that harmonize
Section 4: formulas that clear Heat
Section 5: formulas that warm the Interior
Section 6: formulas that restore (tonify)
Section 7: formulas that astringe
Section 8: formulas that calm the mind
Section 9: formulas that resuscitate
Section 10: formulas that regulate Qi
Section 11: formulas that regulate blood
Section 12: formulas that eliminate Dampness
Section 13: formulas that dissipate Phlegm
Section 14: formulas that expel Wind
Section 15: formulas that moisten Dryness
Section 16: formulas that relieve food retention

Section 3 Common Dosage Forms of Herbal Formulas

Constructing the herbal formula in accordance with the principles of composition is not the last step of the physician's responsibility. The herbal formula should also be prepared in an appropriate physical form based on the needs of a patient and the characteristics of the herbs. The different types of prepared form of the formulas are called dosage forms. In this section, some common types of dosage forms are discussed. There are many other forms available and new forms continue to be devised as new technology becomes available. The most commonly used dosage forms are the following.

I Decoctions

The herbs are soaked in water, a mixture of wine and water, or some other suitable solvent. They are boiled for a specified period of time. After some cooling, the liquid is strained from the herbs.

Decoctions are mostly taken by oral, but may be used externally for washing, steaming or oral rinsing.

Advantages: Decoctions are usually absorbed rapidly. Their effects are strong and immediate. It is especially easy to modify the formula in response to changes in the illness. The decoction is especially suitable for patients with acute and severe illnesses or for those whose illness is still in changing.

Disadvantages: The decoction tends to have a large volume. The active principles of herbs may be difficult to extract or may dissipate rapidly. Decoctions may be difficult or time-consuming to prepare, and are unsuited for mass production. They are not portable. They often have a bad taste.

II Powders

The herbs are ground, mixed and sifted into a relatively uniform powder.

Powders may be ingested or applied externally. Bioactive herbal ingredients for ingestion are generally prepared as a fine powder and are taken directly or with warm water. Some are prepared as coarse-grained powders and are boiled in water when needed for ingestion. Powders for external application are mainly used for disorders of the skin, throat or eyes. These should be ground finely to avoid irritating the injured tissues.

Powders can be prepared ahead of time and their preparation is less wasteful. They are usually absorbed quickly. They can be stored for a long time and are easily portable.

Powders are not decocted with the other herbs, but are taken with warm water or with the strained supernatant from decoctions.

III Pills

The herbs are ground into a fine powder, or extracts of the herbs are concentrated. A viscous medium is then added, and the suspension is formed into firm round pills.

Advantages: Pills tend to have a longer duration of action. Being less wasteful to prepare they tend to have a lower cost. They are convenient to store and to administer. Pills are especially suitable for illnesses that progress slowly or are due to deficiency.

Disadvantages: Pills tend to be absorbed more slowly. However, certain ingredients in pill form do have fast and potent action; they are mostly composed of aromatic or highly toxic herbs that are not suitable for decoction.

The most common types of pills are made with honey, water, paste, or from concentrates.

Pills, like powders, are taken directly with warm water or with the strained supernatant from decoctions.

IV Soft Extracts

The herbs are decocted in water or vegetable oil, and the supernatant is then simmered until the concentrate has a syrupy or gummy consistency. Soft extracts can be used internally or externally. Internally used soft extracts include syrups from prolonged decoction, liquid extractions, and semi-solid extracts. Externally used soft extracts include hard and soft medicinal plasters.

V Medicinal Wines

The herbs are soaked in rice or millet wine for a specified period of time. Wine is of warm nature. It mobilizes blood circulation and unblocks channels and meridians, has dispersing actions, and is generally able to enhance the actions of herbs. Thus, wine is a suitable vehicle for drugs intended for dispersing Wind-Cold, unblocking channels, and tonification.

Externally applied medicinal wines are often used to disperse Wind from the Exterior, mobilize blood circulation, relieve pain and reduce swelling.

Section 4 Drug Administration

I Decocting Herbs

Of the many formulas of herbs, the dosage form of decoction is the most commonly used in CM.

Equipment: The pot for boiling should be made of ceramic or earthenware. China and stainless steel pots are also suitable. Iron or aluminum is unsuitable, as these materials may chemically interact with the chemical ingredients. The pot should be of an appropriate size, and it should have a tight-fitting lid.

Water: Any clean and fresh water is acceptable. Sometimes other liquids are used, such as a mixture of wine and water. The amount of water is based on the amounts and types of herbs and the boiling time. In general, use enough to cover the herbs by about one and a half inches. The strained liquid of the decoction should be 100–150 mL (3–5 oz).

Type of Fire: There are two types of fire for cooking herbs: the high flame fire and the low flame fire. Usually the decoction is brought to a boil using a high flame fire, then cooked on a lower flame. The type of fire chosen is based on the nature of the herbs and the duration of cooking. For herbs to release the Exterior or to drain downward use high flame, a small amount of water, with a short decocting time. For herbs that restore (tonify) use lower flame, a large amount of water and a long cooking time.

Duration: Let the herbs soak for 20–30 min, then cook for 20–30 min. For herbs that have special usages in decocting the special handling is usually mentioned in the prescription.

Decocted First: Two types of herbs should be decocted first. The first type comprises herbs that are toxic. These herbs should be cooked first for 30–60 min. The second type comprises herbs that are minerals or shells. These herbs should be cooked for a long time so as to extract their bioactive components from the herbs.

Decocted Last: Two types of herbs should be added near the end of cooking. One type comprises aromatic herbs. They should be added to the decoction 3–5 min before the end. The other group comprises herbs that have a much stronger effect if added near the end.

Decocted in Gauze: Some herbs, mainly those that stimulate the throat or digestive tract, should be wrapped in gauze during cooking.

Decocted Separately: Very expensive herbs are usually decocted separately.

Dissolved Separately: Highly viscous herbs cannot be decocted with the others. They are dissolved separately in a small bowl and the solution added to the strained decoction.

II Methods of Administration

1 Timing of Administration

The timing of taking the herbal preparation affects its effectiveness.

After Meals: In general, herbs for treating disorders in the upper-jiao should be taken after meals, as should herbs containing chemical ingredients that irritate the stomach.

Before Meals: In general, herbs for treating disorders of the middle and lower-jiao should be taken before meals, as should herbs that restore or drain.

Hour of Sleep: Herbal formula for calming the mind should be taken shortly before sleep.

For acute disorders it should be taken whenever needed. But for chronic disorders they should be taken at regular intervals.

2 Arrangement of Administration

In general, each decoction is intended for the entire day. It is taken in two or three portions throughout the day. The schedule in specific situations may vary depending upon the clinical purposes. Some formulas may be taken several times throughout the day.

Decoctions may be taken warm or cool – cool for illnesses of Heat and warm for illnesses of Cold. If taking of the decoction induces nausea and vomiting, it is advisable to take a small amount of ground ginger with the decoction or add it to the decoction. Alternately, the decoction may be taken in small portions in succession.

Great care must be taken when oral administration that is toxic or strong. In general, start with a small dose and slowly increase the dosage until the desired effect is obtained. As soon as this occurs, discontinue this herbal preparation.

Guidance for Study

I Aim of Study

This chapter introduces the learners to the basic principles governing the construction of the herbal formulas of the complex prescriptions and their pharmaceutical preparation and administration.

II Objectives of Study

Upon completion of this chapter, the learners will

1. Be familiar with the basic organizing principles for the construction of formulas of complex herbal prescriptions;
2. Understand the importance, motivation and consequences of modifying either the composition or the relative amounts of ingredients of an formula.

III Exercises for Review

1. Explain the organizing principles of a complex prescription of herbs.
2. Explain the importance, motivation and clinical consequences of modifying either the composition or the relative amounts of ingredients of an herbal formula.

II Objectives of Study

Chapter 9
Commonly Used Herbal Formulas

In this chapter 84 of the most commonly used complex herbal formulas are discussed. According to the functions of the formulas, they are classified into the following groups in this textbook:

Section 1:	formulas that release exterior
Section 2:	formulas that drain downward
Section 3:	formulas that harmonize
Section 4:	formulas that clear Heat
Section 5:	formulas that warm the interior
Section 6:	formulas that restore (tonify)
Section 7:	formulas that astringe and stabilize
Section 8:	formulas that calm the mind
Section 9:	formulas that open orifices (resuscitate)
Section 10:	formulas that regulate Qi
Section 11:	formulas that regulate blood
Section 12:	formulas that eliminate Dampness
Section 13:	formulas that dissipate Phlegm
Section 14:	formulas that dispel Wind
Section 15:	formulas that relieve Dryness
Section 16:	formulas that relieve accumulations

Section 1 Formulas That Release Exterior

Exterior-releasing formulas comprise all those constructed around herbs that are acrid, light and volatile. These herbs have the ability to induce sweating, release the superficies and penetrate rashes. Exterior-releasing formulas are used to treat illnesses affecting exterior. Among the Eight Methods they belong to the Method of Diaphoresis.

The word exterior refers to the superficies of the body. It is the outer layer that serves as the defensive barrier for the body. When the six exogenous pathogenic

Z.W. Liu and L. Liu (eds.), *Essentials of Chinese Medicine: Volume 2*,

evils first attack a person, an exterior syndrome will manifest. The key symptoms of exterior include: cold-intolerance, headache, fever with or without sweating, a thin tongue coating and a floating pulse.

Because attacks by exogenous evils may be basically of Cold or Heat nature, the exterior-releasing formulas can be separated into two large categories in accordance with their clinical application: acrid-warm exterior-releasing and acrid-cool exterior-releasing. Regardless of which category it may belong to, the ability of a formula to induce sweating and release exterior is primarily due to its efficacy in facilitating the movement of lung-Qi, normalizing the Nutritive and the Defensive Levels, unblocking openings and channels, and facilitating blood circulation. In clinical practice, there are occasions when the patient's illness requires combining in the same formula both acrid-cool and acrid-warm herbs that release exterior in order to enhance their action of releasing exterior.

If an illness of exterior is not treated, or is treated incorrectly, the pathogenic evil cannot be eliminated from exterior but may penetrate into interior. In that case, the illness may transform into a different illness, with different symptoms.

Formulas for releasing exterior contain mostly herbs that are light and volatile. These must not be overcooked to avoid reducing their therapeutic effects. Also, when administering an exterior-releasing formula it is appropriate to avoid exposure to wind or cold and to bundle up to help induce sweating. However, when inducing sweating to release the exterior, it is best to induce a slight amount of sweating. It is not desirable for the sweating to cover only a part of the body or for it to be excessive. If the sweating does not cover the entire body the pathogenic evil cannot be completely dispelled. If the sweating is excessive then genuine Qi may be injured. If severely excessive it may lead to the collapse of Yang or Yin.

Moreover, if the exterior has not been fully released yet symptoms of interior appear, then it is necessary to release exterior first before treating interior, or release exterior and interior simultaneously. Once the pathogenic evils has passed into interior, it is inappropriate to continue administering an exterior-releasing formula.

I Mahuang Tang (Ephedra Decoction)

1 Source: Shang Han Lun (Treatise on Cold-Attack)

2 Composition

Chief Herb: mahuang (*Ephedra sinica*) 6 g

Deputy Herb: guizhi (*Cinnamomum cassia*) 4 g

Assistant Herb: xingren (*Prunus armeniaca*) 9 g

Envoy Herb: fried gancao (*Glycyrrhiza uralensis*) 3 g

3 Application

Actions: induces sweating, releases exterior, facilitates lung functions, and stops wheezing.

Indications: illnesses of Wind–Cold in the exterior.

Main Symptoms: chills and fever, absence of sweating; headache and body ache; labored breathing; a thin white tongue coating; and a floating and tight pulse.

4 Analysis of the Formula

Mahuang is acrid–bitter in flavor, warm in nature and has affinity for the Lung and Bladder Meridians. It is quite effective in stimulating the body's Yang-Qi. It acts to open pores, facilitate the lung and regulate Qi. It serves as the chief herb.

Guizhi can penetrate both Defensive and Nutritive Levels. As deputy herb it warms the channels and disperses Cold. It also aids mahuang to induce sweating, eliminate evil Qi and harmonize defensive and nutritive Qi.

Xingren lowers lung-Qi. When teamed with mahuang, one facilitates and the other suppresses lung-Qi. Together they are stronger in soothing the lung and relieving labored breathing. It is the assistant herb.

Fried gancao harmonizes the facilitating and lowering actions of mahuang and xingren. It also blunts the harshness of the team of mahuang and guizhi, so that the induced sweating does not become so excessive as to injure genuine Qi. It is the envoy herb.

These four herbs act in concert to release exterior of Cold, mobilize Lung-Qi and resolve all the symptoms.

5 Comments

Mahuang Tang uses mahuang and guizhi together and has vigorous action to release exterior by dispelling exogenous pathogenic evil and induce sweating. Its ability to induce sweating is very strong, and for that reason it is not appropriate to prescribe for patients who have bleeding, epistaxis, sores, urethritis, a delayed pulse or a parched throat. Great care must be taken when it is used in the elderly or those with a weak constitution.

Many formulas have been derived from Mahuang Tang. The following are examples.

Da Qing Long Tang is obtained by increasing the amount of mahuang and adding shigao (gypsum), shengjiang (*Zingiber*), and dazao (*Ziziphus*) to Mahuang Tang. It is designed to treat severe syndrome of Wind–Cold in exterior and Heat in interior, with the following key symptoms: severe fever and chills without sweating, body aches, irritability, and a floating and tight pulse.

Mahuang Jia Zhu Tang is obtained by adding baizhu (*Atractylodes*) to Mahuang Tang. It releases the exterior by inducing sweating and dispelling Cold and Dampness. It is designed to treat rheumatism induced by Wind–Cold–Dampness, with heaviness in the body and absence of sweating.

Ma Xing Yi Gan Tang is obtained by replacing guizhi with yiyiren (*Coix*). It dissipates Dampness to release the exterior, and cures rheumatism with generalized body aches and fever that worsens in the afternoon. The illnesses are caused by Wind–Cold attacking a patient already with chronic Dampness. It is particularly effective at dispelling Cold and dissipating Dampness.

San Ao Tang is obtained by removing guizhi from Mahuang Tang. It soothes the lung and releases exterior; and is designed to treat acute Wind causing nasal congestion, laryngitis, cough and chest tightness. It is particularly effective at dispelling Wind–Cold from the lung.

6 Case Study: Influenza in a Young Adult Male

The patient was a miner and had a very strong constitution. He developed an acute illness with strong chills and high fever, but no sweating. He had cold-intolerance, headache and generalized body aches. His nose was congested with much discharge. His tongue coating was white, and his pulse floating and tight.

He had been treated with **Jing Fang Bai Du San**, with poor results. Then, Mahuang Tang was prescribed for one package per day. After 3-day treatment, he sweated, his fever subsided and his physical condition improved.

(Source: *Journal of New Chinese Medicine*, 1975, 4:32.)

II Guizhi Tang (Cinnamomum Decoction)

1 Source: Shang Han Lun (Treatise on Cold-Attack)

2 Composition

Chief Herb: guizhi (*Cinnamomum cassia*) 9 g

Deputy Herb: shengjiang (fresh ginger) (*Zingiber officinale*) 9 g

Assistant Herbs: baishaoyao (*Paeonia lactiflora*) 9 g
dazao (*Ziziphus jujuba*) 3 pieces

Envoy Herb: fried gancao (*Glycyrrhiza uralensis*) 3 g

3 Application

Actions: acrid-warm release of the exterior and the superficies, induction of sweating and harmonization of the Nutritive and Defensive Levels.

Indications: illnesses of exogenous Wind–Cold in a weakened exterior condition.

Main Symptoms: fever with headache; sweating with wind-intolerance; dry heaves; absence of thirst; a white tongue coating; and a floating and slow or a floating and feeble pulse.

4 Analysis of the Formula

Guizhi is the chief herb. It enhances defensive Yang-Qi, unblocks the channels, releases exterior and dispels Wind from the exterior.

Baishaoyao is the deputy herb. It augments Yin and safeguards the Nutritive Level, preventing leakage from it. When guizhi and baishaoyao are teamed, they regulate defensive and nutritive Qi, so that exterior is released of the pathogenic evils and the Defensive and Nutritive Levels are harmonized.

Of the assistant herbs, shengjiang is acrid and warm while dazao is sweet and warm. Shengjiang helps guizhi release exterior and settle the stomach to stop vomiting. Dazao augments stomach-Qi, strengthens the spleen and generates fluids.

Fried gancao harmonizes the actions of the other herbs. It assists guizhi to augment Yang and consolidate the Defensive Level, and it assists baishaoyao to augment Yin and harmonize the Nutritive Level. It is both assistant and envoy herb.

5 Comments

In the clinical application of Guizhi Tang it is important to accurately identify the illness and indications of the patient. Its action in releasing the exterior is not as strong as that of Mauang Tang. Also, the formula uses double the usual amount of gancao and includes shengjiang and dazao. Thus, in addition to releasing the exterior of Wind–Cold and augmenting defensive Qi, it also strengthens the spleen and the stomach and supports weakened nutritive Qi. Disharmony of the Defensive and Nutritive Levels is an important indication for its use.

It is also important to pay close attention to the extent of sweating. The best is a slight amount of sweating over the entire body. If the sweat comes like flowing water, then the illness will not be eliminated. This is a guideline shared by all diaphoretic formulas.

Although Guizhi Tang is an exterior-releasing formula, it differs from the other diaphoretic formulas in that it teams guizhi with baishaoyao to regulate Yin and with shengjiang and dazao to normalize the interior. It may even be used after the illness has been eradicated, following childbirth, or in illnesses in which the Defensive and the Nutritive Levels are in disharmony. The last condition manifests mild intermittent chills and fever, with sweating and a slow pulse.

6 Case Study: Fever in an Adult Female

For about a year the patient had fever and sweating 2–3 times a day. Her food and drink intake, her bowel and urine functions and her sleep pattern were all normal. She was treated for Yin deficiency, but showed no improvement even after more than 20 packages of herbs. On examination her pulse was slow and soft and her tongue was pale with a white coating.

Diagnosis: Disharmony between the Nutritive and the Defensive Levels.

Treatment: Two packages of Guizhi Tang was prescribed. After 2-day treatment the fever no longer recurred and the sweating stopped.

(Source: *Popular Lectures on the Shang Han Lun*.)

7 Case Study: Excessive Sweating in a Young Adult Male

A young fisherman went to sea on a summer day despite much sweating. Subsequently, he continued to have profuse spontaneous sweating regardless of the season or night or day. He was treated on various occasions with Yu Ping Feng San with added longgu (fossil bone), muli (*Ostrea*) and mahuang root, and Guizhi Tang with added huangqi (*Astragalus*). Following each treatment he improved temporarily, but soon relapsed. Over the year he became more and more fatigued. His skin turned pallid, his sweat pores enlarged and his extremities became numb. He had frequent dizzy spells. His urine volume decreased, but he had no thirst. His food and drink intake was normal. His pulse was floating, slow and forceless on pressure.

Diagnosis: Disharmony of nutritive and defensive Qi.

Treatment: Unmodified Guizhi Tang was prescribed. After 3 days, his entire body felt warmer and his limbs comfortable. The sweating stopped. He was treated with two additional doses of Guizhi Tang with added huangqi (*Astragalus*) 15 g, following which he recovered completely.

(Source: *Fujian Chinese Medicine*, 1964, 5:35.)

III Jiu Wei Qianghuo Tang (Nine-Ingredient Qianghuo Decoction)

1 Source: Ci Shi Nan Zhi (Hard-Won Knowledge)

2 Composition

Chief Herb: qianghuo (*Notopterygium incisum*) 6 g

Deputy Herbs: fangfeng (*Saposhnikovia divaricata*) 6 g
cangzhu (*Atractylodes lancea*) 6 g

Assistant Herbs: chuan xiong (Rhizoma Chuanxiong) 3 g
xixin (*Asarum heterotropoides*) 2 g
baizhi (*Angelica dahurica*) 3 g
shengdihuang (*Rehmannia glutinosa*) 3 g
huangqin (*Scutellaria baicalensis*) 3 g

Envoy Herb: fried gancao (*Glycyrrhiza uralensis*) 3 g

3 Application

Actions: acrid-warm release of exterior; elimination of Wind and Dampness; and clearing of interior Heat.

Indications: exogenous Wind–Cold–Dampness, with Heat in interior.

Main Symptoms: chills and fever; headache; absence of sweating; generalized aches and pain; a bitter flavor in the mouth and slight thirst; a white or slightly yellow tongue coating; and a floating pulse.

4 Analysis of the Formula

Qianghuo is an essential herb that enters the Taiyang Meridians and dispels Cold–Wind–Dampness from the exterior. It improves the joints and relieves numbness and pain of the limbs. It is the chief herb.

Fangfeng is acrid–sweet and warm. It is efficacious in dispelling Wind to end fever and in dispersing Cold to stop pain. It is the moistening herb among herbs that disperse Wind. Cangzhu is aromatic, acrid–bitter, warm and dry. It induces sweating and dissipates Dampness. Fangfeng and cangzhu together help qianghuo to disperse Wind–Cold–Dampness and to relieve numbness and pain of the limbs. They are the deputy herbs.

Among the assistant herbs, xixin, baizhi and chuanxiong form a group. They dispel Cold and Wind, soothe numbness and stop headaches and body aches. Shengdihuang and huangqin, belonging to another herbal group, purge Heat from the interior and prevent injury to the fluids by the acrid-warm and drying herbs.

Fried gancao, which harmonizes the actions of the other herbs, serves as the envoy herb.

These herbs acting in concert not only eliminate Wind–Cold–Dampness but also harmonize interior and exterior. Thus, Jiu Wei Qianghuo Tang dissipates Dampness by diaphoresis and purges Heat from the interior.

5 Comments

This formula is designed for curing acute illnesses caused by Wind, Cold and Dampness evils in all seasons. It is commonly used in illnesses in which the pathogenic evil is strong in exterior but without sweating and in which there is no Heat in the interior. The key symptoms are the following: fever with cold-intolerance, headache, absence of sweating, aches and pains in the body and limbs, and bitterness in the mouth with mild thirst.

In the formula, raising and dispersing herbs are combined with Heat-cooling herbs. It should be noted, however, that it emphasizes acridity, warming and drying. Therefore, it is not appropriate for use in illnesses of Wind–Heat in the exterior or deficiency-Heat in the interior.

6 Clinical Study: Acute Wind–Cold Illness

In a clinical study, Jiu Wei Qianghuo Tang, with appropriate modifications, was used to treat 149 patients with acute Wind–Cold illnesses. The main criteria for inclusion were cold-intolerance and fever, with less fever than chills, headaches and body aches. Some patients had additional symptoms of acute Wind–Cold illness: a floating pulse, a white tongue coating, nasal congestion, cough and indigestion. Of the 149, 120 returned for revisit and follow-up.

Results: One hundred and three patients showed a good response and nine showed some improvement, for a rate of 93%. Eight patients showed no response, for a rate of 7%.

(Source: *Fujian Chinese Medicine*, 1964, 5:13.)

IV Xiao Qing Long Tang (Little Green Dragon Decoction)

1 Source: Shang Han Lun (Treatise on Cold-Attack)

2 Composition

Chief Herbs: mahuang (*Ephedra sinica*) 9 g
guizhi (*Cinnamomum cassia*) 9 g

Deputy Herbs: ganjiang (*Zingiber officinale*) 6 g
xixin (*Asarum heterotropoides*) 6 g

Assistant Herbs: wuweizi (*Schisandra chinensis*) 6 g
baishaoyao (*Paeonia lactiflora*) 9 g
banxia (*Pinellia ternata*) 9 g

Envoy Herb: fried gancao (*Glycyrrhiza uralensis*) 6 g

3 Application

Actions: releases exterior and dispels Cold; warms the lung and dissolves congealed fluids.

Indications: Wind–Cold binding exterior, with Rheum accumulating in interior.

Main Symptoms: chills and fever without sweating; cough and wheezing; copious thin sputum or thick sputum that is difficult to expectorate; and chest tightness and inability to lie down. Or, heaviness and pain in the body; puffiness of the head, face and limbs; a white and smooth tongue coating; and a floating pulse.

4 Analysis of the Formula

In this formula, mahuang and guizhi induce sweating to release exterior, dispel Cold and mobilize lung-Qi and relieve labored breathing. They are the chief herbs.

Ganjiang and xixin are acrid and warm. They dissolve Rheum and aid mahuang and guizhi to dispel Cold and release the exterior. They are the deputy herbs.

There are three assistant herbs in this formula. Baishaoyao nourishes nutritive Qi and conserves Yin. Teamed with guizhi it can harmonize the Nutritive and the Defensive Levels, and can prevent mahuang and guizhi from inducing excessive sweating. Teamed with fried gancao it can generate fluids. Wuweizi conserves lung-Qi, stops cough, and prevents damage of lung-Qi by the acridity and warmth of the deputy herbs. Banxia dissolves sputum, dissipates Rheum, regulates the stomach and stops vomiting.

Fried gancao augments stomach-Qi and regulates the middle-jiao. It also harmonizes the actions of the other herbs, and is the envoy herb.

This formula combines herbs that disperse and herbs that astringe. If only acrid and dispersing herbs are used to release the exterior, lung-Qi may be injured and there is a risk that Yin and the fluids may be damaged. Wuweizi is included to conserve Qi and baishaoyao to augment Yin, so that the pathogenic evils can be expelled without injury to lung-Qi and genuine Qi.

5 Comments

Xiao Qing Long Tang is designed to treat illnesses caused by exogenous Wind–Cold and internally accumulated Rheum. The key symptoms for which it is indicated are: chills and fever, absence of sweat, cough or wheezing, copious thin sputum, a white and smooth tongue coating, and a floating pulse. Since the actions of those acrid-dispersing and warm-dissolving herbs are strong, the physician must ascertain that the illness does involve a struggle between fluids and Cold in the lung and that the patient's constitution is strong enough before applying it.

For illnesses of Yin deficiency with a dry cough, or relatively strong Phlegm and Heat, this formula is not appropriate. If Cold in the exterior is predominant, omit guizhi and replace plain mahuang with honey-roasted mahuang. Where interior Heat causes restlessness, add shigao (gypsum) to purge Heat and calm restlessness. Where interior Heat causes thirst, omit banxia and add tianhuafen (*Trichosanthes*) to purge Heat and generate fluids. Where interior Heat causes dyspnea and wheezing add xingren to mobilize lung-Qi and stop wheezing.

6 Clinical Study: Bronchial Asthma

In a clinical study, 24 patients with bronchial asthma induced by Cold or Heat were treated with higher dosage Xiao Qing Long Tang. The composition was: honey-roasted mahuang 15 g, guizhi 9 g, wuweizi 9 g, ganjiang 9–15 g, banxia 30 g, baishaoyao 30 g, xixin 6–9 g and gancao 9–15 g. Modifications were made on the basis of specific symptoms. If the asthma was induced by Cold and was associated with thick and sticky sputum, xuanfuhua (*Inula britannica*), jiezi (*Sinapis alba*), laifuzi (*Raphanus*) and zisuzi (*Perilla*) were added. If the asthma was induced by Heat, shigao (gypsum) was added. If Heat and Phlegm were congealed in the lung, yuxingcao (*Houttuynia*), beimu (*Fritillaria*) and danzhuli (*Phyllostachys nigra*) were added.

Result: In 20 patients the wheezing subsided following one dose. In some the wheezing disappeared completely within half an hour of administration. In the remaining four patients, complete response occurred after treatment with 6–10 packages of herbs, one package per day.

(Source: *Research Journal of Prepared Chinese Formulas*, 1983, 12:21.)

V Ma Xing Shi Gan Tang (Ephedra, Almond, Gypsum and Licorice Decoction)

1 Source: Shang Han Lun (Treatise on Cold-Attack)

2 Composition

Chief Herbs: mahuang (*Ephedra sinica*) 6 g
shigao (gypsum) 18 g

Deputy Herb: xingren (*Prunus armeniaca*) 9 g

Assistant and Envoy Herb: gancao (*Glycyrrhiza uralensis*) 6 g

3 Application

Actions: facilitates lung-Qi movement; cools Heat and stops wheezing.

Indications: Heat in the lung causing cough and wheezing, with pathogenic evil not cleared from the exterior.

Main Symptoms: persistent fever; wheezing with nasal flaring; thirst; with sweat or without; a thin white or yellow tongue coating; and a floating and rapid pulse.

4 Analysis of the Formula

Mahuang is acrid–sweet and warm. It facilitates lung-Qi movement, releases the exterior and stops wheezing. Shigao is acrid–sweet and strongly cold. It purges Heat from the lung and the stomach, and generates fluids. With shigao to help, mahuang unblocks the lung and stops wheezing without aggravating Heat. With mahuang to help, shigao purges Heat from the lung without producing Cold. Thus, they restrain each other without losing their main therapeutic functions of mobilizing lung-Qi and purging Heat. They are chief herbs together.

Xingren is bitter; it mobilizes lung-Qi and stops wheezing. It helps mahuang to suppress the abnormal rising of lung-Qi. It helps shigao to cool and clear the lung. It is the deputy herb.

Fried gancao augments Qi and harmonizes the middle-jiao. It also mediates the cooling and warming, the facilitating and suppressing actions of the other herbs. It is the envoy herb.

These herbs acting together form a formula that facilitates lung-Qi, purges Heat and stops wheezing.

5 *Comments*

When mahuang and shigao are used in concert, they preserve their ability to mobilize lung-Qi and to purge lung-Heat. By using a larger amount of shigao the warming action of mahuang is restrained, so that the entire formula retains its acrid flavor and cool nature.

6 *Case Study: Measles in a 3-Year-Old Girl*

The patient had fever for 5 days and a rash for 2. The fever suddenly rose very high. She became restless and irritable. Her face became flushed and her eyes red. She coughed incessantly and had dyspnea with nasal flaring Her lips became dark purple and her feces were watery and her urine scant and red. The rash was dark red. The tongue was red and dry, with a yellow and dry coating. The pulse was surging and rapid.

Diagnosis: Heat and toxin accumulating in the lung and extending to the Nutritive Level.

Therapeutic Principle: Mobilize lung-Qi, dissolve sputum, purge Heat from the Nutritive Level, cool blood and eliminate rash by promoting full eruption.

Treatment: Ma Xing Shi Gan Tang, with additions, was prescribed. The modified formula include: mahuang 5 g, xingren 10 g, lianqiao (*Forsythia*) 10 g, shigao (cooked first) 30 g, shengdihuang (*Rehmannia*) 15 g, Zhejiang beimu (*Fritillaria*) 8 g, taoren (*Prunus persica*) 8 g, chishaoyao (*Paeonia*) 8 g, gegen (*Pueraria*) 12 g, Tibetan honghua (*Carthamus*) 4 g and fried gancao 4 g. After 3-day treatment (one package of herbs per day) the cough decreased. The child became more alert and the temperature began to fall. After an additional 3-day treatment, the cough and dyspnea were relieved. Further treatment to purge Heat and dispel the pathogenic evil was continued to consolidate the response, until there was complete recovery.

(Source: *Journal of New Chinese Medicine*, 1993, 11:43.)

VI Sang Ju Yin (Mulberry and Chrysanthemum Drink)

1 Source: Wen Bing Tiao Bian (Analysis of Febrile Illnesses)

2 Composition

Chief Herbs: sangye (*Morus alba*) 9 g
juhua (*Chrysanthemum morifolium*) 9 g

Deputy Herbs: xingren (*Prunus armeniaca*) 6 g
jiegeng (*Platycodon grandiflorum*) 6 g

Assistant Herbs: lianqiao (*Forsythia suspensa*) 5 g
bohe (*Mentha haplocalyx*) 5 g
lugen (*Phragmites communis*) 15 g

Envoy Herb: gancao (*Glycyrrhiza uralensis*) 3 g

3 Application

Actions: releases exterior; dispels Wind- Heat; mobilizes lung-Qi and stops cough.

Indications: initial stages of illnesses caused by exogenous Wind–Heat.

Main Symptoms: cough; slight fever with discomfort and thirst; a floating and rapid pulse.

4 Analysis of the Formula

Sangye is sweet–bitter in flavor and cool in nature. It clears Wind–Heat from the upper-jiao. Also, it has a high affinity for the Lung Meridian, and can clear Heat from the lung and stop cough. Juhua is acrid–sweet in flavor and cold in nature. It disperses Wind–Heat, clears the head and the eyes and restrains abnormally risen Lung-Qi. They are together the chief herbs.

Xingren and jiegeng mobilize lung-Qi and stop cough. They are the deputy herbs.

Lianqiao clears Heat and vents the exterior. Lugen is sweet and cold. It cools Heat, generates fluids and stops cough. Bohe disperses Wind–Heat from the upper-jiao. These three herbs are the assistant herbs.

Gancao harmonizes the actions of all the herbs, and is the envoy herb. It also acts in concert with jiegeng to soothe the throat.

These herbs all work together to dissipate Wind and Heat from the upper-jiao and mobilize lung-Qi. By doing so all the exterior symptoms can be relieved and the cough stopped.

5 Comments

Sang Ju Yin is a commonly used formula for treating cough due to exogenous Wind–Heat. The key symptoms are cough, mild fever, mild thirst and a floating and rapid pulse.

The formula is composed of four types of herbs: acrid-cool herbs that release the exterior, herbs that purge Heat and remove poison, herbs that stop cough and dissolve sputum, and herbs that purge Heat and generate fluids. Hence the main functions of the formula are to disperse Wind–Heat, mobilize lung-Qi and stop cough.

Sang Ju Yin is not appropriate for illnesses caused by exogenous Wind–Cold.

The main herbs in the formula are light and volatile in nature. They must not be overcooked during preparation of the decoction.

6 Case Study: Exogenous Wind–Heat Illness in a 26-Year-Old Male

The patient had a chronically weak constitution and frequently fell ill to exogenous illnesses. A month prior, he was exposed to Wind and Cold, but did not seek treatment. At the time of examination, he had a dry and sore throat, thirst with a desire to drink, headache, fever, chest tightness and pain, and a worsening cough that produced a small amount of viscous blood-streaked sputum. His tongue was red, with a thin, white but dry coating, and his pulse was floating and rapid.

Diagnosis: This was originally an illness of exogenous Wind and Cold, but because of negligence and lack of proper treatment, the endogenous Heat arose and attacked the lung.

Therapeutic Principle: Release the exterior with acrid-cool formulas to clear Heat and mobilize lung-Qi.

Treatment: Modified Sang Ju Yin was prescribed, with the following composition: sangye 9 g, juhua 9 g, lianqiao 9 g, Zhejiang beimu (*Fritillaria*) 9 g, xing ren 9 g, jiegeng 4.5 g, raw gancao 3 g, shegan (*Belamcanda*) 6 g, qianhu (*Peucedanum*) 6 g, beishashen (*Glehnia*) 9 g and dry lugen 15 g. After 3-day treatment (one package of herbs per day) the cough stopped and the other symptoms improved. The patient was then prescribed three doses of another herbal formula that restores Yin, after which he recovered completely.

(Source: *Shanghai Journal of Chinese Medicine*, 1965, 6.)

VII Yin Qiao San (Lonicera and Forsythia Powder)

1 Source: Wen Bing Tiao Bian (Analysis of Febrile Illnesses)

2 Composition

Chief Herbs: jinyinhua (*Lonicera japonica*) 15 g
lianqiao (*Forsythia suspensa*) 15 g

Deputy Herbs: bohe (*Mentha haplocalyx*) 6 g
niubangzi (*Arctium lappa*) 6 g
jingjie (*Schizonepeta tenuifolia*) 4 g
dandouchi (*Glycine max*) 5 g

Assistant Herbs: danzhuye (*Lophatherum gracile*) 4 g
lugen (*Phragmites communis*) 4 g
jiegeng (*Platycodon grandiflorum*) 6 g

Envoy Herb: gancao (*Glycyrrhiza uralensis*) 5 g

3 Application

Actions: releases exterior with acrid and cold herbs; clears Heat and relieves poison.

Indications: initial stages of Heat-induced febrile illnesses.

Main Symptoms: fever, no sweating or sweating in limited areas (on the upper part of the body); headache, thirst, cough with sore throat; a red tongue tip and a thin white tongue coating; and a floating and rapid pulse.

4 Analysis of the Formula

The chief herbs, jinyinhua and lianqiao, release exterior, cool Heat and remove poison.

Bohe and niubangzi are acrid in flavor and cool in nature. They disperse Wind and Heat, clear the head and the eyes, release exterior and soothe the throat. Jingjie and dandouchi are acrid and slightly warm. They assist the chief herbs in dispersing exogenous pathogenic evils from exterior and in venting Heat. Though jingjie and dandouchi are acrid-warm, when teamed with large amounts of acrid-cool herbs they can enhance the dispersing actions. These four are the deputy herbs.

Danzhuye clears Heat from the upper-jiao. Lugen clears Heat and generates fluids. Jiegeng mobilizes lung-Qi and stops cough. These three are the assistant herbs.

Gancao not only harmonizes the actions of the herbs in the formula, but also settles the stomach and aids jiegeng in soothing the throat. It serves as both assistant and envoy herb.

5 *Comments*

The composition of Yin Qiao San has two characteristics. One is the inclusion of small amounts of acrid-warm herbs among the acrid-cool herbs; this helps to vent exogenous pathogenic evils without thwarting the beneficial effects of the acrid-cool herbs. The other is the combination of herbs that disperse Wind with herbs that purge Heat and remove poison. Thus, the complete herbal formula has several actions: the dispersing of Wind and Heat, the releasing of the exterior, and the purging of Heat and its poison. In clinical practice this combination of purging and dispersal is usually used at the initial stages against febrile illnesses caused by Wind and Heat. The key symptoms are fever and mild aversion to Cold and Wind, sore throat, thirst, and a floating and rapid pulse.

Yin Qiao San is not appropriate for use in illnesses of exogenous Wind–Cold or in the initial stages of Dampness–Heat illnesses.

6 *Clinical Study: Acute Exogenous Wind–Heat Illnesses*

Yin Qiao San was used to treat 115 patients with acute exogenous Wind–Heat illnesses. The main symptoms were mild aversion to wind and cold, fever, spontaneous sweating, headache, thirst or no thirst but with cough, a white tongue coating, and a floating pulse.

For most of the patients the fever subsided with 1-day treatment with one package of herbs. All patients recovered after 2- to 4-day treatment.

(Source: *Guangdong Journal of Chinese Medicine*, 1962, 5:25.)

VIII Section Summary

Exterior-releasing herbal formulas are used mainly for illnesses in exterior caused by exogenous pathogenic evils. On the basis of their effects the seven formulas selected in this section can be grouped in two categories: acrid-warm release of exterior and acrid-cool release of exterior.

1 *Acrid-Warm Release of Exterior*

Herbal formulas in this category are appropriately used in treating illnesses in exterior caused by exogenous Wind and Cold.

Mahuang Tang teams mahuang and guizhi together. It is particularly powerful in inducing sweating and in dispersing Cold, but it also mobilizes lung-Qi and stops wheezing. It is the strongest acrid-warm exterior-releasing formula, and is appropriate for treating illnesses of exogenous Wind and Cold in exterior, with chills and fever, cold-intolerance, wheezing and absence of sweating.

Guizhi Tang teams guizhi and baishaoyao together. Its ability to release exterior by inducing sweating is weaker than that of Mahuang Tang, but it can harmonize the Nutritive and Defensive Levels. Among the acrid-warm exterior-releasing herbal formulas it is the one with gentle action and is particularly suitable for treating illnesses of exogenous Wind–Cold with fever, sweating but with wind-aversion, and all illnesses of disharmony between the Defensive and the Nutritive Levels.

Jiu Wei Qianghuo Tang has stronger action to induce diaphoresis and dissipate Dampness, and it also clears Heat from interior. It is used for illnesses of exogenous Wind–Cold with Dampness, manifested by chills and fever, body aches without sweating, a bitter taste in the mouth with mild thirst, and other symptoms of Heat.

Xiao Qing Long Tang is particularly effective at releasing exterior and dispelling Cold, warming the lung and dissolving Rheum. It is suitable for treating illnesses caused by exogenous Wind–Cold affecting patients who already have accumulation of Cold-Rheum. These patients manifest chills and fever, cough with much clear sputum, and distention and tightness in the chest.

Ma Xing Shi Gan Tang mobilizes stagnant lung-Qi, cools Heat and stops wheezing. It is suitable for treating illnesses of Heat in the lung causing cough and wheezing.

2 *Acrid-Cool Release of Exterior*

Formulas in this category are appropriately used in treating exterior illnesses caused by exogenous Wind or Heat, or the initial stages of Wind–Heat illnesses.

Yin Qiao San is stronger in releasing the exterior and can also purge Heat and remove poison. It is appropriate for treating illnesses of Wind and Heat invading the Defensive Level, in which there is more fever than chills, cough and sore throat, and thirst. It is a mild acrid-cooling herbal formula.

Sang Ju Yin is weaker in its releasing action, but is stronger in mobilizing lung-Qi and stopping cough. It is suitable for treating milder illnesses of Wind and Heat, with these pathogenic evils in the Lung Meridian and cough as the principal symptom. It is the mildest of the acrid-cool releasing herbal formulas.

In clinical practice, care should be exercised in choosing between Sang Ju Yin and Yin Qiao San.

Section 2 Formulas That Drain Downward

In general, this group comprises herbal formulas that rely on herbs which have the actions of facilitating defecation, purging Heat, breaking up accumulations and dispersing fluids, and which are used to treat illnesses of the interior. Among the Eight Methods, they belong to the Method of Catharsis.

There are a variety of pathogenic evils that can attack interior, and correspondingly there are many illnesses that can result, including conditions of Heat accumulation, Cold accumulation, Dryness accumulation, fluid accumulation and many others. At the same time, there are also differences in the patient's body constitution.

In clinical application, it is essential not to prescribe these formulas until the pathogenic evil has departed from the exterior and has lodged in interior. If the exterior has not been cleared when the interior becomes affected, the physician must either treat exterior before the interior or treat both exterior and interior simultaneously, depending on the relative severity of interior and exterior symptoms.

Downward-draining formulas are not appropriate for patients who are elderly or constitutionally weak; for women who may be pregnant, have very recently given birth, or when they are menstruating; or for those who have depletion of fluids or loss of blood caused by their illness.

Furthermore, because downward-draining herbal formulas can easily damage stomach-Qi, their administration must be discontinued as soon as they have taken effects. While taking such formulas it is important to eschew greasy or fatty foods to avoid aggravating any damage to stomach-Qi.

I Da Cheng Qi Tang (Potent Purgation Decoction)

1 Source: Shang Han Lun (Treatise on Cold-Attack)

2 Composition

Chief Herbs: dahuang (*Rheum palmatum*) 12 g

Deputy Herbs: mangxiao (*Mirabilite*) 6 g

Assistant and Envoy Herbs: houpo (*Magnolia officinalis*) 24 g
zhishi (*Citrus aurantium*) 12 g

3 Application

Actions: removes accumulated Heat caused by catharsis.

Indications and Main Symptoms: (1) Illnesses of exogenous pathogenic evil in the *fu* organs of the Yangming Meridian. Main symptoms: severe constipation with flatulence; distention of the abdomen that is tender and firm to touch; or high fever with delirium, much sweating on the hands and feet; a tongue coating that is yellow, dry and rough, or black, dry and fissured; and a pulse that is deep and replete. (2) Heat accumulation leading to fecal impaction with encopresis. Main symptoms: diarrhea of clear green fluid; peri-umbilical pain, with firm abdominal mass upon palpation; dry mouth and tongue; and a slippery and firm pulse. (3) interior Heat causing collapse, convulsion or delirium.

4 Analysis of the Formula

The chief herb, dahuang, has a bitter flavor and a cold nature. It cools Heat, purges Fire, breaks up and purges accumulated Heat. The deputy herb, mangxiao, has a salty flavor and a cold nature. It moistens the dry and softens the hard, and purges Heat. When dahuang and mangxiao are teamed, their ability to purge accumulated Heat is enhanced.

Both houpo and zhishi facilitate Qi movement and reduce diet accumulations and abdominal distention. They assist dahuang and mangxiao in removing congealed pathogenic evils and accelerate the catharsis of accumulated Heat. They both serve as assistant and envoy herbs.

In this herbal formula the amount of houpo is twice that of dahuang. The reason is that the formula is designed for conditions of exogenous Heat joining with the dry feces to cause the illness. Dahuang has a cold nature to purge Heat and a bitter flavor to facilitate defecation. Houpo, on the other hand, is bitter and warm; hence it can facilitate Qi movement and reduce abdominal distention, but cannot purge Heat by catharsis. Thus it is only the assistant herb.

5 Comments

Da Cheng Qi Tang is designed for rapid purgation while preserving Yin. It is indicated in patients who have not defecated for many days, with distention of the abdomen, a tongue coating that is thick, yellow and dry, or black, dry and fissured, and a pulse that is deep, rapid and forceful.

The key clinical feature is that though the pathogenic evil is strong the genuine Qi is not weakened. If genuine Qi is manifestly weakened – as in Qi deficiency with damage to Yin but only moderate Heat accumulation, or weak constitution in an

Table 9.1 Da Cheng Qi Tang and its derived formulas

	Composition	Preparation	Actions
Da Cheng Qi Tang	Dahuang Mangxiao Houpo Zhishi	Da huang added near end of decocting; mangxiao dissolved in strained decoction	Vigorously purges accumulated Heat in the Interior
Xiao Cheng Qi Tang	Dahuang Houpo Zhishi	Three herbs decocted together	Moderately purges accumulated Heat
Tiao Wei Cheng Qi Tang	Dahuang Mangxiao Fried gancao	Dahuang and fried gancao cooked together; mangxiao dissolved in strained decoction	Mildly purges accumulated Heat
Zeng Ye Cheng Qi Tang	Dahuang Mangxiao Xuanshen Maimendong Shengdihuang	Dahuang added near end of decocting; mangxiao dissolved in strained decoction	Nourishes Yin, generates fluids, drains Heat, unblocks bowels

elderly patient, or pregnancy in a woman, etc. – then the formula must be used with great caution, or with modifications.

If Heat accumulation is accompanied by Qi deficiency, renshen (*Panax*) may be added to augment Qi in order to avoid collapse of Qi due to catharsis. If Heat accumulation is accompanied by Yin deficiency, xuanshen (*Scrophularia*), shengdihuang (*Rehmannia*) and other herbs may be added to nourish Yin and moisten Dryness.

In clinical practice, this formula is generally used for simple uncomplicated intestinal blockage, acute cholecystitis, acute pancreatitis, and Heat-induced illnesses at the stage of high fever, delirium, semi-coma, or sudden fainting, indicating that the pathogenic evil is strong in the Yangming Meridian.

A number of other formulas are derived from Da Cheng Qi Tang through modification. In Table 9.1, three are compared with Da Cheng Qi Tang.

6 Case Study: Acute Dysentery in a 47-Year-Old Male

On a mid-summer day the patient developed severe abdominal cramps, accompanied by mucoid and bloody diarrhea, more blood than mucus, and tenesmus. In one single night he had diarrhea over 30 times. He had a stout body and a flushed but dirty and greasy complexion. He was thirsty, preferring cold fluids. His urine was scanty and dark. His lips were red and dry, tongue red at the tip, and tongue coating thick and yellow. His pulse was slippery, rapid and forceful.

Diagnosis: Heat accumulation in the Yangming Meridian.

Therapeutic Principle: Purge accumulated Heat from the stomach and the intestines.

Treatment: Modified Da Cheng Qi Tang was prescribed, with the following composition: dahuang 15 g, houpo 9 g, zhishi 9 g, and mangxiao 12 g. The herbal formula was decocted in water, and was administered in two portions. After one dose, the symptoms improved. After a second dose, all symptoms improved further. The patient was then prescribed Gegeng Huangqin Huanglian Tang to eradicate the illness. All symptoms resolved, and the patient regained complete health.

(Source: *Journal of Chinese Medical Education*, 1977, 2:28.)

II Wen Pi Tang (Spleen-Warming Decoction)

1 Source: Bei Ji Qian Jin Yao Fang (Essential Prescriptions for Emergency)

2 Composition

Chief Herbs: dahuang (*Rheum palmatum*) 15 g
fuzi (*Aconitum carmichaeli*) 6 g

Deputy Herbs: mangxiao (*Mirabilite*) 9 g
ganjiang (*Zingiber officinale*) 9 g

Assistant Herbs: renshen (*Panax ginseng*) 6 g
danggui (*Angelica sinensis*) 9 g

Envoy Herbs: gancao (*Glycyrrhiza uralensis*) 6 g

3 Application

Actions: purges accumulated Cold and warms spleen-Yang.

Indications: abdominal pain due to Cold accumulation.

Main Symptoms: constipation with abdominal pain and cramps below the umbilicus; cold limbs that are slow to warm; aversion to cold, with preference for heat; a white tongue coating, but no thirst; and a deep, taut and slow pulse.

4 *Analysis of the Formula*

Fuzi and dahuang serve together as chief herbs. The formula uses the strong acrid flavor and hot nature of fuzi to warm and replenish spleen-Yang and to dissipate congealed Cold. Fuzi complements dahuang, which purges accumulated Cold.

For deputy herbs the formula uses ganjiang to aid fuzi in warming interior and dispelling Cold, and mangxiao to soften the hard and moisten the intestines.

They are further assisted by danggui and renshen. Danggui also softens the hard and moistens the intestines. Renshen augments spleen Qi and neutralizes dahuang's tendency to induce diarrhea and damage genuine Qi.

Gancao both helps renshen to augment Qi and harmonizes the actions of the other herbs. It serves as the envoy herb.

This formula is an especially fine prescription for dual emphasis – the warming replenishment of spleen-Yang and the purging of accumulated Cold.

5 *Comments*

Wen Pi Tang is a frequently prescribed warm-purging herbal formula. The key symptoms for its use are abdominal pain, constipation, cold extremities, aversion to cold and preference for warmth, a white tongue coating, and a deep, taut but slow pulse.

When prescribing this formula modify it in accordance with the actual situation. If the abdominal distention and pain are prominent, houpo and muxiang (*Aucklandia*) should be added to mobilize Qi and stop pain. If the abdomen is tender and cold, rougui (*Cinnamomum*) and wuzhuyu (*Evodia*) should be added to enhance the ability to warm the middle-jiao and disperse Cold.

6 *Case Study: Cold Accumulation in a 78-Year-Old Male*

The patient was elderly and had a weak constitution. For several days, he could not eat or drink as any eating precipitated vomiting. His complexion was sallow and emaciated. His abdomen was distended like a drum. On palpation it was hard, tender and cold to the touch. He had not defecated for 14 days, and had difficulty urinating. He was irritable and moaned much. His voice was weak and he appeared fatigued. His tongue was gray and dark, and the coating gray and greasy. His pulse was deep, taut and tight.

Diagnosis: Failure of spleen-Yang to act and Yang-Qi to warm, so that Cold accumulates and blocks the stomach and the intestines. This is an illness of abdominal distention due to deficiency of genuine Qi and strength of evil Qi.

Therapeutic Principle: Warm and mobilize spleen-Yang and purge the accumulated Cold.

Treatment: Modified Wen Pi Tang was prescribed, with the following composition: fuzi 30 g (cooked first for 1 h), ganjiang 10 g, renshen 9 g (cooked separately), gancao 4 g and raw dahuang 9 g (ground into powder and added to the decoction). After one dose (a package of herbs), the abdomen was still distended, with periodic pain, but bowel sounds returned and the patient was able to pass flatus. The prescription was continued, but with the addition of muxiang (*Aucklandia*) 6 g, houpo 10 g and binglang (*Areca*) 12 g. After one dose of the expanded formula the patient was able to defecate, producing 5 or 6 pieces of dry feces. His urine also came more easily and the abdominal distention and pain eased. The patient's condition thus changed, but he still manifested the following symptoms: spontaneous sweating, fatigue, a sallow complexion without luster, emaciation, and a pale red tongue with a thin, greasy and slightly yellow coating. Therefore, the therapeutic approach was changed to one of supporting genuine Qi and warming Yang in order to normalize spleen and stomach functions. With this new approach the patient recovered fully.

(Source: *Guangxi Journal of Chinese Medicine*.)

In this case, 30 g fuzi was prescribed, but this is not a normal dosage. Normally the dose of fuzi is below 15 g in one prescription.

III Dahuang Mudanpi Tang (Rhubarb and Tree Peony Decoction)

1 Source: Jin Gui Yao Lue (Essentials of the Golden Cabinet)

2 Composition

Chief Herbs: dahuang (*Rheum palmatum*) 12 g
mudanpi (*Paeonia suffruticosa*) 9 g

Deputy Herbs: mangxiao (*Mirabilite*) 9 g
taoren (*Prunus persica*) 12 g

Assistant and Envoy Herb: dongguazi (*Benincasa hispida*) 30 g

3 Application

Actions: purges Heat, breaks up blood stasis, dissipates masses and reduces swelling.

Indications: early stages of acute appendicitis.

Main Symptoms: pain and tenderness in the right lower abdomen, or right hip pain eased by flexion and aggravated by extension. In more severe cases: localized swelling in the right lower abdomen, with intermittent fever, spontaneous sweating and cold-intolerance. The tongue coating is thin, greasy and yellow, and the pulse slippery and rapid.

4 Analysis of the Formula

Bitter-cold dahuang has the ability to purge accumulated and congealed Heat in the intestines, and to detoxify poisons and mobilize blood circulation. Bitter–acrid mudanpi cools blood and clears Heat from the Blood and the Nutritive Levels, mobilizes blood and dissipates accumulations. When these two herbs are used together, their bitter and acrid flavors enable them to promote downward movement and they are particularly effective in draining accumulated Heat and impurities. They are the chief herbs.

Mangxiao is salty in flavor and cold in nature. It aids dahuang in attacking accumulated Heat and purging it, and aids mudanpi in softening the hard and dissipating stagnation. Taoren has the ability to break up blood stasis and can also moisten the intestines and facilitate bowel movement. It is included to assist the principal herbs in dissipating congealed stagnation and draining downward.

Dongguazi clears Dampness and Heat from the intestines, drains pus and dissolves abscesses. It is an essential herb for treating abscesses in the Interior.

Acting in concert these herbs have the ability to drain downward and remove accumulated and congealed Dampness and Heat in the body, and to mobilize blood circulation and dissipate accumulations and swellings.

5 Comments

Dahuang Mudanpi Tang is designed for treating illnesses of Dampness and Heat congealing together in the lower-jiao. In clinical practice it is suitable in treating those illnesses in which genuine Qi is not deficient but the pathogenic evil is strong. In conditions of both deficiency of genuine Qi and strength of pathogenic evil it is inappropriate.

If the illness manifests mainly Heat strength, it is appropriate to enhance the formula's action to clear Heat and eliminate poison. Pugongying (*Taraxacum*), jinyinhua (*Lonicera*), baijiangcao (*Patrinia*) or other herbs may be added. If the illness manifests mainly blood stasis, it is appropriate to enhance the formula's action to mobilize blood circulation and remove blood stasis. Ruxiang (*Aucklandia*), moyao (*Commiphora*) or other herbs may be added.

6 Case Study: Acute Appendicitis in a 21-Year-Old Male

The patient had acute abdominal pain for 2 days. The pain began in the right lower abdomen, and gradually worsened. It was accompanied by mild fever (38°C = 100.4°F). AT another hospital this was diagnosed as acute appendicitis that had perforated and had led to generalized peritonitis. Surgical operation was advised, but the patient and his family refused surgery and insisted on treatment with Chinese herbal medicine.

On examination, his abdomen was distended, hard and tender. He had not defecated for 5 days. His tongue was deep red, with a thick, yellow and greasy coating. His pulse was taut and rapid.

Diagnosis: Exogenous Heat and blood stasis in the Yangming Meridian.

Therapeutic Principle: Urgent unblocking of the interior and purging of accumulated Heat from the intestines and the stomach.

Treatment: The patient was promptly treated with combined Da Cheng Qi Tang and Dahuang Mudanpi Tang, with additions. The overall composition was as follows: dahuang 20 g, zhishi 15 g, houpo 15 g, mangxiao 10 g, mudanpi 10 g, dongguazi 10 g, baijiangcao 20 g, jinyinhua 15 g, pugongying 22 g, sanqi (*Panax pseudoginseng*) 3 g, and gancao 3 g. An hour after administration, the patient defecated. The stool was initially hard, then loose. He followed with six successive stools, all watery. His abdomen promptly became soft and relaxed. Over the next 2 days he was treated with the same herbal prescription, but at reduced dosage, and his fever subsided. Though the abdominal pain had basically resolved, in his right lower abdomen he still had an egg-sized tender mass. This was treated with herbal medicine that mobilized blood circulation and remove blood stasis. A month later the mass disappeared, and the patient recovered completely.

(Source: *Jiangxi Journal of Chinese Medicine*, 1983, 1:7.)

IV Maziren Wan (Cannabis Pill)

1 Source: Shang Han Lun (Treatise on Cold-Attack)

2 Composition

Chief Herb: huomaren (*Cannabis sativa*) 20 g

Deputy Herbs: baishaoyao (*Paeonia lactiflora*) 9 g
xingren (*Prunus armeniaca*) 10 g

Assistant Herbs: dahuang (*Rheum palmatum*) 12 g
zhishi (*Citrus aurantium*) 9 g
houpo (*Magnolia officinalis*) 9 g

Envoy Herb: fengmi (honey) q.s. (quantity sufficient) to make pills.

3 Application

Actions: moistens the intestines, purges accumulated Heat, promotes Qi movement and unblocks the bowels.

Indications: Heat-Dryness in the intestines and the stomach, with depletion of fluids.

Main Symptoms: constipation with hard stool, frequent urination; a dry, yellow tongue coating, and a rapid pulse.

4 Analysis of the Formula

Huomaren is sweet in flavor and even in nature, and has affinity for the Spleen, Stomach and Large Intestine Meridians. It moistens the intestines, clears Dryness from the stomach and the spleen and promotes defecation. It serves as the chief herb, and gives its name to the formula. (Huomaren is an alternate name for maziren.)

Xingren is sweet in flavor and even in nature. It moistens Dryness, facilitates lung-Qi and moistens the large intestine. Baishaoyao is bitter–sour in flavor and cool in nature, and has affinity for the Liver, Spleen and Lung Meridians. It generates blood, augments Yin and stops pain. Xingren and baishaoyao are together the deputy herbs.

Dahuang, zhishi and houpo together constitute Xiao Cheng Qi Tang (Minor Purgation Decoction), which gently drains accumulated Heat downward and removes Dryness-Heat from the stomach and the intestines. Xiao Cheng Qi Tang serves as the assistant ingredient.

Honey is used as the medium for this pill. Its sweet flavor blunts the severity of illness. It is able not only to aid huomaren in moistening the intestines and facilitating defecation but also to moderate the force of Xiao Cheng Qi Tang to drain downward, thereby counteracting its potential to damage genuine Qi. It serves as the envoy herb.

5 Comments

Maziren Wan is an expansion of Xiao Cheng Qi Tang. It contains two groups of herbs, one group primarily for catharsis and the other primary for moistening, but the overall emphasis is on catharsis. It is commonly used for constipation caused by Dryness and Heat in the stomach and the intestines, which is commonly seen as habitual constipation in elderly persons, constipation following childbirth, and constipation following hemorrhoid surgery.

Because it does contain herbs that induce catharsis and break accumulations, it is not appropriate for repeated use in elderly patients with a weak constitution or with reduced fluids and blood. Such repeated use may damage Qi and blood. In addition, it must be used with utmost caution during pregnancy.

If constipation is due primarily to fluid deficiency, **Wu Ren Wan** (Five-Seed Pill) is a more appropriate formula. Wu Ren Wan is composed of taoren (*Prunus persica*), xingren (*Prunus armeniaca*), baiziren (*Biota orientalis*), songziren (*Pinus koraiensis*) and yuliren (*Prunus japonica*), with chenpi (*Citrus tangerina*) as envoy herb. Its main action is to moisten the intestines, thereby facilitating defecation. Its principal indication is constipation due to insufficiency of fluids, manifested by constipation, a dry mouth with strong thirst, a dry and dehydrated tongue, and a threadlike and impeded pulse. It is frequently prescribed for constipation following childbirth or an illness, or in elderly persons.

There are prominent differences between Wu Ren Wan and Maziren Wan. Wu Ren Wan acts primarily to moisten the intestines and facilitate defecation, whereas Maziren Wan acts primarily to purge Heat and augment Yin.

6 Clinical Study: Post-surgical Constipation

Five hundred patients with constipation following hemorrhoid surgery were treated with Maziren Wan. Four hundred and seventy nine had soft feces that were easy to expel and 21 had no response, for an efficacy rate of 95.8%. Of the 21 cases that did not respond, 16 had habitual constipation. Maziren Wan was quite effective in preventing pain and bleeding.

(Source: *Journal of Chinese Medicine*, 1965, 10:40.)

V Section Summary

Four herbal formulas have been selected to represent those that drain downward. Their principal actions may be grouped into the following three categories: Cold-purgation, Heat-purgation, and catharsis by moistening.

By teaming dahuang, mangxiao, zhishi and houpo, with the amount of houpo twice that of dahuang, **Da Cheng Qi Tang** is specially designed to purge accumulated Heat. It is representative of formulas that treat Heat gelling in the stomach and the intestines, and is indicated for illnesses of exogenous pathogenic evil in the *fu* organs of the Yangming Meridian. These conditions are characterized by all four of the major symptoms (localized mass or swelling, distention, Dryness, and constipation).

Dahuang Mudanpi Tang is designed to purge accumulated Heat, and is the principal formula for treating intestinal abscesses (such as appendicitis).

Wen Pi Tang is the typical formula for purging accumulated Cold. It warms spleen-Yang, and is indicated for constipation with abdominal pain caused by insufficiency of spleen-Yang and gelling of Cold.

Maziren Wan is the typical formula for moistening the intestines and unblocking the bowels. It is constructed by adding intestine-moistening herbs to Xiao Cheng Qi Tang; hence it is capable of purging gelled Heat and is indicated for treating constipation due to Heat-Dryness in the stomach and the intestines with depletion of spleen fluids.

Section 3 Formulas That Harmonize

All formulas in this section that harmonize the Shaoyang Meridian, regulate the liver and the spleen, and harmonize cold and heat are classified as formulas that harmonize. These formulas are designed for treating illnesses of the Cold evil in Shaoyang, dissociation in the functions of the liver and the spleen, mixed fevers and chills, or both interior and exterior similarly affected. Among the Eight Methods of therapy, these formulas belong in the category of the Method of Mediation.

Harmonizing formulas are designed to treat conditions in which the Cold evil has entered the Shaoyang Meridian. Shaoyang belongs to the Gallbladder Meridian, and is located between exterior and interior, so-called "half-interior, half-exterior." In therapy, neither diaphoresis nor vomiting or catharsis is appropriate; only the method of mediation is the most suitable.

The gallbladder and the liver are intimately linked as an exterior–interior dyad. Illness in the Gallbladder Meridian can affect the liver, just as illness in the Liver Meridian can affect the gallbladder. Moreover, illness in the liver and gallbladder can also affect the spleen and the stomach, causing disharmony between the liver and the spleen.

If central Qi is weak, then Cold and Heat can intermingle; that can also lead to disharmony between the stomach and the intestines. If illness in exterior has not resolved yet acute interior symptoms have developed, then using only release of exterior leaves the interior symptoms untouched, whereas using only purging of the interior cannot eliminate the evil from exterior. For these reasons, herbal formulas that harmonize are applied to harmonize the liver and the spleen in order to treat an overactive liver and a weakened spleen, as well as to harmonize in order to cure illnesses in the Shaoyang Meridian.

In general, if the pathogenic evil is in exterior and has not entered Shaoyang, or the disease evil has internalized but Yangming is vigorous, then it is inappropriate to apply a harmonizing herbal formula.

I Xiao Chaihu Tang (Minor Bupleurum Decoction)

1 Source: Shang Han Lun (Treatise on Cold-Attack)

2 Composition

Chief Herb: chaihu (*Bupleurum chinense*) 12 g

Deputy Herb: huangqin (*Scutellaria baicalensis*) 9 g

Assistant Herbs: banxia (*Pinellia ternata*) 9 g
shengjiang (fresh ginger) (*Zingiber officinale*) 9 g
renshen (*Panax ginseng*) 9 g
dazao (*Ziziphus jujuba*) 4 pieces

Envoy Herb: fried gancao (*Glycyrrhiza uralensis*) 6 g

3 Application

Actions: harmonizes and clears the Shaoyang Meridian.

Indications: illnesses of Cold in the Shaoyang Meridian.

Main Symptoms: alternating chills and fever; chest and subcostal fullness; no desire to speak; loss of appetite; irritability with frequent nausea and vomiting; a bitter taste in the mouth with a dry throat; blurred vision; a white and thin tongue coating; and a taut pulse.

4 Analysis of the Formula

Xiao Chaihu Tang is the principal formula for harmonizing the Shaoyang Meridian and removing pathogenic factors from it. In the formula, chaihu and huangqin are used together: one disperses and the other purifies. Together they clear exterior of pathogenic evils (the "half-exterior" part) and clear the interior of Heat (the "half-interior" part); hence they are capable of harmonizing the Shaoyang Meridian.

Banxia and shengjiang both regulate stomach-Qi, suppress abnormally rising Qi and stop vomiting. Renshen, gancao and dazao augment Qi and harmonize the middle-jiao, so they are capable of supporting genuine Qi and helping to dispel pathogenic evils as well as strengthening the interior and preventing penetration by pathogenic evils.

Fried gancao as envoy herb harmonizes the actions of the other herbs.

With these seven herbs, the formula combines herbs with a cold nature and herbs with a warm nature, regularizes the upward and downward movement of Qi, supports genuine Qi and repels pathogenic evils. By so doing it achieves smooth functional coordination of the sanjiao and smooths Qi movement. In this way, all symptoms of such illnesses can be relieved.

5 *Comments*

This is the principal formula for treating illnesses of disharmony in the Shaoyang Meridian. In the clinical analysis of illnesses of Shaoyang, it is important to focus on the key symptoms in order to determine the diagnosis. It is not necessary for all related symptoms to be present.

Also, for Shaoyang illnesses, the physician must avoid such therapeutic methods as diaphoresis, vomiting or catharsis. These methods are appropriate for treating Taiyang and Yangmind illnesses but not Shaoyang illnesses. Instead, the physician must aim only to harmonize Shaoyang in order to avoid precipitating complications.

II Da Chaihu Tang (Major Bupleurum Decoction)

1 *Source: Jin Gui Yao Lue (Essentials of the Golden Cabinet)*

2 *Composition*

Chief Herb: chaihu (*Bupleurum chinense*) 12 g

Deputy Herbs: huangqin (*Scutellaria baicalensis*) 9 g
dahuang (*Rheum palmatum*) 6 g
zhishi (*Citrus aurantium*) 9 g

Assistant Herbs: baishaoyao (*Paeonia lactiflora*) 9 g
banxia (*Pinellia ternata*) 9 g

Envoy Herbs: dazao (*Ziziphus jujuba*) 10 pieces
shengjiang (*Zingiber officinale*) 15 g

3 *Application*

Actions: harmonizes and clears Shaoyang; and purges accumulated Heat from the interior.

Indications: concurrent Shaoyang and Yangming illnesses.

Main Symptoms: alternating chills and fever; chest and subcostal fullness; persistent nausea and vomiting; depression with mild irritability; epigastric tightness or pain; constipation or diarrhea; a yellow tongue coating; and a taut, rapid and forceful pulse.

4 Analysis of the Formula

Chaihu is the chief herb because it specifically penetrates Shaoyang, where it disperses pathogenic evils through the exterior.

Huangqin is bitter in flavor and cold in nature, and has the ability to clear heat in Shaoyang meridian. Chaihu and huangqin together can harmonize Shaoyang. In small amounts dahuang purges Heat and unblocks the *fu* organs. Zhishi facilitates Qi movement and breaks up stagnant Qi. Dahuang and zhishi together can purge accumulated Heat from the interior.

Baishaoyao, banxia and shengjiang are the assistant herbs in the formula. Baishaoyao replenishes blood, softens the liver, and reduces abdominal cramps. Banxia harmonizes stomach-Qi and lowers abnormally rising stomach-Qi. Shengjiang is used in large amount, half as assistant herb and half as envoy herb. It is particularly effective in stopping vomiting.

Dazao, the other envoy herb, regulates defensive and nutritive Qi. Dazao and shengjiang together harmonize the actions of the other herbs.

5 Comments

Catharsis therapy alone is prohibited in Shaoyang illnesses. However, accumulated Heat in Yangming must be purged by catharsis. In concurrent Shaoyang and Yangming illnesses, it is appropriate and convenient to harmonize Shaoyang and purge Yangming simultaneously. Doing so does not contradict the principle of avoiding catharsis therapy in Shaoyang illness while purging the accumulated Heat.

From its formula it is clear that Da Chaihu Tang is constructed by combining Xiao Chaihu Tang and Xiao Cheng Qi Tang, with some additions and subtractions. As the pathogenic evil in Shaoyang extends into the interior, Heat accumulates in Yangming. In such illnesses, the following generally apply. Because genuine Qi is not diminished, renshen and gancao of Xiao Chaihu Tang are removed. Because vomiting is more severe, the dosage of shengjiang is doubled. Though Heat accumulates in Yangming, it causes tightness and pain only in the epigastrium, not in the entire abdomen, indicating that it is relatively mild. Hence dahuang is reduced in amount, houpo is removed and shaoyao is added to the Xiao Cheng Qi Tang portion. With these modifications, not the formula's cathartic effect is reduced and it also stops pain.

In clinical application, the key symptoms calling for this formula are the following: alternating chills and fever; tightness and pain in the chest, flank and epigastrium; vomiting; a yellow tongue coating; and a taut and rapid pulse.

6 Clinical Study: Acute Pancreatitis

One hundred and thirty-two patients with acute pancreatitis were treated using Da Chaihu Tang as the basic prescription. One hundred and twenty-nine had acute edematous pancreatitis, and three had acute gangrenous pancreatitis.

After treatment three patients with gangrenous pancreatitis all died, but those with edematous pancreatitis all recovered. On average the abdominal pain resolved in 4.2 days and the urine amylase level returned to normal in 3.9 days.

(Source: *Liaoning Journal of Chinese Medicine*, 1986, 2:21.)

III Hao Qin Qing Dan Tang (Artermisia-Scutellaria Gallbladder-Clearing Decoction)

1 Source: Chong Ding Tong Su Shang Han Lun (Popular Treatise on Exogenous Febrile Illnesses, Revised Edition)

2 Composition

Chief Herbs: qinghao (*Artemisia annua*) 6 g
huangqin (*Scutellaria baicalensis*) 6 g

Deputy Herbs: zhuru (*Phyllostachys nigra*) 9 g
banxia (*Pinellia ternata*) 6 g
chenpi (*Citrus tangerina, reticulata*) 5 g
zhiqiao (*Poncirus trifoliata*) 6 g

Assistant and Envoy Herbs: Bi Yu San 9 g
fuling (*Poria cocos*) 9 g

Note: Bi Yu San is itself a powder made of herbal formula comprised of huashi (talcum), gancao (*Glycyrrhiza*), and qingdai (*Baphicacanthus cusia*).

3 Application

Actions: clears the gallbladder, dissipates Dampness, harmonizes the stomach and dissolves Phlegm.

Indications: Dampness–Heat in the Shaoyang Meridian.

Main Symptoms: relapsing fever, with mild chills but high fever; a bitter taste in the mouth; chest tightness; regurgitation of sour and bitter fluids, or vomiting of viscous and yellow mucus. In severe cases: dry heaves with persistent hiccup; tightness and pain in the chest and flanks; a red tongue with white coating; and a rapid but dissociated pulse that is slippery in the right wrist but taut in the left wrist.

4 Analysis of the Formula

Hao Qin Qing Dan Tang is designed for illnesses of Heat in the gallbladder, with Dampness–Heat and thick Phlegm in the Shaoyang Meridian.

The two chief herbs, qinghao and huangqin, used together are especially efficacious for clearing away exogenous evils from the half-interior and half-exterior illnesses of Shaoyang.

The deputy herbs, zhuru, chenpi, zhiqiao and banxia, clear the stomach, stop vomiting and lower abnormally rising stomach-Qi.

Fuling and Bi Yu San are used as assistants to direct Heat downward from the gallbladder, leach out Dampness, and harmonize the herbs. Together they drain Heat from Shaoyang and dissipate Dampness and Phlegm.

5 Comments

Hao Qin Qing Dan Tang and Xiao Chaihu Tang both harmonize and clear illnesses from the Shaoyang Meridian, and are used to treat illnesses in Shaoyang manifesting alternating chills and fever, and chest and subcostal tightness. There are differences between them. Xiao Chaihu Tang contains renshen, which augments and supports genuine Qi as it harmonizes. It is therefore particularly suitable for treating disharmony of the gallbladder and the stomach, in which stomach-Qi is weakened but rising abnormally. Hao Qin Qing Dan Tang, on the other hand, uses qinghao, huashi and fuling to harmonize Shaoyang while purging Heat, dissipating Dampness and dissolving Phlegm. In clinical application, the key is Dampness–Heat in Shaoyang with more Heat than Dampness.

6 Case Study: Exposure to Summer Heat with Dampness, Erroneously Treated, in a 48-Year-Old Woman

The patient suffered from fever at dusk and coldness at dawn, without sweating. She had mild cold-aversion, a mildly dry mouth without thirst and preference for warm drinks, a cough that produces yellow and sticky sputum, mild hoarseness, loss of appetite, aches and weakness in the knees, oliguria, and soft feces. Her tongue was red, with a yellow and greasy coating, and her pulse was threadlike and moderately rapid.

Diagnosis: Summer Heat with Dampness, complicated by erroneous treatment. Heat had penetrated the Blood Level though Cold remained at the Nutritive Level.

Therapeutic Principle: Clear Heat from the Blood Level and dispel Cold from the Nutritive Level.

Treatment: Hao Qin Qing Dan Tang, with modifications, was prescribed. The modified composition was: xiangru (*Mosla chinensis*) 4.5 g, chantui (*Cryptotympana*) 3 g, qinghao 10 g, huangqin 6 g, banxia 6 g, chenpi 6 g, zhuru 10 g, xingren 9 g, mudanpi (*Paeonia suffruticosa*) 9 g and Liu Yi San (Six-One Powder) 10 g. Liu Yi San is composed of 6 parts of talc to one part of gancao (*Glycyrrhiza*).

Two packages of herbs were prescribed each day. The decoction of each package of herbs was divided into three portions, and one portion was administered every 4 h. On return visit the following day, there was improvement in the symptoms. The decision was made to continue with the same formula, except for adding yuxingcao (*Houttuynia*) 12 g, at the same dosage and schedule. On return visit on the third day, the fever and the coldness were relieved. Treatment was changed to Jian Pi Wan with Qing Luo Yin, with modifications, to secure complete recovery.

(Source: *Fujian Chinese Medicine.*)

IV Xiao Yao San (Carefree Powder)

1 Source: Tai Ping Hui Min He Ji Ju Fang (Prescriptions from the Taiping Benevolent Pharmaceutical Bureau)

2 Composition

Chief Herb: chaihu (*Bupleurum chinense*) 9 g

Deputy Herbs: baishaoyao (*Paeonia lactiflora*) 9 g
danggui (*Angelica sinensis*) 9 g

Assistant Herbs: baizhu (*Atractylodes macrocephala*) 9 g
fuling (*Poria cocos*) 9 g
gancao (*Glycyrrhiza uralensis*) 5 g
bohe (*Mentha haplocalyx*) q.s.
shengjiang (*Zingiber officinale*) q.s.

Envoy Herb: (chaihu)

3 Application

Actions: unblocks the liver and removes accumulations; and generates blood and strengthens the spleen.

Indications: spleen insufficiency due to stagnant liver-Qi and blood deficiency.

Main Symptoms: flank pain; headache and blurred vision; dry mouth and throat; lassitude and appetite; and a pulse that is taut and depletive. Or, alternating chills and fever. Or, irregular menses with distended and painful breasts.

4 Analysis of the Formula

Xiao Yao San uses chaihu as chief herb, which unblocks the liver and removes accumulation, so that liver-Qi is mobilized.

Baishaoyao is sour–bitter and cool. It generates blood, conserves Yin and softens the liver. Danggui is sweet–acrid–bitter and warm. It generates and harmonizes blood. When danggui and baishaoyao are used together with chaihu, they nourish the liver and strengthen its functions. As blood circulates and acts normally the liver functions normally, and as blood is ample the liver is soft. Hence these two herbs serve as deputy herbs.

Overabundance of the Wood Element leads to restriction of the Earth Element. Hence, illness of an overactive liver Qi (Wood Element) easily leads to dysfunction of the spleen (Earth Element). For this reason, baizhu, fuling and gancao are used as assistant herbs in order to strengthen the spleen and to invigorate Qi. Not only do they strengthen the Earth Element in order to restrain the Wood Element, but they also provide a source for the generation of blood. They are the assistant herbs. A small amount of bohe is added to mobilize blocked liver-Qi and roast shengjiang is added to suppress abnormally rising Qi and harmonize the interior.

Chaihu has the ability to guide other herbs into the Liver Meridian. Though the chief herb in this formula it also serves as the envoy herb.

Acting in concert these herbs can break up accumulations in the liver, generate and replenish depleted blood and revitalize the weakened spleen. In so doing both Qi and blood are nourished and both liver and spleen are regulated.

5 Comments

Xiao Yao San is the classic herbal formula for regulating the liver and the spleen. Not only does it mobilize the liver and remove stagnation, it also strengthens the spleen and generates blood. In clinical application, it is suitable for many conditions, such as in regulating abnormal menstrual functions in females and in treating chronic liver diseases.

If dihuang is added to Xiao Yao San, the prescription becomes Hei Xiao Yao San (Black Carefree Powder). Dihuang has the ability to enrich Yin and generate blood, so the expanded formula is appropriate in illnesses amenable to treatment with Xiao Yao San but with more pronounced insufficiency of blood. Dihuang may be processed (shudihuang) or raw (shengdihuang). If blood insufficiency has given rise to endogenous Heat, shengdihuang is more appropriate. If blood insufficiency itself is more pronounced, then shudihuang is more appropriate.

For illnesses of stagnation in the liver with blood deficiency, leading to the formation of endogenous Heat or Fire, add mudanpi (*Paeonia*) and zhizi (*Gardenia*) to purge Fire. The augmented formula, Dan Zhi Xiao Yao San (Carefree Powder with Paeonia and Gardenia), is principally used for treating illnesses of stagnation in the liver Qi, blood insufficiency and accumulation of Fire.

6 *Case Study: Breast Mass in a 33-Year-Old Female*

The patient always had irregular menses. She was married but had never conceived. A month earlier, she found a hard mass in her right breast, lateral to the nipple. At first it was the size of a soybean (about 1/4 in.), but rapidly grew to the size of an egg. It was movable, but mildly tender. She also suffered from fatigue, dizziness, reduced appetite, and dry and irritated eyes. These symptoms began after she had become depressed from the breast mass. She consulted a surgeon, who advised prompt surgery. The patient declined and turned to a CM physician. Her tongue coating was found to be thin and pale, and her pulse taut.

Diagnosis: Breast mass caused by stagnation of liver-Qi and concomitant strong pathogenic evil and weak genuine Qi.

Therapeutic Principle: Mobilize liver-Qi and blood to dissipate the mass.

Treatment: The patient was treated with oral and topical medications. For oral treatment, Xiao Yao San with modifications was prescribed. The modified composition was: danggui 5 g, baishaoyao 6 g, fuling 10 g, baizhu 10 g, shengdihuang 10 g, sigualuo (*Luffa cylindrica*) 3 g, quanxie (*Buthus*) 5 pieces, zhizi 5 g, wugong (*Scolopendra*) 2 pieces and gancao 3 g. The dosage was one decoction a day, taken in several portions, for 5 days. For external application, the medication was: raw tiannanxing (*Arisaema consanguineum*, *erubescens*) 30 g and zhangnao (*Cinnamomum camphora*) 30 g mixed with vinegar and a small amount of vaseline. This ointment, not to be taken in the mouth, was applied directly to the mass, and changed twice daily.

After 5-day treatment, the symptoms improved. After 10-day treatment, the mass began to shrink. After a total of 1-month treatment, the mass disappeared altogether. Her vitality and appetite also returned to normal.

(Source: *Guangdong Journal of Chinese Medicine*, 1965, 3.)

V Banxia Xie Xin Tang (Stomach-Fire-Draining Pinellia Decoction)

1 *Source: Shang Han Lun (Treatise on Cold-Attack)*

2 *Composition*

Chief Herb: banxia (*Pinellia ternata*) 12 g

Deputy Herbs: ganjiang (*Zingiber officinale*) 9 g
huangqin (*Scutellaria baicalensis*) 3 g
huanglian (*Coptis chinensis*) 9 g

Assistant Herbs: renshen (*Panax ginseng*) 9 g
dazao (*Ziziphus jujuba*) 4 pieces

Envoy Herb: fried gancao (*Glycyrrhiza uralensis*) 9 g

3 Application

Actions: calms and mediates simultaneous Cold and Heat; eliminates masses and dissipates accumulations.

Indications: local swellings due to concurrent gelling of Cold and Heat.

Main Symptoms: epigastric distention without tenderness; or, vomiting and diarrhea with borborygmus; and a slightly yellow and greasy tongue coating.

4 Analysis of the Formula

Banxia Xie Xin Tang uses acrid-warm banxia as chief herb. It acts to dissipate masses, eliminate accumulations, suppress abnormally rising Qi and stop vomiting.

For deputy herbs, the formula uses ganjiang to warm the middle-jiao and dispel Cold, and huangqin and huanglian to cool Heat and reduce swellings. These three herbs acting in concert with the chief herb are capable of calming and mediating simultaneous Cold and Heat in the middle-jiao.

The gelling of intermixed Cold and Heat in the middle-jiao can also result from deficiency and stagnation of Qi in the middle-jiao. To prevent or reverse this, renshen and dazao are included to augment middle-jiao-Qi. When these two herbs are used to complement banxia, the rising and descending functions of the spleen and stomach could be restored.

Gancao is included both to strengthen the spleen and to harmonize the actions of the other herbs.

5 Comments

Localized masses usually result from rising and descending Qi not cooperating harmoniously in the middle-jiao, so that there is blockage and accumulation of Qi. The condition is generally caused by insufficiency of central Qi, allowing Cold and Heat to congeal together and block middle-jiao-Qi from rising or descending of Qi. Hence, in clinical application the principal task is to restore the functions of rising and descending. Doing so restores the proper circulation of middle-jiao-Qi.

Banxia Xie Xin Tang is designed to treat accumulation in the epigastrium. It is the essential formula for harmonizing the intestines and the stomach. The special feature in its construction is the simultaneous employment of bitter-and-acrid, cold-and-warm, and tonification-and-catharsis. Structurally, the composition of the formula is derived from Xiao Chaihu Tang by subtracting chaihu and shengjiang and adding huanglian and ganjiang. These changes convert a formula for calming and mediating Shaoyang into one for calming and mediating simultaneous Cold and Heat. It is used widely to treat illnesses in which Cold and Heat are present simultaneously and are intermixed, so that ascending and descending functions of Qi are both disturbed.

Appropriate modifications can further broaden the range of clinical application of this formula. Three are briefly described here.

Shengjiang Xie Xin Tang (Stomach-Fire-Draining Ginger Decoction): To obtain this formula the amount of ganjiang is reduced to 3 g and shengjiang 12 g is added. The aim of using the large amount of shengjiang is to disperse accumulated fluids and eliminate masses, to treat the gelling of intermixed fluids and Heat in the middle-jiao or abnormal ascending and descending of the spleen and the stomach.

Gancao Xie Xin Tang (Stomach-Fire-Draining Licorice Decoction): This formula is obtained from Banxia Xie Xin Tang by increasing the amount of gancao to 12 g. Gancao, which tonifies deficient middle-jiao-Qi, is teamed with herbs that use acridity to open channels and bitterness to suppress the abnormally rising of Qi. The new formula is effective for treating severe deficiency of stomach-Qi and intermixed gelling of Cold and Heat.

Huanglian Xie Xin Tang: This is obtained from Banxia Xie Xin Tang by removing huangqin, increasing 15 g huanglian and adding guizhi (*Cinnamomum*). This formula is used for illnesses caused by Heat in the chest and Cold in the stomach.

While they differ from one another in one or two ingredient and in the amounts of some of them, all four formulas have the key actions of acrid-opening of channels, bitter-lowering of the abnormally rising of Qi and harmonization of Cold and Heat. Nonetheless, each has its principal applications. Banxia Xie Xin Tang aims at the gelling of intermixed Cold and Heat. Shengjiang Xie Xin Tang aims at accumulations of water and Heat. Gancao Xie Xin Tang aims at accumulations due to deficiency of stomach-Qi. Huanglian Xie Xin Tang aims at cooling Heat in the upper body and warming Cold in the lower.

6 Case Study: Vomiting in a 36-Year-Old Male

The patient was long addicted to wine. He suffered from epigastric distention, with periodic nausea and vomiting and 3–4 bowel movements a day producing unformed feces. He had been treated with a variety of herbal prescriptions, without any benefit. On examination, his tongue coating was white and his pulse taut and slippery.

Diagnosis: Cold–Heat gelling in the middle-jiao.

Therapeutic Principle: Clear Heat, dispel Cold, and harmonize the stomach.

Treatment: Modified Banxia Xie Xin Tang was prescribed. It contained banxia 12 g, ganjiang 6 g, huanglian 6 g, dangshen (*Codonopsis*) 9 g, fried gancao 9 g and dazao 7 pieces. After one dose, his feces contained much whitish mucus and his nausea and vomiting were reduced by about 70%. After another dose, the epigastric distention and the diarrhea were alleviated. After two additional doses, all symptoms resolved.

(Source: *Popular Commentaries on Shang Han Lun*.)

VI Tong Xie Yao Fang (Essential Formula for Painful Diarrhea)

1 Source: Yi Xue Zheng Zhuan (Records of Orthodox Medicine)

2 Composition

Chief Herb: baizhu (*Atractylodes macrocephala*) 6 g

Deputy Herb: baishaoyao (*Paeonia lactiflora*) 6 g

Assistant Herb: chenpi (*Citrus tangerina, reticulata*) 6 g

Envoy Herb: fangfeng (Saposhnikovia divaricata) 3 g

3 Application

Actions: strengthens the spleen, softens the Liver, dries Dampness and stops diarrhea.

Indications: painful diarrhea due to stagnant liver-Qi and spleen insufficiency.

Main Symptoms: borborygmus, watery diarrhea, abdominal pain associated with an urge to defecate and subsiding when done; a thin and yellow tongue coating; and a pulse that is taut and slow but dissociated in the two wrists.

4 Analysis of the Formula

Tong Xie Yao Fang uses baizhu to strengthen the spleen and to dry Dampness. It is the chief herb. Baishaoyao, the deputy herb, softens the liver and stops pain. The team of baizhu and baishaoyao controls the Wood Element (liver) and nurtures the Earth Element (spleen).

Chenpi harmonizes the functions of the middle-jiao and helps baizhu strengthen the spleen and dry Dampness. It is the assistant herb. Fangfeng in small amounts has the ability to raise and disperse. Used with baizhu and baishaoyao, its acridity can overcome an overactive liver Qi and its aromaticity soothes Spleen-Qi. It also has the ability to dry Dampness and assist in stopping diarrhea, and to facilitate the Spleen Meridian. It is both assistant and envoy herb.

These four herbs used in concert are capable of strengthening the spleen, overcoming Dampness and stopping diarrhea. They strengthen the spleen by softening the liver, regulating Qi and stopping pain, so that the liver and the spleen cooperate in harmony. The painful diarrhea is then resolved spontaneously.

5 Comments

Tong Xie Yao Fang is one of the principal formulas for treating abdominal pain and diarrhea due to an overactive liver Qi that weakens the spleen Qi. It acts to suppress the liver and strengthen the spleen, reduce pain and stop diarrhea.

For the five *zang* organs, working with each organ's nature would result in strengthening it, whereas working against its nature would result in weakening it. Chenpi and fangfeng work with the liver's nature (Wood Element), so they strengthen the liver. At the same time, they normalize its Qi and functions, so that the Wood (liver) does not disturb the Earth (spleen). In that way they weaken the (overactive) liver. Once the liver is normalized, it no longer overpowers the spleen, and the painful diarrhea can stop.

6 Case Study: Diarrhea in a 30-Year-Old Male

For over a year the patient suffered from recurrent borborygmus and pain in the abdomen. Diarrhea always followed the pain. The feces were unformed and contained undigested grains. His urine was clear but scanty. His pulse was taut and slow, strong in the left wrist but weak in the right. His tongue coating was thin but white and greasy.

Diagnosis: Disharmony of the functions of liver and spleen, with an overactive liver Qi that weakens the spleen Qi.

Therapeutic Principle: Soften the liver and strengthen the spleen; eliminate Dampness and stop diarrhea.

Treatment: Tong Xie Yao Fang with modification was prescribed. The modified composition was as follows: stir-fried baizhu 6 g, chenpi 3 g, chuanxiong (*Ligusticum*) 3 g, fangfeng 3 g, fresh baishaoyao 4.5 g and fresh maiya (*Hordeum*) 4.5 g. This was administered at the dosage of once a day for 2 days. The symptoms improved noticeably. After five more packages of herbs the patient recovered completely.

(Source: *Case Studies of Famous Physicians*.)

VII Section Summary

The six formulas included in this section have somewhat different actions and indications.

Xiao Chaihu Tang is the representative formula for harmonizing the Shaoyang Meridian. It is designed to treat illnesses of Cold in Shaoyang manifesting alternating chills and fever, chest and subcostal fullness, dry throat, a bitter or sour taste in the mouth, dizziness, irritability, and vomiting.

Hao Qin Qing Dan Tang is another representative formula for harmonizing the Shaoyang Meridian. Its principal action is to clear Heat from the gallbladder, dry Dampness, harmonize stomach-Qi and dissolve Phlegm. It is mainly indicated for treating congealed Heat–Dampness in the Shaoyang Meridian, manifested by persistent chills alternating with pronounced fever, a bitter taste in the mouth, chest tightness, regurgitation of bitter or sour fluids, thirst with or without a desire to drink, and a thick and greasy tongue coating.

Xiao Yao San is a representative formula for regulating the spleen and the liver. Its main uses are for treating illnesses due to hyperactivity of the liver with blood insufficiency and spleen weakness, manifested by flank pain, headache with blurred vision, reduced appetite, somnolence and lassitude, irregular menses and other symptoms.

Tong Xie Yao Fang strengthens the spleen and softens the liver, though it is mainly aimed at the spleen. It is used principally to treat the painful diarrhea caused by an overactive liver Qi weakening the spleen.

Banxia Xie Xin Tang is the representative formula for regulating fever and chills and is suitable for treating gelling of intermixed Cold and Heat in the middle-jiao, with impairment of the lowering and raising functions. Its principal actions are to settle the stomach, suppress abnormally rising Qi, remove blockage and dissolve accumulations.

Da Chaihu Tang is a representative formula for dispelling pathogenic evil from both interior and exterior. It is suitable for treating illnesses in which the interior and the exterior are simultaneously affected. Its principal actions are to harmonize Shaoyang and purge gelled Heat in the interior. Its main application is the treatment of concurrent illnesses of Shaoyang and Yangming, with the key symptoms of alternating chills and fever, tightness and pain in the chest and flanks, persistent vomiting, epigastric distention or pain, constipation, a yellow tongue coating and a taut and rapid pulse.

Section 4 Formulas That Clear Heat

Heat-clearing formulas are constructed with Heat-cooling herbs, which have the ability to eliminate Heat and purge Fire, to cool blood and remove poison. They are used to treat illnesses caused by Heat in interior. Among the Eight Methods they belong to the Method of Cooling.

In clinical practice, interior Heat may be in the Qi or Blood Levels, of exogenous (strength) or endogenous (deficiency) origin, or in different visceral organs. Accordingly Heat-clearing formulas could be classified into several categories:

Formulas that clear Heat from the Qi Level
Formulas that clear Heat from the Nutritive Level and cool blood
Formulas that clear Heat and eliminate poison

Formulas that clear Heat from the *zang–fu* viscera
Formulas that clear deficiency Heat
Formulas that counteract Summer Heat

Heat-cooling formulas may be prescribed only where symptoms in exterior have resolved, the Heat evil has entered interior, but though interior Heat is strong it has not yet congealed. If exterior has not been released, an exterior-releasing formula should be used. If Heat has gelled in interior, a downward-draining formula should be used. If exterior has not been released but Heat has entered interior, both exterior and interior should be treated simultaneously. If Heat is in the Qi Level but treatment is aimed at the Blood Level, then pathogenic evils may be conducted into the interior. If Heat is in the Blood Level but treatment is aimed at the Qi Level, then Heat will be difficult to eliminate.

In addition, the clinical application of Heat-clearing formulas is guided by four principles. (1) Ascertain the location of the illness and especially the direction in which the illness is changing. (2) Determine whether the symptoms are true or false manifestations of Heat evil. (3) Differentiate those Heat illnesses due to strength of exogenous Heat from those due to endogenous Heat due to deficiency (of Qi or Yin, etc.). (4) Pay attention to the protection of the spleen and the stomach, to avoid their being injured by the bitter-cold herbs.

I Bai Hu Tang (White Tiger Decoction)

1 Source: Shang Han Lun (Treatise on Cold-Attack)

2 Composition

Chief Herb: shigao (gypsum) 50 g

Deputy Herb: zhimu (*Anemarrhena asphodeloides*) 18 g

Assistant Herb: jingmi (*Oryza sativa*) 9 g

Envoy Herb: fried gancao (*Glycyrrhiza uralensis*) 6 g

3 Application

Actions: clears Heat from the Qi Level and generates fluids.

Indications: illnesses of strong Heat in the Qi Level and in the Yangming Meridian.

Main Symptoms: high fever with facial flushing; restlessness; severe thirst; profuse sweating with intolerance of warmth; and a surging and forceful pulse.

4 *Analysis of the Formula*

Shigao is selected to be the chief herb for its acrid–sweet flavor and strong cold nature. These properties enable it to cool and purge strong Heat from the Qi Level and the Yangming Meridian. Zhimu, the deputy herb, has a bitter flavor and cold nature; it has the ability to purge Fire, moisten Dryness and augment Yin. Jingmi and gancao are added to protect the stomach and regulate the middle-jiao, and they serve as the assistant and envoy herbs respectively.

This formula does not use bitter-cold herbs to purge Fire directly because the Heat evil is very strong and the fluids are damaged, so that Yin is already deficient. Hasty and direct application of bitter-cold herbs will unavoidably injure Yin and aggravate Dryness. It also avoids using bitter-cold herbs to induce catharsis because though interior Heat is strong it has not yet gelled. Hasty application of bitter-cold herbs to drain downward will injure the fluids where there is no illness.

5 *Comments*

Bai Hu Tang is designed to treat illnesses of blazing Heat at the Qi Level in the Yangming Meridian. These illnesses are characterized by the "four bigs": big (high) fever, big thirst, big (profuse) sweating, and a big (surging and forceful) pulse.

In an illness of blazing Heat at the Qi Level in Yangming, if both Qi and fluids are clearly injured, manifested by sweating and fever that are mild and a pulse that is large but not forceful, add renshen (*Panax*) to Bai Hu Tang to augment Qi and generate fluids. This is **Bai Hu Jia Renshen Tang** (White Tiger plus Ginseng Decoction).

In illnesses of interior Heat causing mainly exterior symptoms, such as fever without chills and bone and joint aches, add guizhi (*Cinnamomum*) to disperse pathogenic evil from the exterior. This is **Bai Hu Jia Guizhi Tang** (White Tiger plus Cinnamomum Decoction).

In illnesses of Dampness–Heat with Heat stronger than Dampness, manifested by fever, tightness in the chest, profuse sweating, and a red tongue with a white and greasy coating, add cangzhu (*Atractylodes*) to strengthen the spleen and dry the Dampness. This is **Bai Hu Jia Cangzhu Tang** (White Tiger plus Atractylodes Decoction).

The illnesses treated with these four formulas all have strong Heat at the Qi Level in Yangming; but some differences should be noted. Bai Hu Tang is aimed at cooling strong Heat at the Qi Level in Yangming. Bai Hu Jia Renshen Tang is better where the strong Heat has injured Yin. Bai Hu Jia Guizhi Tang is more suitable where the strong Heat is intermixed with another exogenous pathogenic evil. Bai Hu Jia Cangzhu Tang is best where the strong Heat is intermixed with Dampness. In clinical practice, careful diagnosis is necessary to choose among these herbal formulas.

6 *Case Study: Seasonal Febrile Illness in a 54-Year-Old Male*

The patient suffered from the common cold with gradually rising fever. He took western anti-fever formulas. Though the fever would respond it would soon recur. He had thirst, sweating, and a slight sore throat. On examination, his temperature was 38°C (100.4°F). His tongue coating was thin and yellow, and his pulse was floating and forceful.

Diagnosis: Heat in Yangming at the Qi Level.

Therapeutic Principle: Clear Heat with sweet-cold herbs.

Treatment: Modified Bai Hu Tang was prescribed. The modified composition was: shigao 60 g, zhimu 12 g, jingmi (*Oryza*) 12 g, fresh lugen (*Phragmites*) 30 g, fresh maogen (*Imperata*) 30 g, lianqiao (*Forsythia*) 9 g, and fried gancao (Glycyrrhiza) 6 g. The decoction was administered warm in two portions, in the afternoon and at night. After one dose the patient's fever was reduced. After two more doses, the body temperature became normal. The amount of shigao was reduced to 45 g. After two doses of the modified formula all symptoms resolved.

(Source: *Cases Records of Dr. Yue Meizhong*.)

7 *Case Study: Heatstroke in a 38-Year-Old Female*

The patient worked on a farm. At the time of examination she had fever for 2 days and had been comatose for 3 h. Her overall nutritional status was normal. Her entire body was covered with profuse sweat. Her temperature was 40.5°C (104.9°F). The hands and feet were cold, and the mouth parched. The tongue coating was white and thin. The pulse was very rapid, slippery and forceful. The abdomen was firm and tender without guarding.

Upon admission, she was given 100 mL of 25% glucose solution intravenously and one dose of Bai Hu Tang orally. Six hours later the patient complained of thirst. She was given a small amount of cold boiled water. The following day her mental status was normal, but she had headache and weakness. Her temperature was 38.5°C (101.3°F). Bai Hu Tang was continued, with gradual improvement. On the third day, her temperature was normal. Five more days later, she was completely recovered.

(Source: *Journal of Chinese Medicine*, 1984, 11:22.)

II Qing Ying Tang (Nutritive-Clearing Decoction)

1 *Source: Wen Bing Tiao Bian (Analysis of Febrile Illnesses)*

2 *Composition*

Chief Herb: shuiniujiao (*Bubalus bubalis*) 30 g

Deputy Herbs: shengdihuang (*Rehmannia glutinosa*) 15 g
maimendong (*Ophiopogon japonicus*) 9 g
xuanshen (*Scrophularia ningpoensis*) 9 g

Assistant and Envoy Herbs: jinyinhua (*Lonicera japonica*) 6 g
lianqiao (*Forsythia suspensa*) 9 g
danzhuye (*Lophatherum gracile*) 3 g
huanglian (*Coptis chinensis*) 5 g
danshen (*Salvia miltiorrhiza*) 6 g

3 *Application*

Actions: clears Heat from the Nutritive Level, removes poison, vents Heat and augments Yin.

Indications: exogenous Heat at the Nutritive Level.

Main Symptoms: high fever that worsens at night; irritability and insomnia; intermittent delirium; there may or may not be thirst; faint macular and papular rashes; a scarlet and dry tongue; and a rapid pulse.

4 *Analysis of the Formula*

The chief herb, shuiniujiao, is bitter and salty in flavor and cold in nature. It is capable of eliminating Heat and poison from the Nutritive Level.

Shengdihuang, maimendong and xuanshen augment Yin and generate fluids. These actions complement the elimination of Heat and poison, so these herbs serve as deputies.

Between jinyinhua and lianqiao, one has the ability to assist in cooling Heat at the Nutritive Level and eliminating poison, and the other to penetrate the Nutritive Level and pushing the Heat evil back to the Qi Level, where it can be more easily vented. Huanglian assists in cooling the heart and removing poison. Danshen mobilizes blood and reduces swellings. Zhuye clears Heat from the heart meridians. These serve as assistant and envoy herbs.

Used together these herbs have three main actions. One is to clear Heat and its poison from the Nutritive Level. Another is to augment Yin that has been damaged by Heat. The third is to penetrate Heat and mobilize Qi so that the Heat evil at the Nutritive Level can be pushed back to the Qi Level and be further eliminated.

5 Comments

In the clinical application of Qing Ying Tang, the diagnostic key is a crimson and dry tongue. The formula is suitable for treating illnesses of Heat wherein the Heat evil has entered the Nutritive Level but not yet the Blood Level. The main symptoms are the following: fever that worsens at night, restlessness with insomnia, faint macular and papular rashes, a crimson and dry tongue, and a rapid pulse.

In constructing this formula the emphasis is on eliminating Heat from the Nutritive Level. That is the reason for using shuiniujiao as the chief herb. (In former times, rhinoceros horn was used. Today it is replaced by shuiniujiao, water buffalo horn.) At the same time, the herbs also nourish Yin and generate fluids. By combining the actions of the dispersal of Heat and the mobilization of blood, the formula achieves the goal of purging Heat from the Nutritive Level before it can reach the Blood Level.

6 Case Study: Heat at the Nutritive Level in a 17-Year-Old Female

The patient suffered from intermittent but persistent fever for 21 months, with body temperature fluctuating between 37.2–40°C (100–104°F). During fever there were also headache, vomiting and weakness. She was variously treated at several hospitals for tuberculosis, rheumatism and cholecystitis, all without effect. Many clinical tests were performed to establish the diagnosis, but they showed no unusual findings. She was treated with several courses of antibiotics, including anti-tuberculosis formulas, and Chinese herbs, again without effect. The only formula that had any effect at all was prednisone, but as soon this was discontinued the fever recurred.

On admission to hospital again, her body temperature was 37°C (98.6°F) in the morning, but it was 39–40°C (102.2–104°F) between 2 and 11 p.m. She was restless and was unable to sleep. Her mouth was dry, without much thirst. She had headaches and blurred vision. Her body was not emaciated. Her tongue was red or crimson, with a thin yellow coating.

Diagnosis: Heat at the Nutritive Level, incompletely eliminated.

Therapeutic Principle: Clear the Nutritive Level and purge Heat by forcing it outward.

Treatment: Modified Qing Ying Tang was prescribed, with the following formula: shuiniujiao 50 g (boil first), shengdihuang 25 g, xuanshen 20 g, zhuye 10 g, maidong 20 g, danshen 25 g, huanglian 10 g, jinyinhua 25 g, lianqiao 25 g, shigao 100 g (boil first for 45 min), banlangen (*Isatis*) 50 g, pugongying (*Taraxacum*) 50 g, zibeitiankui (*Senecio nudicaulis*) 15 g and zhimu (*Anemarrhena*) 15 g. The decoction of the herbs prescribed was given once every 3 h. After three doses the fever gradually subsided and the symptoms alleviated. Three more doses were administered, with further improvement. The treatment was then discontinued for observation, and there was no recurrence.

(Source: *Heilongjiang Journal of Chinese Medicine*.)

III Huanglian Jie Du Tang (Coptis Detoxification Decoction)

1 Source: Wai Tai Mi Yao (Essentials of Medical Secrets from Imperial Library)

2 Composition

Chief Herb: huanglian (*Coptis chinensis*) 9 g

Deputy Herb: huangqin (*Scutellaria baicalensis*) 6 g

Assistant Herb: huangbai (*Phellodendron chinense*) 6 g

Envoy Herb: zhizi (*Gardenia jasminoides*) 9 g

3 Application

Actions: drains Fire and relieves poison.

Indications: strong Heat and poisonous Fire in the sanjiao.

Main Symptoms: high fever with irritability; dry mouth and throat; incoherent speech and insomnia; or, vomiting of blood and nosebleeds; or, high fever with associated rash and diarrhea. In addition, there is jaundice from Dampness–Heat; the tongue is red with yellow coating and the pulse rapid and forceful.

4 Analysis of the Formula

The formula was designed to treat illnesses caused by Fire that burns the sanjiao, with spillover effects in both the upper and the lower body and in both the interior and the exterior.

Huanglian is used in the formula as the chief herb because of its strong bitter flavor and strong cold nature, and its ability to purge Fire from the heart and the middle-jiao. Huangqin is selected as the deputy herb for its ability to purge Fire from the upper-jiao. They are assisted by huangbai to purge Fire by catharsis from the lower-jiao. The envoy herb, zhizi, has the ability to induce catharsis of all sanjiao, to conduct Heat downward and to remove it by that pathway.

With these four herbs acting in concert, the formula has a bitter flavor and a cold nature, and it acts to expel the Fire evil and eliminate the poison produced by the Heat evil.

5 *Comments*

In the construction of this formula, large amounts of bitter and cold herbs are included to purge Fire from the upper, the middle and the lower jiao. Thus, the formula has a powerful ability to purge Fire and remove poison. For its clinical application, the key symptoms are high fever, restlessness, dry mouth and throat, a red tongue with yellow coating, and a rapid and forceful pulse.

This formula clearly differs from those designed for purging strong Heat by catharsis, but in clinical practice the physician needs not follow rules rigidly. In addition to the key symptoms, if the patient has constipation due to the strong Heat, dahuang may be added to unblock the organs and purge Heat by expelling the Heat evil in the feces.

Because this formula is bitter and cold, its prolonged administration can easily injure the stomach and the intestines. It must be suspended as soon as the illness has been effectively treated. It is inappropriate to use for blazing Fire due to Yin deficiency.

6 *Case Study: Biliary Infection in a 35-Year-Old Male*

The patient was a farmer with a past history of cholecystitis. He developed persistent pain in the right upper abdomen. The pain was also referred to the right shoulder. He had fever and dry heaves. The sclerae of his eyes were slightly jaundiced. His pulse was taut and rapid.

Diagnosis: Dampness–Heat in the liver and the gallbladder.

Therapeutic Principle: Purge Heat and release the gallbladder.

Treatment: Modified Huanglian Jie Du Tang was prescribed, with added zhiqiao (*Poncirus*), muxiang (*Aucklandia*), dahuang (*Rheum*) and yinchenhao (*Artemisia*). After 3-day treatment, the abdominal pain diminished and the patient defecated twice in 1 day. The formula without dahuang was continued for three more doses, and all symptoms resolved.

(Source: *Zhejiang Journal of Chinese Medicine*, 1977, 2:33.)

IV Qing Wen Bai Du Yin (Drink for Clearing Pestilential Illness and Detoxification)

1 Source: Yi Zhen Yi De (Successes in Pestilential Rashes)

2 Composition

Chief Herb: shigao (gypsum) 30 g

Deputy Herbs: zhimu (*Anemarrhena asphodeloides*) 10 g
gancao (*Glycyrrhiza uralensis*) 6 g
danzhuye (*Lophatherum gracile*) 6 g

Assistant Herbs: huanglian (*Coptis chinensis*) 9 g
huangqin (*Scutellaria baicalensis*) 9 g
zhizi (*Gardenia jasminoides*) 9 g
lianqiao (*Forsythia suspensa*) 12 g
shengdihuang (*Rehmannia glutinosa*) 12 g
mudanpi (*Paeonia suffruticosa*) 12 g
chishaoyao (*Paeonia lactiflora*) 12 g
xuanshen (*Scrophularia ningpoensis*) 12 g

Envoy Herb: jiegeng (*Platycodon grandiflorum*) 15 g

(Note: a wide range of amounts for each herb is used in this formula. When this formula is prescribed, the amount of each herb must be based on clinical requirements.)

3 Application

Actions: clears Heat and eliminates poison; cools blood and purges Fire.

Indications: pestilence illness with Heat poison in both the Qi and the Blood Levels.

Main Symptoms: high fever with strong thirst; severe splitting headache; dry heaves; and delirium. Or, there may be a rash, hematemesis, tetany in the limbs, or fainting. The pulse may be deep, threadlike and rapid, or deep and rapid, or floating, large and rapid. The tongue is red with scant coating, and the lips parched.

4 Analysis of the Formula

Qing Wen Bai Du Yin is constructed by merging Bai Hu Tang, Xijiao Dihuang Tang and Huanglian Jie Du Tang, with some additions and subtractions.

Shigao in large amount is used as the chief herb to purge Fire and expel Heat. Its teaming with zhimu, gancao and danzhuye is built according to the principles of Bai Hu Tang and intended for expelling Heat and protecting fluids. The inclusion of huanglian, huangqin, zhizi and lianqiao is built according to the principles of Huanglian Jie Du Tang, which emphasizes the purging of Fire and the elimination of its poison. Xijiao (rhinoceros horn) and shengdihuang are teamed with mudanpi, chishaoyao and xuanshen in imitation of Xijiao Dihuang Tang, with its main actions of purging Heat and cooling blood, removing poison and dissolving stasis.

Jiegeng is included as the envoy herb to conduct the other herbs upward. These herbs together achieve the expulsion of Heat, the removal of poison, the cooling of blood and the purgation of Fire.

5 Comments

Qing Wen Bai Du Yin is designed to treat pestilence with Heat poison in both the Qi and the Blood Levels. The key symptoms are intense fever, thirst, dry heaves, splitting headache, agitation and delirium or coma; or rashes; or hematemesis, epistaxis, with tetany of the limbs or convulsion. The pulse is deep, threadlike and rapid, or floating, large and rapid. The tongue is crimson with parched lips.

Prior to prescribing this formula, the physician must first ascertain whether the illness is caused by Heat or Cold, the location of the pathogenic evil (exterior or interior), and the relative severity of the Cold and the Heat.

6 Clinical Study: Ecephalitis B

Qing Wen Bai Du Yin was prescribed in 78 cases of encephalitis B. Of these 78 cases, 17 were mild, 28 moderate, 22 severe, and 11 acute.

The formula was modified as follows. For patients with illness primarily at the Defensive and Qi Levels, xijiao and mudanpi were omitted, jinyinhua and daqingye were added, and lianqiao and zhuye were increased in amount. For patients with illness primarily at the Defensive and Nutritive Levels, lianqiao and zhuye were omitted, and maimendong, lingyangjiao, gouteng and quan xie were added.

On average, 6.8 doses were administered. Some patients were also prescribed An Gong Niuhuang Wan or Zhi Bao Dan.

Results: Sixty-nine patients recovered completely. Five improved. Four died. The overall effective rate was 94.9%.

(Source: *Journal of the Hunan School of Chinese Medicine*, 1988, 3:55.)

V Dao Chi San (Red-Conducting Powder)

1 Source: Xiao Er Yao Zheng Zhi Jue (Key to Children's Illnesses)

2 Composition

Chief Herb: chuan mutong (*Akebia quinata, trifoliata*) 9 g

Deputy Herb: shengdihuang (*Rehmannia glutinosa*) 9 g

Assistant and Envoy Herbs: danzhuye (*Lophatherum gracile*) 9 g
gancao (*Glycyrrhiza uralensis*) 9 g

3 Application

Actions: clears the heart, nourishes Yin and promotes urination.

Indications: Fire searing the Heart Meridian.

Main Symptoms: feverishness and irritation in the chest; thirst with desire for cold drinks; facial flushing; ulcers in the mouth and on the tongue; or, feverishness in the heart moving to the small intestines, with sharp dysuria, difficulty with urination and red urine; a red tongue, and a rapid pulse.

4 Analysis of the Formula

Dao Chi San is primarily indicated for Fire searing the Heart Meridian. The formula uses shengdihuang to cool blood and augment Yin in order to reduce Fire in the heart meridian, and uses mutong to purge Fire from the Heart Meridian and drive Heat downward to the small intestines. Together these two herbs augment Yin and promote diuresis; they also can stimulate Yin to reduce Fire in the heart meridian. They thus serve as chief and deputy herbs respectively.

Danzhuye clears the heart and relieves restlessness. It alleviates Dampness and promotes urination and can push Heat from the heart downward to the small intestines. Gancao eliminates Heat and poison, unblocks the urinary pathway and stops pain. It also harmonizes the other herbs in the formula. These two serve as both assistant and envoy herbs.

5 Comments

Red is the color of the heart. "Dao chi" ("conducting the red") means moving the Heat evil out from the Heart Meridian by promoting diuresis; hence the name of the formula.

In clinical application of the formula, the key symptoms for its indication are feverishness and irritation in the chest, thirst, ulcers in the mouth and tongue; or, impeded and painful urination with red urine; a red tongue and a rapid pulse.

If the Heat in the Heart Meridian is very strong, huanglian (*Coptis*) may be added to purge Fire and calm the heart. If Heat has transferred to the small intestines, causing difficulty with urination, cheqianzi (*Plantago*) and fuling (*Poria*) may be added to enhance the Heat-clearing and urine-promoting actions.

6 Clinical Study: Painful and Impeded Urination

Dao Chi San was used to treat 15 cases of painful and impeded urination. In five patients the painful urination was due to sand in the urine, in seven to Qi impedance, and in three to blood in the urine. All 15 had reduced urine output and grating pain on urination, the pain also referring to the umbilicus. In some it was severe enough to lead to pain and swelling in the waist, with a white and greasy or thin and yellow tongue coating and a rapid pulse that is taut or threadlike.

Dao Chi San was the basic herbal formula selected. For those with sand in the urine haijinsha (*Lygodium*), bianxu (*Polygonum aviculare*) and jinqiancao (*Glechoma*) were added. For those with blood in the urine baimaogen (*Imperata*), raw cebaiye (*Platycladus orientalis*) and xiaoji (*Cephalanoplos*) were added. For those with Qi impedance Sichuan houpo (*Magnolia*) and xiangfu (*Cyperus*) were added.

Results: Nine patients had completely recovered, and the other six improved.

(Source: *Guangxi Journal of Chinese Medicine*, 1965, 2:17.)

VI Longdan Xie Gan Tang (Liver-Clearing Gentiana Decoction)

1 Source: *Yi Fang Ji Jie (Explanation of Collected Prescriptions)*

2 Composition

Chief Herb: longdancao (*Gentiana scabra, triflora*) 6 g

Deputy Herbs: huangqin (*Scutellaria baicalensis*) 9 g
zhizi (*Gardenia jasminoides*) 9 g

Assistant Herbs: cheqianzi (*Plantago asiatica*) 6 g
chuan mutong (*Akebia quinata, trifoliata*) 6 g
zexie (*Alisma plantago-aquatica, orientale*) 6 g
shengdihuang (*Rehmannia glutinosa*) 6 g
danggui (*Angelica sinensis*) 3 g
chaihu (*Bupleurum chinense, scorzonerifolium*) 6 g

Envoy Herb: gancao (*Glycyrrhiza uralensis*) 6 g

3 Application

Actions: clears Fire from the liver and the gallbladder and purges Dampness–Heat from the lower-jiao.

Indications and Main Symptoms: (1) Fire blazing upward from the liver and gallbladder. Symptoms: headache with red eyes; subcostal pain; a bitter taste in the mouth; ear swelling with loss of hearing; a red tongue with yellow coating; and a taut, rapid and forceful pulse. (2) Dampness–Heat in the liver and gallbladder with downward movement. Symptoms: scrotal swelling or itch; cold sweat; difficult and painful urination; a red tongue with yellow and greasy coating; and a taut, rapid and forceful pulse. In women, there may be vaginal discharge that is yellow and malodorous.

4 Analysis of the Formula

Longdancao is extremely bitter and extremely cold. It is capable of upward expulsion of Fire from the liver and gallbladder and downward purgation of Dampness–Heat from the liver and gallbladder. It is the chief herb.

Huangqin and zhizi are both bitter and cold. They have affinity for the Liver, Gallbladder and Sanjiao Meridians. Hence they can purge Fire and remove poison, dry Dampness and clear Heat. They serve as the deputy herbs to enhance the chief herbs' action to eliminate Heat and Dampness.

In the illness for which this formula is designed the lower-jiao is blocked by congealed Dampness–Heat. Cheqianzi, mutong and zexie, which eliminate Dampness and expel Heat, are included to conduct Dampness and Heat downward for elimination by the urinary pathway. They serve as assistant herbs. However, the liver is the storehouse for blood, so strong Fire in the Liver Meridian can easily injure Yin and blood. Moreover, the chief and deputy herbs are all bitter and cold and have the capability of drying Dampness and promoting urination. In other words, they can injure Yin. Therefore, shengdihuang and danggui are included, one to augment Yin and the other to generate blood. Although the substance of the liver belongs to Yin, its function belongs to Yang. By its nature, the liver prefers to act freely and detests being constrained. When the Fire evil lodges in the liver liver-Qi cannot move freely. Large amounts of bitter and cold herbs can promote diuresis, but can also aggravate the constraint on liver and gallbladder Qi. To avoid this aggravation chaihu is included to facilitate movement of liver and gallbladder Qi and to guide the other herbs into the Liver and Gallbladder Meridians. When chaihu and huangqin are teamed, they can not only dispel Heat from the liver and the gallbladder but also facilitate its upward expulsion. These six herbs – cheqianzi, mutong, zexie, shengdihuang, danggui and chaihu – together serve as assistant herbs.

Gancao is included as the envoy herb for two purposes. It blunts the actions of bitter and cold herbs to minimize injury to the stomach, and it can harmonize the actions of the other herbs.

From the selection of herbs one can see that the formula is characterized by its ability to tonify as it purges, to raise up as it suppresses, to avoid injuring genuine Qi as it dispels pathogenic evils, and to avoid attacking the stomach as it purges Fire. It forces Fire down and dispels Heat, so that Dampness and other impurities can be eliminated and all the symptoms from the affected meridians can be resolved.

5 Comments

Longdan Xie Gan Tang is representative of formulas that clear the Liver Meridian of strong Fire and purge the liver and the gallbladder of strong Heat. It is suitable for all illnesses in which liver-Fire blazes upward or Dampness and Heat in the Liver Meridian oppress downward. It uses longdancao to purge Fire–Dampness–Heat, and at the same time it employs herbs that promote fluid movement and urination, to ensure that there is a pathway for the Dampness–Heat–Fire to be expelled downward.

This formula is very bitter and cold. In clinical application, be careful to stop its administration as soon as the illness is substantially improved, in order to avoid bitter-cold injury to the stomach.

6 Clinical Study: Hepatitis

Thirty-two patients with hepatitis were treated. The basic herbal formula was Longdan Xie Gan Tang modified by omitting danggui and shengdihuang and adding tianjihuang (*Hypericum japonicum*). The dosage was one decoction of the formula daily, administered in two separate portions, for 1 month.

The patients were followed for a period of time ranging from 3 months to 6 years. Twenty-seven recovered completely and were able to resume normal work. Four improved but had relapse in association with over-exertion or incidental common cold. One did not respond.

The basic formula was further modified as needed.

For flank pain chuanlianzi (*Melia*) and yanhusuo (*Corydalis*) were added.

For obvious abdominal distention zhiqiao (*Poncirus*), chenpi (*Citrus*), Sichuan houpo (*Magnolia*) and foshou (*Citrus medica L. v. sacrodactylis*) were added.

For vomiting processed banxia (*Pinellia*), chenpi (*Citrus tangerina*), zhuru (*Phyllostachys nigra*) and huoxiang (*Agastache*) were added. For diarrhea baizhu (*Atractylodes*) and fuling (*Poria*) were added.

For patients in whom Dampness was more severe than Heat doukou (*Amomum kravanh*), caoguo (*Amomum tsao-ko*), huoxiang (*Agastache*), yinchenhao (*Artemisia*), huashi (talcum) and yiyiren (*Coix*) were added.

For blood stasis danshen (*Salvia*), honghua (*Carthamus*) and taoren (*Prunus persica)* were added.

(Source: *Journal of New Chinese Medicine*, 1978, 529.)

VII Shaoyao Tang (Peony Decoction)

1 Source: Su Wen Qi Yi Bao Ming Ji (Collection on Pathogenesis for Preserving Life)

2 Composition

Chief Herb: baishaoyao (*Paeonia lactiflora*) 12 g

Deputy Herbs: huangqin (*Scutellaria baicalensis*) 9 g
huanglian (*Coptis chinensis*) 9 g

Assistant Herbs: dahuang (*Rheum palmatum*) 6 g
muxiang (*Aucklandia lappa*) 5 g
binglang (*Areca catechu*) 5 g
danggui (*Angelica sinensis*) 9 g

Envoy Herbs: rougui (*Cinnamomum cassia*) 3 g
gancao (*Glycyrrhiza uralensis*) 6 g

3 Application

Actions: dispels Heat, dries Dampness, regulates Qi and harmonizes blood.

Indications: dysentery due to Dampness–Heat.

Main Symptoms: abdominal pain, diarrhea with pus and blood, tenesmus, a burning sensation in the anus; dark and scanty urine; a greasy and yellow tongue coating, and a taut and rapid pulse.

4 Analysis of the Formula

This formula is designed to treat dysentery caused by congealed Dampness and Heat. For the chief herb it uses baishaoyao for its bitter and sour flavor and cool nature, and for its ability to soften the liver, regulate the spleen, harmonize Qi and blood, and stop abdominal pain and dysentery.

For deputy herbs the formula uses huanglian and huangqin, both of which are bitter and cold. They dispel Heat and dry Dampness to purge Heat-poison from the intestines, thereby curing the cause of the dysentery.

There are four assistant herbs. Dahuang is bitter and cold. It acts to purge Heat and break up accumulations. By dissolving stagnant blood the dysentery can stop. Muxiang and binglang facilitate Qi movement and eliminate its obstruction. Danggui softens the liver and harmonizes blood. Danggui and dahuang together can dissolve stagnation, so that Qi and blood can both circulate freely. As blockage is removed the tenesmus would resolve.

Two herbs serve as envoys. Rougui is acrid and hot. Used in conjunction with bitter and cold herbs it can prevent the bitterness and coldness from damaging the stomach, and used in conjunction with herbs that facilitate blood circulation it enhances that effect. Gancao is sweet and mild. It aids the stomach and the middle-jiao, and it harmonizes the actions of the other herbs. In conjunction with baishaoyao it also relieves abdominal pain and tenesmus.

Acting in concert the herbs together purge Heat and dry Dampness, regulate Qi and facilitate blood circulation, soften the liver and regulate the spleen, dissolve stagnation and stop dysentery.

5 Comments

Clinical application of this herbal formula requires the key symptoms of dysenteric feces with mucus and blood, abdominal pain with tenesmus, and a tongue coating that is yellow and greasy. Its use is not appropriate where dysentery has just begun and is accompanied by symptoms of the exterior.

The formula is constructed by teaming herbs that purge Heat, remove poison and dry Dampness with those that regulate Qi and promote blood circulation, in order to achieve the capability of clearing Heat and poison and simultaneously stimulating blood and Qi circulation. In clinical practice it is often prescribed for bacterial dysentery, amebic dysentery, allergic enteritis and acute enteritis.

VIII Qing Wei San (Stomach-Clearing Powder)

1 Source: Lan Shi Mi Cang (Private Records of the Orchid Cabinet)

2 Composition

Chief Herb: huanglian (*Coptis chinensis*) 6 g

Deputy Herbs: shengma (*Cimicifuga heracleifolia, foetida*) 9 g
shengdihuang (*Rehmannia glutinosa*) 6 g
mudanpi (*Paeonia suffruticosa*) 9 g

Assistant Herbs: danggui (*Angelica sinensis*) 6 g

3 Application

Actions: drains stomach-Fire and cools blood.

Indications: stomach-Fire with toothache.

Main Symptoms: toothache radiating to the head; facial flushing; the teeth preferring cold over hot, or gingival bleeding, or pyorrhea; or, swelling of the lips, tongue and cheeks, with foul halitosis; a dry mouth; a tongue that is red and dry; and a slippery and rapid pulse.

4 Analysis of the Formula

This is the main formula for treating toothache due to stomach-Fire. It uses the bitter and cold huanglian as chief herb to purge Fire from the stomach.

Shengma dispels Heat and removes poison. With shengma as complement huanglian can purge Fire without the risk of inducing Cold; with huanglian as complement shegnma can disperse Fire without the risk of the Fire blazing upward. Heat or Fire in the stomach always injures Yin-blood. For that reason shengdihuang is included to cool blood and augment Yin, and mudanpi is included to cool blood and dispel Heat. These three all serve as deputy herbs.

Danggui enriches and harmonizes blood, and serves as the assistant herb. Shengma guides other herbs into the meridians, so it also serves as the envoy herb.

5 Comments

The main application of Qing Wei San is for stomach-Fire blazing upward along the Yangming Meridian, not for Heat accumulation in the *fu* organ of the Yangming Meridian. Thus, it applies the method of using bitter-cold herbs to clear Heat from the stomach, rather than the method of using bitter-cold herbs to purge downward. If the illness also manifests constipation due to dry intestines, dahuang may be added to drive the Heat out by catharsis. In clinical practice Qing Wei San is often used to treat illnesses of stomach-Fire attacking upward, such as stomatitis, periodontitis, and trigeminal neuralgia.

6 Clinical Study: Acute Periodontitis

Acute periodontitis is characterized by inflammation of the periodontal tissues, sometimes with bleeding and purulent drainage. It is often accompanied by fever, thirst, halitosis, constipation, red and scant urine. The tongue is red, with a thick yellow coating. The pulse is surging and rapid.

Therapeutic Principle. Clear Heat from the stomach and cool blood.

Fifty-six cases were treated. The prescription was Qing Wei San with additions. The composition was as follows: huanglian 6 g, zhuye (*Phyllostachys nigra*) 6 g, shengdihuang 12 g, lianqiao (*Forsythia*) 12 g, mudanpi 10 g, shengma 10 g, danggui 10 g, dahuang (*Rheum*) 10 g, shigao (gypsum) 30 g (boiled first), and tianhuafen (*Trichosanthes*) 15 g. This was administered at one dose per day. Most of the patients took 3–5 doses.

Results: Of the 54 cases, 32 (57%) recovered completely, 19 (34%) improved substantially, 4 (7%) showed some improvement, and 1 (2%) had no improvement.

(Source: *Journal of Traditional Chinese Medicine*, 1985, 7:65.)

IX Qinghao Biejia Tang (Woomwood and Turtle Shell Decoction)

1 Source: Wen Bing Tiao Bian (Analysis of Febrile Illnesses)

2 Composition

Chief Herbs: biejia (*Amyda sinensis*) 6 g
qinghao (*Artemisia annua, apiacea*) 15 g

Deputy Herbs: shengdihuang (*Rehmannia glutinosa*) 12 g
zhimu (*Anemarrhena asphodeloides*) 6 g

Assistant and Envoy Herb: mudanpi (*Paeonia suffruticosa*) 9 g

3 Application

Actions: augments Yin and vents Heat.

Indications: late stages of Heat illnesses, characterized by Heat entrenched at the Yin (Nutritive and Blood) Levels.

Main Symptoms: night fever and morning coolness; absence of sweating as fever subsides; a red tongue with little coating; and a threadlike and rapid pulse.

4 Analysis of the Formula

Biejia augments Yin and generates fluids. It is also efficacious in clearing Heat that is deeply entrenched at the Yin Levels. Qinghao is bitter and slightly acrid in flavor and cold in nature, and is aromatic. It is an essential herb for clearing and venting the Heat evil. When biejia and qinghao are used together, biejia specializes in entering the Yin Levels to augment Yin whereas qinghao specializes in forcing Heat out to the Yang Levels for venting. In this way Yin can be augmented without retention of the pathogenic evil and Heat is vented without injuring genuine Qi. These two are together the chief herbs.

Shengdihuang is sweet and cool, and zhimu is bitter and cold. Both herbs are capable of augmenting Yin and clearing Heat. They enhance the ability of biejia to augment Yin and eliminate deficiency-Heat. They are the deputy herbs.

Mudanpi is acrid–bitter and cool. It can clear Fire lodged at the Blood Level and aid qinghao in clearing the Yin Levels of entrenched Heat. It serves as the assistant herb.

Together these five herbs of the formula augment, clear and vent simultaneously, covering both causes and symptoms, and achieving the result of augmenting Yin and venting Heat.

5 Case Study: Relapsing Fever in a 21-Year-Old Male

For 3 months the patient suffered recurrent cold-intolerance and fever, his body temperature often reaching 40°C (104°F). Blood tests and bone marrow examination did not reveal any abnormality. He was treated with a number of antibiotics and hormones, without any improvement. At the time of admission to hospital, he was emaciated and had alternating chills and fever. The fever was worst in the afternoon, but broke at night with sweating, following which he would be thirsty and drank. His feces were dry and his urine very dark. His tongue was red with a thin coating. His pulse was threadlike and rapid.

Diagnosis: Heat evil entrenched at the Yin Levels, and the high fever has injured fluids.

Therapeutic Principle: Clear Heat and augment Yin, invigorate Qi and generate fluids.

Treatment: The patient was treated with two prescriptions simultaneously. One prescription was modified from Qinghao Biejia Tang and had the following composition: jinyinhua (*Lonicera*) 15 g, lianqiao (*Forsythia*) 12 g, qinghao 12 g, biejia 21 g, qinjiao (*Gentiana*) 12 g, zhimu 9 g, shengdihuang 18 g, maimendong (*Ophiopogon*) 15 g, digupi (*Lycium*) 12 g, and whole danggui (*Angelica*) 9 g. The other prescription was prepared as follows. Renshen (*Panax*) 15 g was decocted, then mixed with shenqu (medicated leaven) and made into pills. These two formulas were administered at one dose each per day, taken at the same time. The fever subsided after 3 days and the temperature returned to normal after 5 days. The formulas were prescribed for 10 more days, to consolidate the response. During subsequent observation for 2 years, he had no recurrence.

(Source: *Journal of the Anhui College of Chinese Medicine*.)

X Section Summary

Nine herbal formulas are included in this section on Heat-clearing formulas. They can be grouped in accordance with their actions into the following six categories:

- Formulas that clear Heat from the Qi Level
- Formulas that clear Heat from the Nutritive Level and cool blood
- Formulas that clear both Qi and Blood Levels
- Formulas that clear Heat and eliminate poison
- Formulas that clear Heat from the *zang-fu* viscera
- Formulas that clear deficiency-Heat

Bai Hu Tang is representative of herbal formulas that clear Heat from the Qi Level. Its action is to clear Heat and generate fluids. It is designed to cure strong Heat at the Qi Level in the Yangming Meridian, manifested by high fever, profuse sweating, restlessness and severe thirst, and a large surging pulse.

Qing Ying Tang is an essential formula for clearing Heat from the Nutritive Level and cooling blood. It acts to clear the Nutritive Level and vent Heat, to augment Yin and stimulate blood circulation, and to facilitate the dispersal of Heat to the Qi Level, where it can be vented. It is designed to cure illnesses in which the Heat evil has just entered the Nutritive Level, as manifested by fever that is worst at night, intermittent delirium, restlessness with insomnia, and faint rashes.

Qing Wen Bai Du Yin is representative of formulas that clear Heat from both the Qi and the Blood Levels. It has three simultaneous actions: to clear Heat at the Qi Level; to clear Heat from the Blood Level and cool blood; and to purge Fire and remove poison. It is designed for curing pestilential poison or Heat suffusing interior and exterior, illnesses that are of Fire at both the Qi and the Blood Levels. The key manifestations of these illnesses are of strong Heat at the Qi and the Blood Levels, abnormal circulation of blood due to the Heat, and Heat poison entrenched in interior.

Huanglian Jie Du Tang is an important formula for clearing Heat and relieving poison. Its action is to purge Fire and remove poison through its bitter flavor and cold nature. It is designed to cure the sanjiao of Fire and its poison, manifested by irritability, delirium, vomiting, nosebleed, rashes and carbuncles.

If Heat in the visceral organs is particularly strong, it is necessary to purge the Heat evil. Four of the formulas fall in this category. **Dao Chi San** is the essential formula for purging Fire from the heart. Its actions are to clear the heart, promote fluid circulation and augment Yin. It is designed to cure illnesses in which there is Heat in the Heart Meridian and the small intestines, manifested by heart palpitation, tightness in the chest, mouth ulcers and painful urination. The main actions of **Longdan Xie Gan Tang** are to purge the liver and the gallbladder of Fire, to suppress the abnormally rising Heat and stop vomiting. The main actions of **Qing Wei San** are to clear Heat from the stomach and to cool blood. It is designed to cure the toothache, headache, periodontal bleeding and painful swelling of the cheeks due to Fire in the stomach attacking upward. The main application of **Shaoyao Tang** is to clear Heat from the large intestines. Its main action is to regulate Qi and blood, and it is designed to cure dysentery with blood and mucus and tenesmus.

Qinghao Biejia Tang is an essential formula for treating deficiency-Heat. Emphasizing equally the augmentation of Yin and the venting of Heat, it is designed for curing illnesses in which the Heat evil has injured Yin, or the Heat evil is entrenched at the Yin Levels. The key symptoms are fever at night and chills in the morning, and the breaking of fever without sweating.

Section 5 Formulas That Warm Interior

Interior-warming formulas comprise all those formulas that are constructed primarily of herbs that are warm or hot in nature and have the ability to warm interior and expel Cold, or to rescue Yang and prevent collapse. These formulas are used to treat Cold in the interior. Among the Eight Methods it belongs to the category of the Method of Warming.

In clinical application it is important first to determine in which *zang–fu* organ Cold is located. In particular, special attention must be paid to differentiating between true and false Heat and between true and false Cold, so as not to be misled by false manifestations. Treating an illness of true Heat and false Cold with an interior-warming formula may aggravate the illness.

Attention must also be paid to the appropriateness of using such a formula in the particular patient, at the particular time and in the particular location (see Volume 1, Part II, Chapter 10, Section 1, Subsection III). In a patient whose body is habitually warmed by Fire, or affected by Yin deficiency and blood loss, or during high summer, or in a southern tropical region, the dosage to be used must be reduced and the treatment should be suspended when the illness is half resolved. On the other hand, if the weather is cold, or the patient's body is chronically deficient in Yang, then the dosage may appropriately be increased. In a patient whose body has been weakened by prolonged insufficiency of Yang-Qi, if treatment with an interior-warming formula has expelled Cold from the interior but Yang-Qi is still deficient, then another warming-nourishing formula must be sought.

If Yin-Cold has been excessive, or there is true Cold and false Heat, there may be vomiting upon taking the medication. This is known as "(medication) rejection"; it can be managed by adding a small amount of an herb that is bitter or salty in flavor and cold in nature. Alternately, the medication may be taken cold. Medication rejection may be avoided by either technique. This is the method of using cold herb to treat Cold illness.

I Li Zhong Wan (Middle-Jiao-Regulating Pill)

1 Source: Shang Han Lun (Treatise on Cold-Attack)

2 Composition

Chief Herb: ganjiang (*Zingiber officinale*) 9 g

Deputy Herbs: renshen (*Panax ginseng*) 9 g

Assistant Herb: baizhu (*Atractylodes macrocephala*) 9 g

Envoy Herb: fried gancao (*Glycyrrhiza uralensis*) 9 g

3 Application

Actions: warms the middle-jiao, disperses Cold, tonifies Qi and strengthens the spleen.

Indications and Main Symptoms: (1) deficiency-Cold in the spleen and stomach. Symptoms: epigastric and abdominal pain, diarrhea; absence of thirst; aversion to cold, cold limbs; vomiting, reduced appetite; a pale tongue with a white coating, and a deep and threadlike pulse. (2) Yang deficiency with blood loss. (3) Infantile convulsion. (4) Somnolence and excessive salivation during convalescence from another illness. (5) Vomiting or diarrhea from cholera.

4 Analysis of the Formula

Ganjiang is acrid and hot, and these properties enable it to warm interior and expel Cold. This formula therefore uses it as the chief herb.

Renshen is sweet and warm. It has the ability to enter the spleen and augment Qi in the middle-jiao. It serves as the deputy herb.

Insufficiency of the spleen leads to ineffective transformation and transport of food and water, which in turn leads to internal stagnation and gives rise to Cold and Dampness. Baizhu, which is sweet and bitter in flavor and warm in nature, is therefore added as assistant herb to dry Dampness and strengthen the spleen.

Gancao is added as the envoy herb because it can nourish Qi and strengthen the spleen as well as harmonize the actions of the other herbs.

This formula contains four herbs, all of which can warm and nourish the middle-jiao. Though the number of herbs is small, the action is concentrated. It is quite effective in dispelling Cold, restoring Yang and augmenting Qi in the middle-jiao. As the spleen's control over transformation and transport is reestablished, all symptoms of deficiency Cold in the middle-jiao will resolve.

5 Comments

Li Zhong Wan is representative of formulas that warm the middle-jiao and dispel Cold. Its principal application is in illnesses of deficiency Cold in the spleen and the stomach causing digestive problems.

It has had considerable influence on the subsequent development of interior-warming formulas, and many formulas that warm centrally are built on its foundation. The following are examples.

Fuzi Li Zhong Wan is obtained by adding fuzi (Aconitum) to Li Zhong Wan. It treats deficiency Cold in the spleen and the stomach with an indistinct pulse, cold limbs, and abdominal pain.

Lian Li Tang is obtained by adding huanglian (*Coptis*) to Li Zhong Wan. It acts to warm the middle-jiao and dispel Cold, and purge liver-Fire. It is used to treat deficiency Cold in both the spleen and the stomach, with vomiting.

Li Zhong Wan favors warming and drying. It is contraindicated in Yin deficiency.

6 Case Study: Spleen Insufficiency with Diarrhea in a 39-Year-Old Male

The patient suffered from diarrhea for over a year. He had frequent watery diarrhea, sometimes as often as 8–9 times in a day. The diarrhea was often accompanied by borborygmus. He had a chronically poor appetite and his feces often contained undigested grains. He had a pallid and lusterless complexion, and was lethargic.

He had moderate abdominal distention, but the discomfort was alleviated by moderate pressure. His tongue coating was yellow, viscous and curd-like. His pulse was threadlike and slow.

Diagnosis: Spleen insufficiency with diarrhea.

Therapeutic Principle: Tonify the middle-jiao and the spleen.

Treatment: The patient was treated with modified Li Zhong Wan, with the following composition: renshen 9 g, stir-fried baizhu 9 g, Heilongjiang ganjiang 7.5 g and fried gancao 6 g. After six consecutive doses he recovered completely.

(Source: *Jiangxi Journal of Chinese Medicine*, 1964, 3:149.)

II Xiao Jian Zhong Tang (Minor Middle-Jiao-Strengthening Decoction)

1 Source: Shang Han Lun (Treatise on Cold-Attack)

2 Composition

Chief Herbs: yitang (maltose) 30 g

Deputy Herbs: guizhi (*Cinnamomum cassia*) 9 g
shaoyao (*Paeonia lactiflora*) 12 g

Assistant and Envoy Herbs: fried gancao (*Glycyrrhiza uralensis*) 6 g
shengjiang (*Zingiber officinale*) 10 g
dazao (*Ziziphus jujuba*) 5 pieces

3 Application

Actions: warms and tonifies the middle-jiao, harmonizes the interior and moderates spasm.

Indications: abdominal pain due to deficiency of spleen-Yang.

Main Symptoms: abdominal pain alleviated by pressure and warmth; palpitation; fever; a lusterless complexion; a pale tongue with white coating; a deep and weak or threadlike and taut pulse. Alternately, the symptoms are palpitation of the heart, agitation and restlessness, and a lusterless complexion; or, hotness in the palms and soles and a dry mouth and throat.

4 Analysis of the Formula

The formula uses yitang as the chief herb for its sweet flavor and warm nature and for its ability to augment spleen-Qi, replenish spleen-Yin, warm the middle-jiao, relieve pain and slow the course of acute conditions.

Of the two deputy herbs, shaoyao nourishes Yin and moderates acute conditions of the liver, whereas guizhi warms Yang in the middle-jiao and dispels deficiency-Cold.

There are three assistant herbs. Gancao augments Qi. It assists yitang and guizhi in augmenting Yang, invigorating Qi, warming the middle-jiao and relieving spasm, and it assists shaoyao in releasing stagnated Yin, softening the liver, nourishing the spleen and regulating Yang. Shengjiang warms the stomach and dazao strengthens the spleen. These two act together to guide Qi in the middle-jiao upward and to regulate Qi at the Nutritive and Defensive Levels.

Acting in concert these six herbs aid the transformations and movement of both Yin and Yang. Together they warm the middle-jiao, replenish what is deficient, and relieve pain and spasm.

5 Comments

Both Xiao Jian Zhong Tang and Li Zhong Wan have the ability to warm the middle-jiao and to augment what is deficient. Li Zhong Wan teams renshen with ganjiang, so that it tonifies as it warms. It is efficacious for treating illnesses of deficiency-Cold in the spleen and stomach and of spleen dysfunction. Xiao Jian Zhong Tang, on the other hand, is constructed by adding guizhi and shaoyao to large amounts of yitang. It tonifies as it warms the middle-jiao, and relieves spasm and pain. Since the two formulas use different complementation they have different applications. Xiao Jian Zhong Tang is mainly used to treat acute illnesses caused by internal deficiency and fatigue. It is aimed at such symptoms as recurrent abdominal pain that is alleviated by warmth and pressure, a pale tongue with white coating, and a pulse that is deep and threadlike.

Adding danggui to Xiao Jian Zhong Tang produces **Danggui Jian Zhong Tang**. This is mainly used to treat postpartum abdominal pain and postpartum complications such as unremitting abdominal pain, rigidity of the lower abdomen with referred pain to the back, and inability to eat or drink.

In clinical application bear in mind that this formula is contraindicated in illnesses of strong Fire in Yin deficiency, repeated nausea and vomiting, especially vomiting of ascarid worms, or distention in the middle-jiao.

6 *Case Study: Abdominal Pain in a Male*

The patient suffered from abdominal pain that was alleviated by pressure. The pain was accompanied by the feeling as though there was cold Qi pressing down from the upper body. His pulse was depletive but taut. He had mild aversion to cold.

Diagnosis: The spleen being constrained by the liver.

Treatment: The patient was successfully treated with modified Xiao Jian Zhong Tang, as follows: guizhi 9 g, shaoyao 18 g, gancao 6 g, shengjiang 3 pieces, dazao 12 pieces and yitang 10 g.

(Source: *Jingfangshiyanlu, Testing and Affirmation of Formulas.*)

III Si Ni Tang (Frigid-Extremities Decoction)

1 *Source: Shang Han Lun (Treatise on Cold-Attack)*

2 *Composition*

Chief Herb: processed fuzi (*Aconitum carmichaeli*) 15 g

Deputy Herb: ganjiang (*Zingiber officinale*) 9 g

Assistant and Envoy Herb: fried gancao (*Glycyrrhiza uralensis*) 6 g

3 *Application*

Actions: rescues Yang and prevents collapse.

Indications and Main Symptoms: (1) Illnesses caused by Cold, in the Shaoyin Meridian. Main symptoms: extremely cold extremities, intolerance of cold; malaise and somnolence; vomiting without thirst; abdominal pain with diarrhea; a pale tongue with white and smooth coating; and an indistinct pulse. (2) Illnesses in the Taiyang erroneously treated by inducing diaphoresis, resulting in Yang collapse.

4 *Analysis of the Formula*

Si Ni Tang is an essential formula for rescuing Yang from collapse. It uses processed fuzi as the chief herb because of its strong acrid flavor and very hot nature. It is the most indispensable herb for the warm-tonification of innate kidney-Yang, and is capable of coursing all 12 meridians. It can reach both interior and exterior, rescue depleted Yang and expel Cold. For these reasons it is the chief herb.

In addition, ganjiang is selected to be the deputy herb. Kidney-Yang is the root of the entire body's Yang. If kidney-Yang is depleted, so will heart-Yang and spleen-Yang. When that happens, neither the *zang–fu* viscera nor the somatic body will function properly, as manifested by such symptoms as malaise, somnolence, abdominal pain with vomiting and diarrhea, and cold intolerance. Ganjiang is acrid and hot. It acts to warm spleen-Yang and disperse interior Cold. It aids fuzi to disperse Yin-Cold and rescue kidney-Yang.

Fuzi is pure Yang and is hot in nature. When aided by ganjiang it is especially harsh. Fried gancao is therefore added to augment Qi and calm the middle-jiao. It not only counteracts the toxic effects of fuzi, but also blunts the harshness of fuzi and ganjiang; and it protects Yin. It enables the formula to rescue Yang and expel Cold without severely damaging Yin-fluid or risk scattering the already depleted Yang.

5 Comments

The "si ni" ("four recalcitrants") of Si Ni Tang refers to the extreme coldness of the four limbs with loss of responsiveness. The coldness of the limbs is due to severe lack of Yang complicated by Yin-Cold. When Yang cannot permeate the limbs, the limbs become cold and dysfunctional. In such circumstances, only herbs of pure Yang nature are capable of countering the devastating effects of Yin-Cold and of re-invigorating Yang. This is the reason for using fuzi and ganjiang together, so that their concerted action can rescue Yang.

When fuzi is used, it is important to add herbs to restrain and blunt its toxic effects.

If Si Ni Tang is modified by doubling the amount of ganjiang, then it becomes **Tong Mai Si Ni Tang** (Channel-Unblocking Si Ni Tang). This augmented formula is used to treat extreme coldness of the four limbs with a pulse that is so indistinct that it is on the verge of ceasing. It exploits ganjiang's ability to warm Yang and preserve the middle-jiao, thereby opening all the channels.

6 Case Study: Coma in a 30-Year-Old Female

The patient was inadvertently drenched with cold water during her time of menstruation. Subsequently she developed shaking chills at night, followed by somnolence and soon by unconsciousness. Her pulse became indistinct and threadlike, as though on the verge of ceasing. All her limbs became cold and unresponsive. She was immediately treated with acupuncture. She regained consciousness briefly, but promptly sank back into coma.

Diagnosis: Extreme Yin-Cold, causing depletion of Yang-Qi and stagnation of Qi and blood.

Therapeutic Principle: Rescue Yang and tonify blood.

Treatment: Large-dose Si Ni Tang was prescribed, as follows: increase baked processed fuzi to 25 g. The formula was decocted in water, and the decoction was divided into four portions. One portion was administered every half-hour. (This was the technique of gradual administration of a potent herb with a large dosage. If the decoction had been administered all at once, there would have been the risk of "violent rebound of the pulse.") Before all four portions had been administered the patient began to show warming of the limbs and strengthening of the pulse. She fully regained consciousness.

(Source: *Analysis of the Essentials of the Treatise on Cold-Attack.*)

IV Danggui Si Ni Tang (Angelica Frigid-Extremities Decoction)

1 Source: Shang Han Lun (Treatise on Cold-Attack)

2 Composition

Chief Herbs: danggui (*Angelica sinensis*) 12 g
guizhi (*Cinnamomum cassia*) 9 g

Deputy Herbs: baishaoyao (*Paeonia lactiflora*) 9 g
xixin (*Asarum heterotropoides, sieboldi*) 3 g

Assistant Herb: tongcao (*Tetrapanax papyriferus*) 6 g

Envoy Herbs: fried gancao (*Glycyrrhiza uralensis*) 6 g
dazao (*Ziziphus jujuba*) 8 pieces

3 Application

Actions: warms the meridians, expels Cold, nourishes blood, and unblocks the blood channels.

Indications: illnesses of deficiency-Cold due to blood depletion and causing frigid extremities.

Main Symptoms: cold hands and feet; absence of thirst; or, pain in the waist, lower back, legs, feet, etc.; a pale tongue with white coating; and a pulse that is deep and threadlike or threadlike and on the verge of ceasing.

4 Analysis of the Formula

Danggui Si Ni Tang is constructed from Guizhi Tang by removing shengjiang, doubling the amount of dazao, and adding danggui, tongcao and xixin. It is an essential herbal formula for warming the Liver Meridian and generating blood.

Depletion of blood allows Cold to accumulate and congeal. Danggui is sweet and warm, and it generates and regulates blood. Guizhi is acrid and warm, and acts to warm and unblock the channels, thereby dispersing the Cold evil that has lodged in the channels and opening the channels for free passage of blood. These two are the chief herbs.

Baishaoyao and xixin serve as the deputy herbs. Baishaoyao generates blood. Working with danggui it augments Yin-blood. Working with guizhi it harmonizes both Qi and blood. Xixin is acrid and warm. In the exterior it warms the meridians and the channels, and in the interior it warms the *zang–fu* organs; in this way the Cold evil can be dispelled from both exterior and interior. Xixin also enhances the ability of guizhi to warm the channels and disperse Cold.

Tongcao is the assistant herb. It acts to unblock the channels.

Gancao and dazao are sweet in flavor. They augment Qi and strengthen the spleen, as well as harmonize the actions of the other herbs. Dazao is used in larger than usual amount both to aid danggui and baishaoyao in generating blood and to counteract the excessive warming and drying by guizhi and xixin so as to avoid damaging Yin-blood. These two serve as the envoy herbs.

Acting in concert the herbs of this formula are warming but not drying. Together they achieve the goal of warming the meridians and unblocking the blood channels, so that Yin-blood can be full, exogenous Cold dispelled, Yang-Qi re-invigorated, the channels unblocked, the limbs warmed and the pulse restored.

5 Comments

The extreme coldness of the limbs treated by this herbal formula is different from that caused by acute exhaustion of Yang and treated by Si Ni Tang. Danggui Si Ni Tang is indicated for attack by exogenous Cold in a patient with chronic deficiency of blood and Yang. This in turn causes impeded circulation of Qi and blood and therefore inability to warm the extremities; hence the cold limbs and the threadlike pulse that is on the verge of ceasing. Proper treatment requires attending to both the expulsion of exogenous Cold through warming and dispersion and the generation of blood with unblocking of the channels; neither must be neglected. Si Ni Tang is called for when the patient is in a state of critical Yang exhaustion.

6 Case Study: Severe Exposure to Cold in a 30-Year-Old Male

The patient was caught in a wind and snow storm. After walking several miles he collapsed. Neighbors discovered him and carried him home. His limbs were extremely cold, and he could not move even in bed.

Diagnosis: Severe cold exposure.

Therapeutic Principle: Rescue Yang and expel Cold.

Treatment: Danggui Si Ni Tang was prescribed, using the temperature of the limbs as the measure of progress. After four doses (one dose per day), he developed walnut-like purplish swellings over the body, which soon turned into chilblain. Treatment was continued. A few days later, he was able to move and turn. A month later he was completely recovered.

(Source: *Case Records of Dr. Yu Meizhong*.)

V Yang He Tang (Yang-Normalizing Decoction)

1 Source: Wai Ke Zheng Zhi Quan Sheng Ji (Treatise on the Diagnosis and Treatment of Surgical Illnesses)

2 Composition

Chief Herbs: shudihuang (*Rehmannia glutinosa*) 30 g
lujiaojiao (*Cervus nippon*) 9 g

Deputy Herbs: charred ganjiang (*Zingiber officinale*) 2 g
rougui (*Cinnamomum cassia*) 3 g

Assistant Herbs: mahuang (*Ephedra sinica*) 2 g
jiezi (*Sinapis alba*) 6 g

Envoy Herbs: gancao (*Glycyrrhiza uralensis*) 3 g

3 Application

Actions: warms Yang, generates blood, dispels Cold and removes stagnation.

Indications: Yin-type ulcers or swellings.

Main Symptoms: subcutaneous swelling without heads, without color change in the overlying skin and without heat; and swellings of the knee joints – all attributable to blood insufficiency and stasis due to Cold.

4 Analysis of the Formula

Yang He Tang uses a large amount of shudihuang to warm and tonify the Nutritive Level and blood, generate essence and nourish the bone marrow. It is complemented by lujiaojiao, which augments kidney-Yang and strengthens the tendons and bones. Used together these two generate blood and support Yang. They serve as the chief herbs.

Internal accumulation of Cold and Dampness can be eliminated only by warmth and dispersal. For that purpose, acrid and warm charred ganjiang and rougui are used as deputy herbs. Charred ganjiang warms the middle-jiao and disperses deficiency-Cold. Rougui disperses deficiency-Cold and facilitates Yang movement. If Cold is in the Nutritive and Blood Levels, rougui has the ability to enter these phases and unblock the channels by warming them.

Mahuang is acrid and warm, and can reach the Defensive Level. It warms the meridians, disperses gelled Cold by facilitating Yang circulation. Jiezi dissipates Cold–Phlegm and dries accumulated Dampness. Together these two not only enhance Qi and blood circulation but also enable shudihuang and lujiaojiao to exert their tonic effects without congealing.

Gancao is used as the envoy herb for its ability to detoxify and to harmonize the actions of the other herbs.

5 Comments

Yang He Tang is an essential formula for all Yin-type exterior illnesses. It is indicated for all types of ulcers and swellings without eruption, heat or redness.

In clinical practice it is important to pay attention as well to the symptoms affecting the rest of the body, in order to avoid erroneous application.

6 Case Study: Osteoma in a 17-Year-Old Male

For several months the patient had an egg-sized mass in the left side of his neck. It was not painful or tender, and was not movable. His complexion was lusterless, and he appeared chronically fatigued. His limbs were cold, his tongue was plump, and his pulse was deep, threadlike and forceless.

Diagnosis: Osteoma caused by deficiency of genuine Qi with gelling of Yin-Cold.

Therapeutic Principle: Warm Yang and disperse Cold, and support genuine Qi and release blood stasis.

Treatment: Yang He Tang with added processed fuzi (*Aconitum*) 10 g was prescribed, at the dosage of one decoction each day, administered in three portions. This was continued for over 50 consecutive days. The mass dissipated completely and all symptoms resolved. The only residual finding was moderate hyperpigmentation of the overlying skin.

(Source: *Journal of the Guiyang School of Chinese Medicine*, 1983, 4:32.)

VI Section Summary

Five formulas are described in detail in this section. They can be grouped by their actions into three categories: those that warm the middle-jiao and dispel Cold; those that rescue Yang and prevent collapse; and those that warm channels and disperse Cold.

Li Zhong Wan and Xiao Jian Zhong Tang are representative of those that warm the middle-jiao and dispel Cold. They are the mainstays for treating Cold in the middle-jiao due to Yang deficiency. **Li Zhong Wan** warms and tonifies the middle-jiao, disperses Cold, and strengthens the spleen. Often also used as a decoction, it is a standard treatment for deficiency Cold in the middle-jiao with abdominal pain, vomiting and diarrhea. **Xiao Jian Zhong Tang** warms the middle-jiao and augments what is deficient, harmonizes interior and moderates spasm. It is a standard treatment for acute interior illnesses as well as palpitations brought on by insufficiency of the *zang* organs of the middle-jiao. It is the mainstay for warming and strengthening these organs.

Si Ni Tang is the representative formula for rescuing Yang and preventing collapse. It is the mainstay for treating illnesses in which Yang has been depleted and Yin-Cold is excessive in the interior, leading to extremely cold limbs and Yang that is on the verge of extinction.

Danggui Si Ni Tang is the principal formula for warming channels and dispersing Cold. Its main actions are to warm and unblock the channels, disperse Cold and generate blood. It is mainly indicated for illnesses of blood insufficiency and Cold causing frigid limbs. It is best for treating Cold that is in the meridians and associated with blood insufficiency. In such conditions the coldness of the limbs is due to a different cause from that treated with Si Ni Tang.

Yang He Tang acts to warm Yang and generate blood, dispel Cold and unblock channels. It is the key formula for treating exterior lesions of the Yin-type.

Section 6 Formulas That Restore (Tonify)

Herbal formulas that restore (tonify) are constructed around herbs with the actions of augmenting or nourishing Qi, blood, Yin or Yang. They are mainly used for curing the many types of deficiency illnesses. Among the Eight Methods of Therapy they fall in the category of the Method of Restoration (Tonification).

Insufficiency of Qi, blood, Yin or Yang may result in an illness of deficiency. A condition of deficiency may be due to innate insufficiency, or to a lack of proper care subsequent to birth. Regardless whether due to innate insufficiency or inappropriate postnatal care, the deficiency condition is closely related to the *zang* organs. For this reason, the principles of therapy of a deficiency condition use Qi, blood, Yin and Yang as woof and the *zang* organs as warp. Such an approach is critically important in the diagnosis and treatment of deficiency illnesses.

In clinical practice, note that the methods of invigorating Qi and of invigorating blood have different emphasis. But Qi and blood are mutually interdependent and are intimately connected. In general, when treating Qi deficiency though the primary herbs augment Qi it is appropriate to complement them with herbs that nourish blood. Similarly, when treating blood deficiency though the primary herbs generate blood it is appropriate to complement them with some that augment Qi.

Similar considerations apply when selecting herbs that nourish Yin or Yang. Yin and Yang are also mutually interdependent. When nourishing Yang in Yang deficiency illnesses, it is appropriate to include herbs that nourish Yin. For Yang is rooted in Yin, so that nourishing Yin provides support for Yang and uses the ability of Yin-herbs to moisten to restrain the ability of Yang-herbs to warm and dry, thereby permitting invigoration of Yang without damaging body fluids. Conversely, when nourishing Yin in Yin deficiency illnesses, it is appropriate to include herbs that nourish Yang. For Yin is rooted in Yang, and the inclusion of Yang-nourishing herbs enables Yin to transform properly. It also exploits the warming action of Yang-herbs to restrain the tendency of Yin-herbs to bring about gelling, so that Yin is invigorated without stagnation. In deficiency of both Yin and Yang it is proper to nourish both.

When prescribing restorative herbal formulas the physician must ascertain whether the state of deficiency or (evil) strength is genuine or only apparent. In illnesses of deficiency that resist invigoration it is appropriate first to regulate the spleen and the stomach. This can be achieved by including appropriate herbs that strengthen the spleen and the stomach as well as those that regulate Qi and promote digestion. Doing so will facilitate the movement of the vital force and permit its invigoration without risk of stagnation.

I Si Jun Zi Tang (Four Nobles Decoction)

1 Source: Tai Ping Hui Min He Ji Ju Fang (Prescriptions from the Taiping Benevolent Pharmaceutical Bureau)

2 Composition

Chief Herb: renshen (*Panax ginseng*) 9 g

Deputy Herb: baizhu (*Atractylodes macrocephala*) 9 g

Assistant Herb: fuling (*Poria cocos*) 9 g

Envoy Herb: fried gancao (*Glycyrrhiza uralensis*) 6 g

3 Application

Actions: replenishes Qi and strengthens the spleen.

Indications: deficiency of spleen and stomach-Qi.

Main Symptoms: pallid complexion; low and soft voice; reduced appetite; shortness of breath; weakness in the limbs; loose feces; a pale tongue with a white coating; and a depletive and feeble pulse.

4 Analysis of the Formula

Renshen is sweet in flavor and warm in nature. It powerfully augments spleen and stomach-Qi, and serves as the chief herb.

Baizhu is bitter in flavor and warm in nature. It strengthens the spleen and dries Dampness, and serves as the deputy herb.

Fuling is slightly sweet in flavor and mild in nature. It strengthens the spleen and dries Dampness, and serves as the assistant herb. When fuling and baizhu are teamed together, their ability to strengthen the spleen and dry Dampness is much enhanced.

Fried gancao has a sweet flavor and warm nature. It enhances Qi and warms the middle-jiao. It also harmonizes the actions of the other herbs in the formula, and serves as the envoy herb.

These four herbs act in concert to invigorate Qi and strengthen the spleen.

5 Comments

This formula is commonly used to strengthen the spleen, to nourish the stomach, and through its sweet flavor and warm nature to enhance Qi.

Many formulas for invigorating Qi are derived from this formula. Examples include Yi Gong San and Liu Jun Zi Tang. The spleen and the stomach are the postnatal sources of Qi, blood, Nutritive and Defensive Qi. Hence the physician who desires to augment Qi must do so by strengthening the spleen and the stomach. **Yi Gong San**, derived from Si Jun Zi Tang by adding chenpi (*Citrus tangerina*), is most effective for curing vomiting and diarrhea, insufficiency of both the spleen and the stomach, and loss of appetite. **Liu Jun Zi Tang**, derived from Si Jun Zi Tang by adding chenpi and processed banxia (*Pinellia*), is most effective for regulating the spleen and settling the stomach. If muxiang (*Aucklandia*) and sharen (*Amomum*) are further added, the formula becomes **Xiang Sha Liu Jun Zi Tang**. This expanded prescription is especially effective in regulating Qi movement and strengthening the spleen.

II Bu Zhong Yi Qi Tang (Middle-Restoring and Qi-Augmenting Decoction)

1 Source: Pi Wei Lun (Treatise on the Spleen and the Stomach)

2 Composition

Chief Herb: huangqi (*Astragalus membranaceus*) 18 g

Deputy Herbs: renshen (*Panax ginseng*) 6 g
baizhu (*Atractylodes macrocephala*) 9 g

Assistant Herbs: danggui (*Angelica sinensis*) 3 g
chenpi (*Citrus tangerina, reticulata*) 6 g
shengma (*Cimicifuga heracleifolia, foetida*) 6 g
chaihu (*Bupleurum chinense, scorzonerifolium*) 6 g
fried gancao (*Glycyrrhiza uralensis*) 9 g

3 Application

Actions: tonifies middle-jiao-Qi and raises sunken Yang.

Indications and Main Symptoms: (1) Deficiency of the spleen and the stomach. Main symptoms: reduced appetite; fatigue and weakness in the limbs; unwillingness to speak much; pallid complexion; scant and watery feces; a large but depletive pulse. (2) Deficient Qi with sunken Yang. Main symptoms: prolapse of the rectum or uterus; chronic diarrhea or dysentery; massive vaginal bleeding; shortness of breath with weakness; a pale tongue; and a depletive pulse. (3) Qi deficiency with fever. Main symptoms: fever; spontaneous sweating; thirst with preference for hot drinks; shortness of breath with weakness; a pale tongue; a depletive and forceless pulse.

4 Analysis of the Formula

Bu Zhong Yi Qi Tang uses a large amount of huangqi to strengthen the middle-jiao, enhance Qi, raise Yang and consolidate the exterior. This makes huangqi the chief herb.

The deputy herbs, renshen and baizhu, enhance Qi and strengthen the spleen. They complement huangqi to enhance the tonification of the middle-jiao and the invigoration of Qi.

Blood is the mother of Qi. When Qi has been deficient for a long time, Nutritive blood also becomes deficient. For this reason danggui is used to generate blood, regulate the Nutritive Level, and assist renshen and huangqi in their action to invigorate Qi and generate blood. Chenpi regulates Qi and the stomach, and aids the other herbs in tonification without stagnation. Thus, danggui and chenpi both serve as assistant herbs. In addition, small amounts of shengma and chaihu are included for their ability to lift Yang and raise the collapsed. They assist the chief herb to raise collapsed middle-jiao-Qi.

Fried gancao harmonizes the actions of the various herbs. In this formula it serves as both assistant and envoy.

Used in concert these herbs nourish what is deficient and lift up what has collapsed. In patients who have fever due to Qi deficiency, treatment with this sweet, warm and Qi-enhancing herbs will remove the fever and make genuine Qi full, so that pure Yang can rise. In this way, all the symptoms will resolve.

5 Comments

Bu Zhong Yi Qi Tang is representative of formulas that nourish Qi, raise sunken Yang and clear Heat by their sweet flavor and mild nature. The key symptoms the formula aims at are fatigue and weakness, shortness of breath and lassitude, a pallid complexion, and a pulse that is depletive and forceless.

The formula is not appropriate for such illnesses as fever due to Yin deficiency or strong internal Heat.

6 Case Study: Postpartum Anuria in a 28-Year-Old Female

For 5 days following giving birth the patient was unable to urinate. Her complexion was pallid. She was short of breath and unwilling to talk. Her perspiration was excessive. She felt tired and was weak, desiring to sleep all day long. She had an urgency to urinate but was unable to do so. Her lower abdomen was distended, and her lochia were pink. Her tongue was pale and marked by indentations from the teeth. Her pulse was deep, feeble and slow.

Diagnosis: Deficiency of Qi and blood, with sinking of central Qi and impedance in the movement of bladder-Qi.

Therapeutic Principle: Augment Qi and nourish blood.

Treatment: She was treated with Bu Zhong Yi Qi Tang with added taoren (*Prunus persica*), honghua (*Carthamus*) and mutong (*Akebia quinata, trifoliata*). She recovered after five doses.

(Source: *Fujian Journal of Chinese Medicine*, 1986, 4:53.)

III Yu Ping Feng San (Jade-Screen Powder)

1 Source: Yi Fang Lei Ju (Classified Prescriptions)

2 Composition

Chief Herb: huangqi (*Astragalus membranaceus*) 6 g

Deputy Herb: baizhu (*Atractylodes macrocephala*) 12 g

Assistant Herb: fangfeng (*Saposhnikovia divaricata*) 12 g

3 Application

Actions: replenishes Qi, consolidates the exterior and stops sweating.

Indications: deficiency affecting the exterior, with spontaneous sweating.

Main Symptoms: aversion to wind; pallid complexion; spontaneous sweating; a pale tongue with white coating; and a pulse that is floating and depletive. Or, a weak body that is highly susceptible to Wind.

4 Analysis of the Formula

Defensive Qi guards the exterior of the body and wards off pathogenic factors. When it is deficient there will be spontaneous sweating and exterior is unable to ward off pathogenic evils, especially invasion by Wind. Treatment should be based on strengthening Qi, firming the exterior and stopping the sweating.

Yu Ping Feng San uses huangqi as the chief herb for its ability to replenish Qi, firm the exterior and stop sweating. Baizhu is the deputy herb; it has the ability to strengthen the spleen and augment Qi and it facilitates huangqi. With these herbs acting in concert Qi is invigorated and the exterior becomes strong, so that sweat does not leak outward and Wind does not invade.

The two herbs are assisted by fangfeng, which dispels Wind. The combined action of fangfeng, huangqi and baizhu expels Wind and augments genuine Qi. In the presence of fangfeng huangqi fortifies the exterior without retaining pathogenic factors. In the presence of huangqi fangfeng dispels Wind without injuring genuine Qi.

The entire formula acts to augment Qi, consolidate the exterior, stop sweating, support the normal Qi and dispel Wind.

5 Comments

Characteristically this formula invigorates in dispersion and disperses in invigoration, so that there is both invigoration and dispersion. Fangfeng guides huangqi to exterior and magnifies its ability to stabilize the exterior. Huangqi makes fangfeng more powerful in dispelling Wind yet does not injure genuine Qi. In addition, there is baizhu to fortify the interior; and fortification of the interior leads automatically to a stronger exterior.

In its actions of invigorating Qi, fortifying the exterior, stopping sweating and dispelling Wind, this formula functions like a barricade yet has dispersing effects. Its name is derived from these actions.

6 Case Study: Cold Urticaria in a 37-Year-Old Female

The patient had a somewhat weak constitution and often caught the common cold. Whenever the season changed, with the coming of cold air she felt chills and developed intensely itchy nodules on many parts of the body. She took western medications intermittently for over a year, without benefit. Her tongue was pale, with a thin and pale yellow coating. Her pulses in all locations were floating and taut.

Diagnosis: Deficiency of Defensive Qi, leading to weakness in the exterior and invasion by Wind.

Therapeutic Principle: Invigorate Qi, fortify the exterior, dispel Wind and stop the itch.

Treatment: She was prescribed Yu Ping Feng San with added jingjie spikes (*Schizonepeta*), chantui (*Cryptotympana*), cangerzi (*Xanthium sibiricum*) and gancao (Glycyrrhiza). After three daily doses, the urticarial nodules on the back disappeared, and those on the head, face and limbs shrank and partially faded. After three additional doses, all symptoms resolved.

IV Sheng Mai San (Pulse-Generating Powder)

1 Source: *Yi Fang Qi Yuan (The Sources of Medicine)*

2 Composition

Chief Herb: renshen (*Panax ginseng*) 9 g

Deputy Herb: maimendong (*Ophiopogon japonicus*) 9 g

Assistant and Envoy Herb: wuweizi (*Schisandra chinensis*) 6 g

3 Application

Actions: replenishes Qi, generates fluids, restrains Yin and stops sweating.

Indications: (1) Qi exhaustion and Yin damage caused by Heat or hot weather. (2) Lung insufficiency and chronic cough due to injury to both Qi and Yin.

Main Symptoms: profuse perspiration with lethargy; fatigue and weakness; shortness of breath with reluctance to speak; dry throat and thirst; a red tongue with scant coating; and a depletive and rapid pulse.

4 Analysis of the Formula

Sweet and warm renshen is the chief herb in this formula. It replenishes Qi and generates fluids, thereby strengthening the lung. When lung-Qi is ample then the Qi of the other visceral organs are also ample.

Maimendong replenishes Yin, clears Heat, moistens the lung and generates fluids. It serves as the deputy herb. The ability to nourish Qi and Yin is enhanced when maimendong is teamed with renshen.

Wuweizi restrains lung-Qi, stops sweating, generates fluids and removes thirst. It is the assistant herb.

With these three herbs acting in concert – one nourishes, one disperses, one restrains – the formula is especially efficacious in augmenting Qi and restoring Yin, generating fluids and stopping sweating, and at the same time restraining Yin and eliminating thirst. By restoring Qi and regenerating fluids, stopping the sweating and preserving Yin, the pulse is animated by full Qi and is rescued; hence the formula is named "pulse-generating."

In illnesses involving injury to both Qi and Yin, leading to lung insufficiency and chronic cough, the formula is prescribed for its ability to replenish Qi and restore Yin, thereby restraining the lung, stopping cough, moistening the lung and generating fluids. This relieves all the symptoms.

5 Comments

Sheng Mai San is a commonly prescribed formula for illnesses involving double injury to Qi and Yin. It is used to treat conditions of excessive sweating due to Summer Heat damaging Qi and fluids. It is also used for lung deficiency and chronic cough due to deficiency of both Qi and Yin. The key requirement for its application is pure deficiency of Qi and fluids without exogenous disease evil.

However, this formula is not a panacea for mid-summer illnesses. If the Summer Heat evil is in the exterior, or if there is no injury to Qi or Yin in the face of excessive Summer Heat, then it is contraindicated.

6 Case Study: Sudden Prostration in a 65-Year-Old Male

The patient had high fever, a cough productive of rust-colored sputum and chest pain. He was admitted to hospital for lobar pneumonia. On the fifth day, after extreme overeating he suddenly developed projectile vomiting, followed by shallow respiration, pallor, profuse cold sweat, cold limbs, a threadlike pulse, and a precipitous drop in blood pressure to 30 mmHg.

Diagnosis: In conference with consultants, the diagnosis of sudden prostration (septic shock in western medical terminology) was reached.

Therapeutic Principle: Augment Qi and generate fluids.

Treatment: The patient was treated with Sheng Mai San, augmented with Korean white renshen (*Panax*) 10 g, maimendong (*Ophiopogon*) 10 g, wuweizi (*Schisandra*) 3 g, processed fuzi (*Aconitum*) 10 g, refined ganjiang (*Zingiber*) 6 g, and fried gancao (Glycyrrhiza) 10 g. After three successive doses, the limbs began to warm and the blood pressure rose toward normal levels. He was treated further, with additions or subtractions depending on the symptoms, and recovered fully.

(Source: *Sichuan Journal of Chinese Medicine*.)

V Si Wu Tang (Four Substances Decoction)

1 Source: Xian Shou Li Shang Xu Duan Bi Fang (Secret Celestial Prescriptions for Wounds and Fractures)

2 Composition

Chief Herb: shudihuang (*Rehmannia glutinosa*) 12 g

Deputy Herb: danggui (*Angelica sinensis*) 9 g

Assistant and Envoy Herbs: baishaoyao (*Paeonia lactiflora*) 9 g
chuanxiong (*Ligusticum chuanxiong*, *wallichii*) 6 g

3 Application

Actions: nourishes and regulates blood.

Indications: insufficiency and stasis of blood at the Nutritive Level.

Main Symptoms: palpitation and insomnia; dizziness with blurred vision; dull and lusterless complexion; in females, irregular menses with little flow or no flow at all; abdominal pain around the umbilicus; a pale tongue; and a pulse that is threadlike and taut or threadlike and impeded.

4 Analysis of the Formula

The chief herb shudihuang nourishes both Yin and blood. The deputy herb danggui tonifies blood, nourishes the liver and regulates blood and menstruation. Two herbs assist them. Baishaoyao nourishes blood, softens the liver and regulates Yin. Chuanxiong facilitates the circulation of blood and Qi.

The special characteristic of this formula is the complementation of two groups of herbs. Shudihuang and baishaoyao are Yin and gentle in action, whereas danggui and chuanxiong are acrid and warm. This enables the formula to generate blood without causing stasis and regulate blood without injuring it. By generating and regulating blood these four herbs working in concert harmonize Nutritive blood, so that the formula is suitable for generating blood in blood insufficiency and mobilizing blood in blood stasis.

5 Comments

Si Wu Tang is the main formula for generating blood as well as the main one for regulating menstruation. It focuses on nourishing and regulating blood. In clinical application, the key symptoms suggesting its use are palpitation of the heart, dizziness, a lusterless complexion, a pale tongue and a threadlike pulse.

For patients who also have Qi deficiency, renshen (*Panax*) and huangqi (Astragalus) may be added to the formula in order to invigorate Qi as well as produce blood. For patients who also have blood stasis, taoren (*Prunus persica*) and honghua (*Carthamus*) may be added. The formula then becomes **Tao Hong Si Wu Tang**, which is used to generate blood, facilitate its movement and resolve stasis, and which is also the main treatment in females for early menstruation, excessive menstrual flow that is purple and mucoid or with clots, or abdominal pain and distention.

For patients who also have endogenous Cold arising from blood insufficiency, refined ganjiang (*Zingiber*) and wuzhuyu (*Evodia*) may be added to warm and open the meridians. For patients who also have endogenous Heat arising from blood insufficiency, huangqi and mudanpi (*Paeonia suffruticosa*) may be added and shudihuang replaced by shengdihuang, in order to purge Heat and cool blood.

VI Gui Pi Tang (Spleen-Restoring Decoction)

1 Source: Ji Sheng Fang (Life-Saving Prescriptions)

2 Composition

Chief Herbs: huangqi (*Astragalus membranaceus*) 12 g
longyanrou (*Dimocarpus longan*) 12 g

Deputy Herbs: renshen (*Panax ginseng*) 6 g
baizhu (*Atractylodes macrocephala*) 9 g
danggui (*Angelica sinensis*) 9 g

Assistant Herbs: fushen (*Poria cocos*) 9 g
suanzaoren (*Ziziphus jujuba*) 12 g
yuanzhi (*Polygala tenuifolia*) 6 g
muxiang (*Aucklandia lappa*) 6 g

Envoy Herbs: fried gancao (*Glycyrrhiza uralensis*) 3 g
shengjiang (*Zingiber officinale*) 5 pieces
dazao (*Ziziphus jujuba*) 1 piece

3 Application

Actions: augments Qi, tonifies blood, strengthens the spleen and nourishes the heart.

Indications and Main Symptoms: (1) Deficiency of both Qi and blood in the spleen and the heart. Main symptoms: palpitation and fearfulness; forgetfulness and insomnia; night sweats of deficiency-Heat; fatigue with reduced appetite; pallid and wan complexion, a pale tongue with a thin and white coating, and a threadlike and feeble pulse. (2) Inability of the spleen to control blood. Main symptoms: hematuria, easy bruising with purpura in the skin; excessive menstrual flow coming earlier than due, with menses that are large in quantity and pale in color, or menses that continue to spot without stopping; a pale tongue and a threadlike pulse.

4 Analysis of the Formula

Gui Pi Tang uses huangqi and longyanrou as chief herbs. Huangqi strengthens the spleen and augments Qi. Longyanrou augments spleen-Qi and nourishes the heart and blood.

Renshen and baizhu are sweet and warm, and they augment Qi. Teaming with huangqi enhances their ability to augment Qi and nourish the spleen. Danggui is acrid–sweet and slightly warm, and it nourishes blood at the Nutritive Level. Teaming with longyanrou enhances their ability to nourish the heart and blood. These three are the deputy herbs.

The assistant herbs fall in two groups. In one group, fushen (fuling grown around a pine root), suanzaoren and yuanzhi nourish the heart and calm the mind. In the other, the sole herb muxiang regulates Qi and stimulates the spleen. Teamed with Qi-augmenting and blood-generating herbs these four ensure that augmenting is not accompanied by impeding, so that as spleen-Qi becomes more ample there is not indigestion.

Fried gancao and dazao augment spleen-Qi and harmonize the actions of the other herbs. They are the envoy herbs.

Used together these herbs make a fine formula for augmenting and generating Qi and blood.

5 Comments

The heart houses the mind and controls the emotions, while the spleen houses thought and controls the circulation of blood. Prolonged brooding exhausts the heart and the spleen. That in turn leads to exhaustion of the spirit, anorexia and insomnia. The spleen and the stomach are the fountainhead of Qi and blood. Spleen deficiency leads to deficiency of blood, so that the heart loses its source of nourishment and becomes even more insufficient; this results in severe palpitations, melancholy and tiredness, as well as forgetfulness and night sweat. Gui Pi Tang re-invigorates the heart and the spleen. As Qi becomes full again, blood can be readily generated and the symptoms of palpitations, melancholy, tiredness, insomnia and others, can all be relieved.

In addition, women in whom Spleen-Qi is deficient and unable to control blood may have excessive menses or metrorrhagia. This can be treated with Gui Pi Tang as well.

VII Ba Zhen Tang (Eight Treasures Decoction)

1 *Source: Zheng Ti Lei Yao (Classification and Treatment of Traumatic Injuries)*

2 *Composition*

Chief Herbs: renshen (*Panax ginseng*) 9 g
shudihuang (*Rehmannia glutinosa*) 9 g

Deputy Herbs: baizhu (*Atractylodes macrocephala*) 9 g
fuling (*Poria cocos*) 9 g
danggui (*Angelica sinensis*) 9 g
baishaoyao (*Paeonia lactiflora*) 9 g

Assistant Herb: chuanxiong (*Ligusticum chuanxiong*, *wallichii*) 9 g

Envoy Herb: fried gancao (*Glycyrrhiza uralensis*) 5 g

3 *Application*

Actions: replenishes Qi and tonifies blood.

Indications: deficiency of both Qi and blood.

Main Symptoms: pallid or sallow complexion; dizziness and blurred vision; fatigue, shortness of breath and unwillingness to speak much; palpitation and melancholy; anorexia: a pale tongue, and a threadlike and feeble or large but depletive and forceless pulse.

4 *Analysis of the Formula*

Ba Zhen Tang is constructed by combining Si Jun Zi Tang and Si Wu Tang. The chief herbs, renshen and shudihuang, replenish Qi and nourish blood. Two of the deputy herbs, baizhu and fuling, strengthen the spleen and dry Dampness, thereby reinforcing the actions of renshen. The other deputy herbs, danggui and baishaoyao, nourish blood and regulate Nutritive Yin, thereby assisting shudihuang in generating blood. As assistant herb chuanxiong mobilizes blood and Qi circulation to prevent stagnation. The envoy herb is fried gancao, which augments and regulates Qi in the middle-jiao and modulates the potency of all herbs in the formula. These herbs together make a formula that augments Qi and generates blood.

5 *Comments*

Ba Zhen Tang is commonly prescribed for concurrent deficiency of Qi and blood, as it combines herbs that generate blood and herbs that augment Qi in order to bring about tonification of both Yin and Yang. In clinical practice it is often used for deficiency of both the spleen and the stomach, atrophy of the muscles, or the deficiency of both Qi and blood from pregnancy or heavy vaginal bleeding.

A number of formulas are based on Ba Zhen Tang. If huangqi (*Astragalus*) and rougui (*Cinnamomum*) are added, the formula becomes **Shi Quan Da Bu Tang**. The augmented herbs are suitable for treating cough due to deficiency and overexertion, spermatorrhea or urethral bleeding in males, and heavy vaginal bleeding or irregular menses in females.

If chuanxiong is removed from Shi Quan Da Bu Tang and wuweizi (*Schisandra*), yuanzhi (*Polygala*), chenpi (*Citrus tangerina*), shengjiang (*Zingiber*) and dazao (*Ziziphus*) are added, the resulting formula is **Renshen Yang Rong Tang**. Renshen Yang Rong Tang nourishes the heart and calms the mind at the same time as it augments Qi and generates blood. It is the mainstay for treating deficiency of both Qi and blood caused by exhaustion and damage from overexertion.

If rougui and fuling are removed from Shi Quan Da Bu Tang and xuduan (*Dipsacus asperoides*), huangqin (*Scutellaria*), sharen (*Amomum*) and nuomi (*Oryza sativa*) are added, the resulting formula is **Tai Shan Pan Shi San**. In addition to its basic function of augmenting Qi and generating blood this formula can also calm the fetus. It is used to treat habitual miscarriages due to deficiency of both Qi and blood.

6 *Clinical Study: Habitual Miscarriage*

The efficacy of Ba Zhen Tang with additions was evaluated in 38 cases of habitual miscarriages, with complete success. The women were all between 25 and 30 years of age. The number of miscarriages ranged from a low of 2 to a high of 5. The basic herbal formula used was Ba Zhen Tang with added sharen (*Amomum*) and zisu (*Perilla*). Additional modifications are as follows.

For those patients with Qi deficiency as well, huangqi (*Astragalus*) was added. For those with blood deficiency, ejiao (*Equus asinus*) was added. For those with vomiting due to strong deficiency-Fire, huangqin (*Scutellaria*) and zhuru (*Phyllostachys nigra*) were added. For those with dryness in the mouth and throat due to deficiency-Fire, shudihuang (*Rehmannia*) was removed and shengdihuang (*Rehmannia*) and yuzhu (*Polygonatum*) were added.

(Source: *Fujian Journal of Chinese Medicine*, 1960, 10:3.)

VIII Liu Wei Dihuang Wan (Six-Ingredient Rehmannia Pill)

1 Source: Xiao Er Yao Zheng Zhi Jue (Key to Therapeutics of Children's Illnesses)

2 Composition

Chief Herb: shudihuang (*Rehmannia glutinosa*) 24 g

Deputy Herbs: shanyao (*Dioscorea opposita*) 12 g
shanzhuyu (*Cornus officinalis*) 12 g

Assistant and Envoy Herbs: zexie (*Alisma plantago-aquatica, orientale*) 9 g
mudanpi (*Paeonia suffruticosa*) 9 g
fuling (*Poria cocos*) 9 g

3 Application

Actions: nourishes and augments kidney-Yin.

Indications: deficiency of kidney-Yin.

Main Symptoms: aching and weakness in the lower back and the knees; dizziness and blurred vision; tinnitus or diminished hearing; night sweat; spontaneous and nocturnal semen emissions; deficiency-fever with recurrent fever, toothache, hotness in the palms and soles; excessive urine; thirst, dry mouth and throat; a red tongue with little coating; and a deep, threadlike and rapid pulse.

4 Analysis of the Formula

Liu Wei Dihuang Tang, which dates from the Song dynasty, uses large amounts of shudihuang to replenish Yin, strengthen the kidney, restore the vital force and nourish the marrow. It serves as chief herb.

Shanzhuyu nourishes the liver and the kidney, and can also slow the flow of semen. Shanyao replenishes spleen-Yin and can also firm up semen. They serve as deputy herbs. Used in concert the chief and deputy herbs effectively nourish the liver, the spleen and the kidney, and are together known as the "three restorative herbs." However, in this formula the amount of shudihuang equals the sum of the amounts of shanzhuyu and shanyao; hence the main action is to invigorate kidney Yin.

Zexie promotes diuresis to leach out Dampness and impurities. It also counteracts the tendency of shudihuang to increase fat and its affinity for certain external pathogenic factors. Mudanpi calms and purges kidney-Fire. It also curbs the warm and astringent nature of shanzhuyu. Fuling leaches out Dampness from the spleen. It also aids shanyao to strengthen the spleen. Together these three herbs are known as the "three cathartic herbs." They overcome the impurities of Dampness, reduce deficiency Fire and curb the excesses of the "three restorative herbs." They serve as the assistant herbs.

5 Comments

Liu Wei Dihuang Wan is the basic herbal formula for treating deficiency of kidney-Yin. The key symptoms requiring its use are weakness and aches in the waist and knees, dizziness with blurred vision, dry mouth and throat, a red tongue with scant coating, and a pulse that is deep, threadlike and rapid. It is contraindicated in diarrhea caused by spleen insufficiency.

The formula uses six herbs, three restoratives and three cathartics. The restoratives are used in larger amounts, so the main activity is to tonify. Though it invigorates Yin in three organs – liver, spleen and kidney – the most important function is to invigorate kidney-Yin. This is the characteristic of the selection and balance of the herbs in the formula.

Many useful formulas are based on Liu Wei Dihuang Wan.

Zhi Bai Dihuang Wan is obtained by adding zhimu (*Anemarrhena*) and huangbai (*Phellodendron*) to Liu Wei Dihuang Wan. In addition to nourishing Yin, it has the ability to subdue Fire. It is used to treat blazing Fire due to Yin deficiency, manifested as deficiency-fever syndrome, anxiety with restlessness, night sweats, aches in the waist and back and spontaneous and nocturnal emissions.

Du Qi Wan is obtained by adding wuweizi (*Schisandra*) to Liu Wei Dihuang Wan. It has the ability to nourish the kidney and stabilize Qi, and is used to treat dyspnea and hiccup caused by deficiency of kidney-Yin.

Mai Wei Dihuang Wan is obtained by adding maimendong (*Ophiopogon*) and wuweizi to Liu Wei Dihuang Wan. This has the ability to restrain the lung and stabilize the kidney. It is used to treat deficiency of lung and kidney Yin, which produces cough, dyspnea, recurrent fever, night sweats and other symptoms.

Qi Ju Dihuang Wan is obtained by adding gouqizi (*Lycium*) and juhua (*Chrysanthemum*) to Liu Wei Dihuang Wan. This has the ability to nourish the kidney and the liver. It is used for treating deficiency of liver and kidney Yin, which causes dizziness and blurred vision, xerophthalmia or tearing on exposure to wind.

Table 9.2 compares Liu Wei Dihuang Wan with its most important derivative formulas.

Table 9.2 Liu Wei Dihuang Wan and its derived formulas

Formula	Composition	Actions	Application
Liu Wei Dihuang Wan	Basic six (see text)	Nourishes Yin, strengthens kidney	Deficiency of kidney-Yin Symptoms: see above
Zhi Bai Dihuang Wan	Basic six + zhimu, huangbai	Nourishes Yin, drains deficiency Fire	Blazing Fire due to Yin deficiency Symptoms: deficiency-fever syndrome, anxiety with restlessness, night sweats, aches in the waist and back, spontaneous and nocturnal emissions
Du Qi Wan	Basic six + wuweizi	Nourishes kidney, improves respiration	Deficiency of kidney-Yin Symptoms: dyspnea, hiccup
Mai Wei Dihuang Wan	Basic six + maimen-dong, wuweizi		Deficiency of lung and kidney Yin Symptoms: cough, dyspnea, recurrent fever, night sweats
Qi Ju Dihuang Wan	Basic six + gouqizi, juhua	Nourishes kidney	Deficiency of liver and kidney Yin Symptoms: dizziness and blurred vision, xerophthalmia or tearing on exposure to wind

6 *Case Study: Chronic Nephritis in a 26-Year-Old Male*

The patient developed chronic nephritis at the age of 16. He basically recovered at that time. One year ago, he was found to have a high blood pressure. Western medications were prescribed to lower his blood pressure and Chinese medications that calm the mind and restrain semen flow. The results were not satisfactory.

He now presented with aches in his waist and weakness in his limbs. He had headaches, restlessness and reduced urine output. On examination he had a pallid complexion and shortness of breath, and was dispirited as though suffering from insomnia. His lower limbs were somewhat swollen, his tongue coating was thin and white, and his pulse was deep and threadlike. His blood pressure was 175/95 mmHg. Radiological study showed that the shape of the renal pelvis was consistent with changes induced by diminished blood flow to the kidney.

Diagnosis: Chronic deficiency of Yin superimposed on already weakened kidney-Yin, resulting in high blood pressure.

Therapeutic Principle: Nourish Yin and strengthen the kidney.

Treatment: Modified Liu Wei Dihuang Wan was prescribed. The composition was: shudihuang 24 g, shanzhuyu 12 g, zexie 4.5 g, danshen (*Salvia*) 12 g, maodongqing (*Ilex pubescens*) 24 g, duzhong (*Eucommia*) 9 g, and tusizi (*Cuscuta*) 12 g.

Following three daily doses, the blood pressure dropped to 142/80 mmHg, and the patient became more alert with alleviation of his symptoms. A differently modified formula was prescribed for ten doses, then changed to the basic Liu Wei Dihuang Wan. After taking it for 6 months the patient recovered completely.

(Source: *Lectures on Selected Chinese Medical Formulas*, The Guangdong Science and Technology Publishing House, 1981.)

IX Fried Gancao Tang (Fried Licorice Decoction)

1 Source: Shang Han Lun (Treatise on Cold-Attack)

2 Composition

Chief Herb: fried gancao (*Glycyrrhiza uralensis*) 12 g

Deputy Herbs: renshen (*Panax ginseng*) 6 g
shengdihuang (*Rehmannia glutinosa*) 30 g
dazao (*Ziziphus jujuba*) 10 pieces
ejiao (*Equus asinus*) 6 g
maimendong (*Ophiopogon japonicus*) 10 g
huomaren (*Cannabis sativa*) 10 g

Assistant and Envoy Herbs: guizhi (*Cinnamomum cassia*) 9 g
shengjiang (*Zingiber officinale*) 9 g

3 Application

Actions: nourishes Yin and blood, replenishes Qi, warms Yang, restores the pulse and stops palpitations.

Indications: illnesses of Yin and blood deficiency.

Main Symptoms: irregular pulse; palpitations; emaciation; shortness of breath; a shiny tongue with little coating.

4 Analysis of the Formula

The chief herb, fried gancao, is sweet in flavor and warm in nature. In large amounts it augments Qi and nourishes the heart.

This formula uses six deputy herbs. Renshen is potent in augmenting genuine Qi. Shengdihuang nourishes Yin-blood. Dazao augments Spleen-Qi and nourishes the heart. Ejiao augments Yin-blood. Maimendong moistens the stomach and the lung. Huomaren nourishes Yin and moistens the intestine.

Guizhi and shengjiang serve as assistant herbs. They warm heart-Yang and unblock blood vessels.

These herbs acting together have the overall effect of replenishing Yin-blood and Yang-Qi. Doing so brings about fullness of Yin and blood and normalizes their flow through the channels. Yin and Yang thereby become balanced, Qi and blood regulated, and heart symptoms resolved.

By adding wine during decoction, the formula gains potency in opening the meridians for freer flow and makes the herbs more efficacious.

5 Comments

Fried Gancao Tang is the principal herb for the treatment of certain types of irregular pulses: slow irregular pulse, consistently irregular pulse, and rapid irregular pulse. It can also be used generally for treating a variety of illnesses, such as: irregular pulse and palpitations due to excessive diaphoresis or blood loss; abnormal heart rate and anxiety due to deficiency of Qi and blood; and prolonged lung insufficiency causing cough and deficiency of both Qi and blood.

By omitting four of the Qi-augmenting-Yang-warming herbs (renshen, dazao, guizhi and shengjiang) and adding the blood-generating-Yin-restraining shaoyao (*Paeonia*), the formula becomes **Jia Jian Fu Mai Tang**. This modification changes the action from augmenting both Yin and Yang to one of nourishing Yin and generating fluids. It is used in treating the late stages of Yin exhaustion due to excessive Heat. (Note: Fu Mai Tang is an alternate name for Fried Gancao Tang.)

6 Case Study: Rheumatic Heart Illness in a 35-Year-Old Female

The patient had rheumatic heart illness for 6 years. For the past 2 months she suffered from sudden dizziness and palpitations, with a rapid and irregular pulse of 150 beats per min. Her tongue coating was thin and white.

Diagnosis: Deficiency and stagnation of Yin-blood, so that the heart loses its nourishment.

Treatment: She was prescribed Fried Gancao Tang. After 21 daily doses, the symptoms gradually decreased, including palpitations. Her appetite also improved.

(Source: *Jiangsu Journal of Chinese Medicine*, 1959, 1:14.)

X Yi Guan Jian (Yin-Generating Liver-Opening Prescription)

1 *Source: Xu Ming Yi Lei An (Supplement to Case Records of Celebrated Physicians)*

2 *Composition*

Chief Herb: shengdihuang (*Rehmannia glutinosa*) 18 g

Deputy Herbs: beishashen (*Radix Glehniae*) 9 g
maimendong (*Ophiopogon japonicus*) 9 g
danggui (*Angelica sinensis*) 9 g
gouqizi (*Lycium barbarum*) 9 g

Assistant and Envoy Herb: chuanlianzi (*Melia toosendan*) 5 g

3 *Application*

Actions: nourishes Yin and unblocks the liver.

Indications: deficiency of kidney and liver Yin, with trapping of liver-Qi.

Main Symptoms: subcostal and chest pain; acid regurgitation; dry or parched mouth and throat, a red and dry tongue; and an depletive and taut pulse.

4 *Analysis of the Formula*

The chief herb, shengdihuang, is used in large amount for its ability to nourish Yin and generate blood, and to strengthen the liver and the kidney.

Beishashen, maimendong, danggui and gouqizi are the deputy herbs. They augment Yin, generate blood and soften the liver, thereby assisting the chief herb in strengthening the liver and contributing to the growth of Yin and Yang. This is important, for the liver is Yin in its substance but is Yang in its activities; it stores blood and facilitates the movement of Qi.

The assistant herb, chuanlianzi, mobilizes constrained liver Qi and clears away Heat. It therefore regulates Qi and stops pain. Chuanlianzi is bitter and cold. If used alone it can damage Yin, but when used with large amounts of sweet and cold herbs that nourish Yin and generate blood the risk of damage to Yin is minimized.

These herbs together nourish the liver and promote the free flow of liver-Qi, so that subcostal pain, chest pain and other symptoms can be relieved.

5 Comments

Yi Guan Jian is clearly constructed by adding a small amount of an herb that unblocks the liver and regulates its Qi (chuanlianzi) to herbs that nourish liver and kidney Yin. It is used mainly for illnesses of Yin deficiency in both the liver and the kidney, so that the liver loses its nourishment and liver-Qi moves erratically.

Since Yin-nourishing herbs are emphasized in this formula, it is inappropriate if the patient has stagnation and accumulation of Phlegm–Rheum.

6 Case Study: Chronic Hepatitis in a 40-Year-Old Female

The patient suffered from chronic hepatitis for several years, with abnormal liver functions and a fluctuating course. It is aggravated whenever she is fatigued from overwork. At the time of presentation she had tenderness in the liver region, abdominal distention, a poor appetite, insomnia with frequent dreams, generalized weakness, pitting edema of the legs in the afternoon, feverishness and sometimes low-grade fever in the afternoon. Her menstrual flow was scanty. Her tongue was red, with scant coating. Her pulse was deep, threadlike and rapid.

Diagnosis: Deficiency of liver and kidney Yin, with Heat.

Therapeutic Principle: Enrich Yin and purge Heat.

Treatment: Yi Guan Jian with the addition of 30 g of danshen (*Salvia*) was prescribed, in order to promote blood circulation and tissue regeneration. This method used facilitation of circulation as the means to nourish. After 27 daily doses, the patient recovered completely and all symptoms disappeared. Her liver functions returned to normal, and she was able to resume her work. She was re-examined a year later and did not have any relapse.

(Source: *Journal of the Shandong College of Chinese Medicine*, 1979, 3, 12.)

XI Baihe Gu Jin Tang (Lily Metal-Solidifying Decoction)

1 Source: Shen Zhai Yi Shu

2 Composition

Chief Herbs: baihe (*Lilium brownii*) 12 g
shengdihuang (*Rehmannia glutinosa*) 9 g
shudihuang (*Rehmannia glutinosa*) 9 g

Deputy Herbs: maimendong (*Ophiopogon japonicus*) 9 g
xuanshen (*Scrophularia ningpoensis*) 9 g

Assistant Herbs: danggui (*Angelica sinensis*) 9 g
beimu (*Fritillaria cirrhosa*) 6 g
jiegeng (*Platycodon grandiflorum*) 6 g

Envoy Herbs: raw gancao (*Glycyrrhiza uralensis*) 3 g

3 Application

Actions: nourishes the kidney, moistens the lungs, stops cough and dissolves Phlegm.

Indications: lung and kidney Yin deficiency with an upward attack by deficiency-induced endogenous Fire.

Main Symptoms: cough productive of blood-streaked sputum; wheezing; dry and sore throat; dizziness and blurred vision; recurrent fever in the afternoon or unremitting fever; a red tongue with little coating; and a threadlike and rapid pulse.

4 Analysis of the Formula

In Baihe Gu Jin Tang, baihe nourishes Yin and purges Heat, moistens the lung and stops cough. Shengdihuang and shudihuang used together can enrich Yin and generate blood as well as purge Heat and cool blood. These three are chief herbs together.

Maimendong is sweet and cold. It acts together with baihe to nourish Yin and purge Heat, to moisten the lung and stop cough. Xuanshen is salty and cold. It aids the two types of dihuang to nourish Yin and augment fluids, thereby purging deficiency-Fire. These two serve as deputy herbs.

Danggui relieves the cough and dyspnea caused by abnormally rising lung-Qi. Shaoyao enriches Yin and invigorates blood circulation. Beimu moistens the lung to dissipate Phlegm and stop cough. Jiegeng guides all herbs upward. It also clears Heat from the throat, dissipates Phlegm and breaks up accumulations. These four together serve as assistant herbs.

Raw gancao purges Heat and Fire, and harmonizes the actions of the other herbs. It serves as envoy herb.

These herbs acting in concert nourish the kidney and protect the lung, so that the Metal and the Water Elements (lung and kidney respectively) are both regulated. Consequently they act to promote the production of Yin-blood, and full Yin-blood brings about dissipation of deficiency-Fire, dissolves Phlegm and stops cough. Through such actions they strengthen and protect lung-Qi. For this reason the formula is named "gu jin" (Metal-solidifying).

5 Comments

Baihe Gu Jin Tang is potent in nourishing Yin and moistening Dryness, particularly replenishing kidney-Yin and moistening lung-Dryness. It is a commonly used herbal formula. In clinical practice, the key symptoms are cough, dry and sore throat, a red tongue with scant coating, and a threadlike and rapid pulse.

Most of the herbs in the formula are sweet and cold. Do not use, or use with great caution, in watery diarrhea and anorexia due to spleen insufficiency.

6 Case Study: Pulmonary Tuberculosis with Hemoptysis in a 34-Year-Old Female

The patient had pulmonary tuberculosis for many years, with concomitant emaciation. Recently, because of failure to adjust to changes in cold and heat, she developed a severe cough. The cough led to hemoptysis, frequent vomiting and constipation. Her tongue was red, with a thin yellow coating, and her pulse was deep, threadlike and rapid.

Diagnosis: Deficiency of lung-Yin and kidney-Fire.

Therapeutic Principle: Nourish Yin and purge Fire.

Treatment: Baihe Gu Jin Tang with additions was prescribed. The composition was: baihe 12 g, shengdihuang 12 g, shudihuang 12 g, xuanshen 12 g, maimendong 12 g, stir-fried baishaoyao (*Paeonia*) 12 g, beimu 10 g, danggui 6 g, jiegeng 8 g, gancao 2 g and raw dahuang (*Rheum*) 5 g.

After three daily doses the hemoptysis was reduced, but the cough was not suppressed. The other symptoms all improved. After three more daily doses, the hemoptysis stopped.

(Source: *Zhejiang Journal of Chinese Medicine*, 1986, 1:31.)

XII Shen Qi Wan (Kidney-Qi Pill)

1 Source: Jin Gui Yao Lue (Essentials of the Golden Cabinet)

2 Composition

Chief Herb: shudihuang (*Rehmannia glutinosa*) 24 g

Deputy Herbs: shanzhuyu (*Cornus officinalis*) 12 g
shanyao (*Dioscorea opposita*) 12 g
processed fuzi (*Aconitum carmichaeli*) 3 g
rougui (*Cinnamomum cassia*) 3 g

Assistant and Envoy Herbs: zexie (*Alisma plantago-aquatica, orientale*) 9 g
fuling (*Poria cocos*) 9 g
mudanpi (*Paeonia suffruticosa*) 9 g

3 Application

Actions: tonifies the kidney and augments Yang.

Indications: deficiency of kidney-Yang.

Main Symptoms: low back pain; weakness of the lower extremities; dysuria or polyuria; a pale and plump tongue; a depletive and feeble pulse that is deep and threadlike at the chi position.

4 Analysis of the Formula

The chief herb, shudihuang, is used in large amount for its ability to augment Yin and strengthen the kidney.

There are four deputy herbs in two groups. One group contains shanzhuyu and shanyao; they strengthen the liver and the spleen and augment the vital force and blood. The other group contains processed fuzi and rougui; they are acrid and hot, and they assist the Vital Gate to warm Yang and facilitate Qi circulation. The chief and deputy herbs facilitate one another to strengthen the kidney and the vital force, as well as to nourish the kidney and to warm Yang. This is the method of bringing forth Yang from Yin.

Zexie and fuling promote fluid circulation, dry Dampness and purge impurities. Mudanpi purges deficiency-Fire. These three herbs are cathartics acting within the context of a group of restorative herbs. They are therefore effective in clearing away pathogenic factors and preventing stagnation that can result from Yin-augmenting herbs.

Used together these herbs warm without producing Dryness, nourish without cloying, augment weak kidney-Yang to circulate water, and overcome Yin deficiency to generate Yang.

5 Comments

There are two special features in the construction of Shen Qi Wan. One is the combination of Yang-augmentation and Yin-augmentation. The formula augments both Yin and Yang, though it acts mainly to augment kidney-Yang. The other is the addition of small amounts of rougui and fuling to warm Yang, with the goal of seeking

Yang within Yin, thereby invigorating kidney-Qi. These are the reasons for the formula's name and for its primary use in treating deficiency of kidney-Qi.

If the patient has prominent deficiency of kidney-Yang, then **You Gui Wan** is more appropriate. The main actions of You Gui Wan are to warm and nourish kidney-Yang, strengthen the vital force and generate blood. Its composition is as follows: shudihuang 24 g, baishaoyao (*Paeonia*) 12 g, shanzhuyu 9 g, gouqizi (*Lycium*) 12 g, lujiaojiao (*Cervus nippon*) 12 g, tusizi (*Cuscuta*) 12 g, duzhong (*Eucommia*) 12 g, danggui (*Angelica*) 12 g, rougui (*Cinnamomum*) and processed fuzi (*Aconitum*). It is used mainly for treating deficiency of primordial Yang, with endogenous Cold due to deficiency of the vital force and blood. The key symptoms are chronic lethargy with somnolence, and intolerance of cold and cold limbs; or loose feces sometimes containing undigested grains; or, urinary incontinence; or, aches and weakness in the waist and knees, with edema of the lower limbs. In males there are testicular atrophy and spermatorrhea, or impotence and infertility.

6 *Clinical Study: Relapsing Mouth Ulcers*

Relapsing mouth ulcers are due to primordial Yang dissociating from Fire of the Vital Gate, so that deficiency-Fire blazes and forces Yang to the exterior. This results in upper body Heat and lower body Cold. The main symptoms are ovoid sores or ulcers appearing on the lips, the tongue and the mouth. These are pale, have light red collars, and are about 1/4 in. They may be mildly or severely painful. They tend to break out when the patient is physically fatigued, and are often accompanied by aversion to cold, cold limbs, lassitude with unwillingness to speak, clear urine and watery feces.

Relapsing mouth ulcers are treated with Shen Qi Wan to warm and nourish the Fire of the Vital Gate, thus guiding Fire to its normal location. If the ulcers have a putrid odor, add digupi (*Lycium*) 10 g, shigao (gypsum) 15 g and increase the amount of mudanpi to 10 g. If thirst is prominent, add shihu (*Dendrobium chrysanthum, nobile*) 20 g and maimendong (*Ophiopogon*) 10 g.

In one study, five patients were treated. In two the condition was cured. In two others there was a cure followed by relapse, but the relapse responded well to repeat treatment. In one patient, the condition was improved but not cured.

(Source: *Hubei Journal of Chinese Medicine*, 1983, 2:11.)

XIII Section Summary

This section describes 12 formulas. They have the ability to replenish Qi, generate blood or to invigorate both Yin and Yang.

Si Jun Zi Tang, **Bu Zhong Yi Qi Tang**, **Yu Ping Feng San** and **Shen Mai San** are representative of herbal formulas that augment Qi. They are the main formulas for treating Qi deficiency, but their indications are different. Si Jun Zi Tang is the basic formula for augmenting Qi and strengthening the spleen. It is especially suitable for treating deficiency of spleen and stomach Qi. Bu Zhong Yi Qi Tang is especially efficacious for augmenting Qi and raising Yang in the middle-jiao. It is appropriate for insufficiency of the spleen and the stomach, with fever resulting from the Qi deficiency or with sunken Qi causing prolapse of the rectum or uterus. Yu Ping Feng San aims narrowly at replenishing Qi, consolidating the exterior and stopping sweating. It is usually used in spontaneous sweating due to deficiency in the exterior. Shen Mai San not only invigorates Qi but also augments Yin, generates fluids, stops sweating, and stops cough by restraining the lung. It is particularly efficacious for treating excessive sweating due to Summer Heat, which damages Qi and Yin, and chronic cough damaging the lung and depleting Qi and Yin.

Si Wu Tang is the basic formula for generating blood. It has the actions of generating blood and regulating the menses. But in illnesses of concurrent deficiency of Qi and blood **Ba Zhen Tang** is more suitable.

Liu Wei Dihuang Wan, **Fried Gancao Tang** and **Yi Guan Jian** all can nourish Yin and are appropriate for treating illnesses of Yin deficiency; but their clinical applications differ. Liu Wei Dihuang Wan is representative of formulas for nourishing Yin and strengthening the kidney. It emphasizes nourishment of kidney-Yin and possesses the ability to replenish fluids and control Fire. It is appropriate in the many conditions of insufficiency of the liver and the kidney, with overactive Yang due to deficient Yin. Fried Gancao Tang acts mainly to augment Qi and nourish Yin, generate blood and restore the pulse. It is mostly used in treating illnesses of deficiency or weakness of Qi and blood, or to calm a restless fetus. Yi Guan Jian nourishes Yin, releases pent-up liver Qi, and generates blood. Its main indication is for Yin deficiency in the liver and the kidney, drying of blood fluids and chest and subcostal pain from pent-up Qi.

Baihe Gu Jin Tang has the ability to nourish the kidney and moisten the lung. It can stop cough and dissolve Phlegm. It is mainly used for cough and dyspnea, with bloody sputum, caused by deficiency of lung and kidney Yin with upward attack by deficiency-induced Fire.

Shen Qi Wan is representative of herbal formulas that nourish kidney-Yang, and is mainly used for treating illnesses of deficiency of kidney-Yang.

Section 7 Formulas That Astringe and Stabilize

Formulas that astringe and stabilize comprise all those that are constructed around astringent herbs. These formulas have the ability to stabilize body processes and prevent abnormal leakage. They are designed to treat illnesses in which Qi, blood, the vital force and the fluids are all at risk of depletion through leakage.

Under normal conditions, Qi, blood, and fluids are in equilibrium between continual consumption and continual replenishment. If the consumption is excessive, or there is unrestrained leakage, they are gradually depleted. In mild cases, it will affect health. In severe cases, it may be fatal. Any loss that exceeds replenishment must be treated with a formula that astringes.

Astringent formulas are designed for illnesses in which genuine Qi is deficient and is leaking from the body. In clinical application it is important to determine the extent to which the patient's Qi, blood, vital force and fluids have been injured and to prescribe an appropriate formula to augment them accordingly, so that both cause and effect are tended to. It must also be noted that astringent formulas are designed for illnesses of deficiency of genuine Qi without an exogenous pathogenic evil. If such exogenous disease evil has not been eliminated, the use of an astringent formula can easily trap the disease evil within the body, where it can injure genuine Qi or cause another illness. Hence, it is important to pay close attention to the illnesses and symptoms for which these formulas are indicated and to the contraindications to their use.

I Si Shen Wan (Four Miracle-Herbs Pill)

1 Source: Nei Ke Zhai Yao (Essentials of Internal Medicine)

2 Composition

Chief Herb: buguzhi (*Psoralea corylifolia*) 12 g

Deputy Herb: roudoukou (*Myristica fragrans*) 6 g

Assistant Herbs: wuweizi (*Schisandra chinensis*) 6 g
wuzhuyu (*Evodia rutaecarpa*) 6 g

Envoy Herbs: shengjiang (*Zingiber officinale*) 12 g
dazao (*Ziziphus jujuba*) 5 pieces

3 Application

Actions: warms the kidney and the spleen, astringes the intestines and stops diarrhea.

Indications: diarrhea due to kidney insufficiency.

Main Symptoms: pre-dawn diarrhea; anorexia, and inability to digest what is eaten; or, abdominal pain and cold limbs; fatigue and lethargy; a pale tongue with a thin white coating; and a deep, slow and forceless pulse.

4 Analysis of the Formula

For chief herb this formula uses buguzhi in large amount. It augments Fire of the Vital Gate, thereby warming the kidney.

Roudoukou is acrid and warm. It warms the spleen and the stomach, astringes the intestines and stops diarrhea. It serves as deputy herb.

Wuweizi is a strong, warm, and astringent herb that strengthens the binding action of roudoukou. Wuzhuyu warms the liver, the spleen and the kidney, and dispels Yin-Cold. They serve together as assistant herbs.

Shengjiang warms the stomach and dispels Cold. Dazao tonifies the spleen and the stomach. These two serve as envoy herbs.

The six herbs together invigorate the spleen and strengthen the Earth Element (to which the spleen belongs), thereby resolving diarrhea induced by kidney insufficiency.

5 Comments

Si Shen Wan is obtained by combining **Er Shen Wan** and **Wuweizi San**, both from the book *Pu Ji Ben Shi Fang*. Er Shen Wan is composed of roudoukou and buguzhi, and acts to cure anorexia by augmenting spleen and kidney Yang. Wuweizi San is composed of wuweizi and wuzhuyu, and acts to stop diarrhea due to kidney insufficiency. By combining those two formulas, Si Shen Wan is particularly effective in warming and strengthening the spleen and the kidney and astringing the intestines to stop diarrhea.

6 Case Study: Hypersensitive Enteritis

The patient suffered from chronic diarrhea for 9 years. He defecated 3–5 times daily, producing feces that were watery and unformed. There was no blood or pus, and he did not have tenesmus. He was repeatedly treated with Chinese or Western formulas, without effect. On examination, he had a pale and plump tongue, and a deep, threadlike and forceless pulse. Radiographic examination of the gastrointestinal tract showed no abnormality.

Diagnosis: Deficiency of kidney-Yang.

Treatment: Si Shen Wan was prescribed at the dosage of 6 g 3 times daily. His diarrhea soon improved. After 20 days of treatment, his defecation pattern returned to normal and his abdominal pain subsided. Treatment was discontinued, and the patient was observed for an additional month. There was no relapse.

(Source: *Shanghai Journal of Chinese Medicine*, 1965, 10:13.)

7 Case Study: Enuresis in a 16-Year-Old Male

The patient had enuresis since childhood, wetting the bed at least twice each night. In cold weather he was often tired from poor sleep. Many treatments were tried, with poor results. On examination, his tongue was pale, with a thin white coating, and his pulse was deep and slow.

Diagnosis: Deficiency of kidney-Yang with dysfunction of bladder-Qi.

Therapeutic Principle: Warm and strengthen the kidney.

Treatment: He was prescribed Si Shen Wan with additions. The composition was as follows: buguzhi 9 g, wuzhuyu 6 g, wuweizi 9 g, roudoukou 7 g, yizhi (*Alpinia oxyphylla*) 7 g, rougui (*Cinnamomum*) 2 g, shichangpu (*Acorus*) 6 g, wuyao (*Lindera*) 9 g, and one pig bladder. The herbs were inserted into the pig bladder, and the bladder neck tied. Several holes were punched in the bladder with a large needle. It was then boiled in 5 L of water for about an hour. The contents were removed and the bladder sliced and eaten in one sitting. After two doses, the enuresis stopped. There was no relapse during an observation period of half a year.

(Source: *Journal of Chinese Medicine*, 1984, 5:80.)

II Zhen Ren Yang Zang Tang (True Man's Zang-Nourishing Decoction)

1 Source: Tai Ping Hui Min He Ji Ju Fang (Prescriptions of the Taiping Benevolent Bureau)

2 Composition

Chief Herb: yingsuqiao (*Papaver somniferum*) 15 g

Deputy Herbs: roudoukou (*Myristica fragrans*) 6 g
hezi (*Terminalia chebula*) 12 g

Assistant Herbs: renshen (*Panax ginseng*) 9 g
baizhu (*Atractylodes macrocephala*) 9 g
danggui (*Angelica sinensis*) 6 g
baishaoyao (*Paeonia lactiflora*) 15 g
rougui (*Cinnamomum cassia*) 3 g
muxiang (*Aucklandia lappa*) 45 g

Envoy Herb: fried gancao (*Glycyrrhiza uralensis*) 6 g

(Note: the use of yingsuqiao is now restricted.)

3 Application

Actions: astringes the intestines, stops diarrhea, warms the middle-jiao and restores deficiency.

Indications: chronic diarrhea and dysentery.

Main Symptoms: unremitting chronic diarrhea or dysentery, sometimes with fecal incontinence. In severe cases, prolapsed rectum and peri-umbilical pain, no desire for food or drink; a pale tongue with white coating; and a deep and threadlike pulse.

4 Analysis of the Formula

For chief herb Zhen Ren Yang Zang Tang uses yingsuqiao in large amount to astringe the intestines and stop diarrhea. For deputy herbs it uses roudoukou and hezi to warm the spleen and the middle-jiao and aid in astringing the intestines and stopping diarrhea.

For assistants there are two groups of herbs. Chronic diarrhea and dysentery damage Qi and blood. The formula uses renshen and baizhu to augment Qi and strengthen the spleen, and danggui and baishaoyao to generate and regulate blood. Baishaoyao also stops diarrhea and relieves abdominal pain. Since the visceral organs are also affected, the formula also includes rougui and muxiang: rougui to warm and strengthen the spleen and the kidney and to dispel Cold; and muxiang to regulate Qi and stimulate the spleen. Together these two herbs prevent the astringent herbs from causing blockage of Qi circulation.

For the envoy the formula uses fried gancao, which harmonizes the actions of the other herbs. It also aids renshen and baizhu to invigorate the middle-jiao and augment Qi, and aids baishaoyao to relieve spasm and pain.

These herbs acting in concert astringe the intestines, stop diarrhea, warm the middle-jiao, boost what has become deficient and nourish visceral organ Qi that has been exhausted.

5 Comments

In the treatment of dysentery in its early stages, when the pathogenic evil is strong, the appropriate method is to drain. Using the method of astringency at this stage would be premature. But if the dysentery becomes chronic and unremitting, the congealed accumulations are gone, whether abdominal pain is absent or present but relieved by pressure, then the visceral organs have become insufficient and unable to avoid further leakage of their Qi. In such conditions, it is necessary to use astringents to stop the diarrhea.

Zhen Ren Yang Zang Tang is designed to treat dysentery that is due purely to spleen and kidney insufficiency. The key symptoms are chronic and unremitting diarrhea, abdominal pain, anorexia, malaise, a pale tongue with white coating, and a threadlike and slow pulse.

Zhen Ren Yang Zang Tang is contraindicated in chronic fungal dysentery with blood and pus.

6 Clinical Study: Post-dysentery Syndrome

The key features for the diagnosis of post-dysentery syndrome are the following: diarrhea, feces with mucus, abdominal pain and tenesmus.

Fourteen patients were studied. They were all young men. Most of them were hospitalized for a long time and showed little response to treatment with other formulas. None had fungal dysentery.

They were treated with Zhen Ren Yang Zang Tang. Thirteen were cured, requiring on average 6.7 days. The frequency of defecation needed on average 2.2 days to return to normal. The feces needed on average 3.2 days to return to normal gross appearance. The abdominal pain needed on average 2.7 days to subside.

(Source: *Medical Journal of the People's Liberation Army*, 1985, 4:325.)

III Jin Suo Gu Jing Wan (Gold Lock Semen-Stabilizing Pill)

1 Source: Yi Fang Ji Jie (Explanation of Collected Prescriptions)

2 Composition

Chief Herb: shayuanzi (*Astragalus complanatus*) 12 g

Deputy Herbs: qianshi (*Euryale ferox*) 12 g
lianzi (*Nelumbo nucifera*) 50 g

Assistant and Envoy Herbs: longgu (fossil bone) 10 g
muli (*Ostrea gigas*, *rivularis*) 10 g
lianxu (*Nelumbo nucifera*) 12 g

3 Application

Actions: nourishes the kidney and astringes the vital force.

Indications: spermatorrhea.

Main Symptoms: spermatorrhea and spontaneous emission; listlessness and fatigue; lumbago and tinnitus; a pale tongue with white coating; and a thread-like and feeble pulse.

4 Analysis of the Formula

Shayuanzi is sweet and warm; and it nourishes the kidney and stabilizes the vital force. It serves as the chief herb.

Qianshi and lianzi are both able to strengthen the kidney, stop the leakage of semen, and assist the chief herb in stabilizing the vital force. Lianzi also keeps the heart (Fire Element) and the kidney (Water Element) in balance. These two serve together as deputy herbs.

The chief and deputy herbs are assisted by longgu and muli, which are salty in flavor and even in nature. These two herbs can astringe semen and stop spermatorrhea. Lianxu is sweet in flavor and even in nature, and is particularly effective as an astringent. These three serve as assistant and envoy herbs.

These herbs acting in concert nourish the kidney, astringe the vital force and stop spermatorrhea. This is truly a formula that aims at both the cause and the effects of the illness.

5 Comments

Spermatorrhea can result from various causes, but is closely related to the liver and the kidney. The kidney stores the vital force, and the liver controls its flow. Deficiency of kidney-Yin permits leakage of the vital force, whereas excessive liver-Yang permits endogenous Fire to blaze; both can lead to spermatorrhea. In general, spermatorrhea associated with dreams is mostly due to blazing endogenous Fire, whereas spermatorrhea not associated with dreams is mostly due to deficiency of kidney-Yin and imbalance of the heart and the kidney.

Jin Suo Gu Jing Wan is suitable for treating spermatorrhea due to deficiency of kidney-Yin, but is inappropriate if it is due to Dampness–Heat.

6 Case Study: Galactorrhea (Milk Production) in a 53-Year-Old Female

For about a month, the patient noticed that her breasts became increasingly swollen and began to produce milk. For 2 weeks, she was able to express 100–150 mL a day of dilute, pale white milk. Occasionally it leaked spontaneously. There was no obvious breast mass. However, she had fatigue, with dizziness and tinnitus, palpitation of the heart, reduced appetite and nocturnal polyuria.

Diagnosis: Galactorrhea due to prolonged stagnation of liver-Qi causing insufficiency of both the spleen and the kidney.

Therapeutic Principle: Strengthen the spleen and the kidney, and astringe the vital force.

Treatment: The patient was prescribed modified Jin Suo Gu Jing Wan, with the following composition: shayuanzi 12 g, lianxu 10 g, chaihu 10 g, qianshi 30 g, refined muli 30 g, maiya (*Hordeum*) 30 g, refined longgu 30 g, huangqi (*Astragalus*) 30 g, qingpi (*Citrus tangerina*) 6 g, fried gancao (*Glycyrrhiza*) 3 g, and hezi (*Terminalia chebula*) 4 pieces. The muli and longgu were decocted first.

The formula was further modified in response to changes in the course of the illness. After six daily doses, she recovered.

(Source: *New Chinese Medicine*, 1986, 5:26.)

IV Gu Chong Tang (Chong Meridian Stabilizing Decoction)

1 Source: Yi Xue Zhong Zhong Can Xi Lu (Discourse on Integrated Chinese and Western Medicine)

2 Composition

Chief Herbs: baizhu (*Atractylodes macrocephala*) 30 g
huangqi (*Astragalus membranaceus*) 18 g

Deputy Herbs: shanzhuyu (*Cornus officinalis*) 24 g
baishaoyao (*Paeonia lactiflora*) 12 g

Assistant and Envoy Herbs: longgu (fossil bones) 24 g
muli (*Ostrea gigas*, *rivularis*) 24 g
charred zonglu (*Trachycarpus fortunei*, *wagnerianus*) 6 g
wubeizi (*Melaphis chinensis*,) 15 g
haipiaoxiao (*Sepiella maindroni*) 12 g
qiancao (*Rubia cordifolia*) 9 g

3 Application

Actions: replenishes Qi, invigorates the spleen, stabilizes the Chong Meridian and stops bleeding.

Indications: deficiency of spleen-Qi and instability of the Chong meridian.

Main Symptoms: massive menstrual bleeding, or heavy menstrual flow that is pale and thin; palpitation of the heart; shortness of breath; lumbar and knee aching and weakness; a pale tongue; and a feeble and indistinct pulse.

4 *Analysis of the Formula*

Gu Chong Tang is designed for uterine bleeding or heavy menstrual flow due to instability of the Chong meridian and deficiency of spleen-Qi. For chief herbs, large amounts of baizhu and huangqi are used to augment Qi and strengthen the spleen. When spleen-Qi is ample then control of menses is effective.

The liver controls the "sea of blood," and the kidney controls the Chong and Ren Meridians. Instability of the Chong and Ren Meridians is likely to make control over blood ineffective. Shanzhuyu and baishaoyao are included as deputy herbs to strengthen the liver and the kidney, nourish blood and astringe Yin.

The six assistant and envoy herbs fall in two groups. One group contains longgu, muli, zonglu and wubeizi; they astringe and stop bleeding. Because stopping bleeding occasionally leads to blood stasis, the herbs of the other group, haipiaoxiao and qiancao, are included to dissolve static blood as well as stop bleeding, so that as bleeding stops there is little risk of inducing blood stasis.

Thus the herbal formula as a whole treats the cause, by augmenting Qi and stabilizing the Chong Meridian, and the symptoms, by astringing and stopping bleeding. It has the capability of binding up and stopping bleeding, including massive uterine bleeding.

5 *Comments*

The Chong Meridian is the "sea of blood." Massive uterine bleeding leads to deficiency and instability in the Chong Meridian. Gu Chong Tang has the capability of augmenting Qi, strengthening the spleen, stabilizing the Chong Meridian and binding up blood.

In clinical application, the key symptoms are excessive bleeding of pale and thin blood, lumbar and knee weakness and aches; a pale tongue and a feeble and indistinct pulse.

Gu Chong Tang is contraindicated in massive uterine bleeding due to Heat in the blood causing it to flow wildly.

6 *Clinical Study: Dysfunctional Uterine Bleeding*

Twenty-two patients with dysfunctional uterine bleeding were treated with Gu Chong Tang. Four patients were 12–20 years of age, nine were 21–45 years of age, and nine were 46 or more years of age. The duration of dysfunctional uterine bleeding ranged from 10 days to 10 years. All the patients had been treated with various Western and Chinese formulas, with little effect.

Gu Chong Tang, with modifications in amounts and the addition of shanyao (*Dioscorea*), was prescribed, as follows: baizhu 25–50 g, huangqi 25–50 g, shanzhuyu 30 g, baishaoyao 20 g, qiancao 20 g, zonglu 20 g, haipiaoxiao 20 g, wubeizi 15 g, muli 25 g, longgu 25 g, and shanyao 25–50 g. During this treatment all other herbs were suspended.

Results: Twenty-one patients recovered completely. One patient showed no benefit.

V Section Summary

Both **Si Shen Wan** and **Zhen Ren Yang Zang Tang** act mainly to astringe the intestines and stop diarrhea. They are used to treat chronic unremitting diarrhea. There are differences between them. The emphasis of Si Shen Wan is on warming the kidney and the spleen to astringe the intestines and stop diarrhea. The emphasis of Zhen Ren Yang Zang Tang is on augmenting Qi and strengthening the spleen; its astringent properties are stronger than those of Si Shen Wan.

The main action of **Jin Suo Gu Jing Wan** is to astringe the vital force and stop seminal emission. It emphasizes the consolidation of the kidney and is used mainly to treat seminal leakage due to insufficiency of the kidney.

Gu Chong Tang is the representative formula for stopping massive uterine bleeding and vaginal discharge. It is mainly used for augmenting Qi, strengthening the spleen, and stabilizing the Chong Meridian to control blood flow. It is indicated for massive uterine bleeding or heavy menstrual flows caused by deficiency of Spleen-Qi and instability of the Chong Meridian.

Section 8 Formulas That Calm the Mind

Tranquilizing herbal formulas are composed primarily of tranquilizing herbs that calm the mind. They are used to treat mental agitation and related illnesses.

Illnesses of the mind are of two main types: excess or deficiency. The excess type is mainly caused by fright, which forces stagnant liver-Qi to transform into Fire. This endogenous Fire in turn causes disturbances of the mind. The deficiency type is mainly caused by deficiency of Yin and blood, so that the mind becomes disturbed by the lack of nourishment.

However, when Fire blazes it often injures Yin, and deficiency of Yin often enables Yang to rise abnormally. This makes the pathology of deficiency illnesses of the mind a complex mixture of deficiency and excess.

In clinical practice, illnesses of the mind are sometimes treated by tranquilization and sometimes by tonification to calm the mind. Careful diagnosis is important.

I Tian Wang Bu Xin Dan (Celestial Emperor's Heart-Nourishing Pill)

1 Source: She Sheng Mi Pou (Exposition on Health Conservation)

2 Composition

Chief Herb: shengdihuang (*Rehmannia glutinosa*) 12 g

Deputy Herbs: tiandong (*Asparagus chochinchinensis*) 9 g
maimendong (*Ophiopogon japonicus*) 9 g
suanzaoren (*Ziziphus jujuba*) 9 g
baiziren (*Biota orientalis*) 9 g
danggui (*Angelica sinensis*) 9 g

Assistant Herbs: renshen (*Panax ginseng*) 5 g
wuweizi (*Schisandra chinensis*) 5 g
fuling (*Poria cocos*) 5 g
yuanzhi (*Polygala tenuifolia*) 5 g
xuanshen (*Scrophularia ningpoensis*) 5 g
danshen (*Salvia miltiorrhiza*) 5 g
zhusha* (cinnabar) 3 g

Envoy Herb: jiegeng (*Platycodon grandiflorum*) 5 g

*Recent research has found that zhusha contains high concentrations of certain heavy metals. It should therefore be used with great caution, or not used at all.

3 Application

Actions: nourishes Yin, generates blood, tonifies the heart and calms the mind.

Indications: mental agitation due to deficiency of Yin and blood.

Main Symptoms: palpitations, insomnia, restlessness and agitation; nocturnal emission of semen; forgetfulness; hotness in the palms and soles; mouth and tongue sores, a red tongue with scant coating; and a threadlike and rapid pulse.

4 Analysis of the Formula

For the chief herb, Tian Wang Bu Xin Dan uses shengdihuang in large amount to nourish Yin and generate blood.

For deputies it uses five herbs. Tiandong and maimendong nourish Yin and clear Heat; suanzaoren and baiziren nourish the heart and calm the mind; and danggui generates blood and moistens the intestines.

For assistants it uses seven herbs. Renshen augments Qi, so that vigorous Qi induces the generation of Yin and blood, and also calms the mind. Wuweizi stimulates Qi and nourishes Yin, both by itself and as aid to the chief and deputy herbs. Fuling and yuanzhi nourish the heart and calm the mind, and can also harmonize the activities of the heart and the kidney. Xuanshen augments Yin and lowers Fire, thereby preventing deficiency-Fire from rising. Danshen cools the heart and stimulates blood circulation, so that tonification does not lead to stasis. Zhusha tranquilizes the mind, and at the same time treats the symptoms of its agitation.

For envoy, the formula uses jiegeng for its ability to conduct the other herbs upward, enabling them to enter the Heart Meridian. It also complements danshen to stimulate the Qi and blood circulation, so that the other herbs can tonify without causing gelling or stagnation.

The whole formula acts to augment Yin, generate blood, nourish the heart and calm the mind. It also augments Yin to lower Fire and enhances the coordination between the heart and the kidney. In consequence, it cures palpitation of the heart, insomnia, forgetfulness and related symptoms.

5 Comments

Insufficiency of the heart and the kidney, brooding, deficiency of Yin and excess of Yang all can cause deficiency-Fire to break out of control. Common manifestations are such symptoms as insomnia with fitful sleep and frequent dreams, palpitation of the heart and forgetfulness. Tian Wang Bu Xin Dan can nourish and regulate both the heart and the kidney, so that all these symptoms can be relieved.

Gui Pi Tang (section 6) and Tian Wang Bu Xin Dan are both formulas that nourish the heart and calm the mind. Both are used to treat forgetfulness, anxiety and insomnia. Tian Wang Bu Xin Dan emphasizes spleen-strengthening and Qi-augmentation, and is appropriate for illnesses of Qi deficiency. Gui Pi Tang, on the other hand, emphasizes the nourishment of Yin and the cooling of Heat, and is more suitable for deficiency of Yin and blood.

II Suanzaoren Tang (Jujube Seed Decoction)

1 Source: Jin Gui Yao Lue (Essentials of the Golden Cabinet)

2 Composition

Chief Herb: suanzaoren (*Ziziphus jujuba*) 15 g

Deputy Herbs: fuling (*Poria cocos*) 6 g
zhimu (*Anemarrhena asphodeloides*) 6 g

Assistant Herb: chuanxiong (*Ligusticum chuanxiong*, *wallichii*) 6 g

Envoy Herb: gancao (*Glycyrrhiza uralensis*) 3 g

3 Application

Actions: generates blood, calms the mind, clears Heat and eliminates agitation.

Indications: agitation with insomnia.

Main Symptoms: insomnia, palpitations, agitation; dizziness and vertigo; a dry throat and mouth; a red tongue; and a taut and threadlike pulse.

4 Analysis of the Formula

Suanzaoren Tang uses a large amount of suanzaoren to enter the Heart and Liver Meridians, to generate blood and nourish the liver, and to calm the heart and the mind. It serves as the chief herb and gives its name to the formula.

Fuling calms the heart and the mind. Zhimu augments Yin and clears Heat. These two serve as deputy herbs. When teamed with suanzaoren they enhance the action of calming the mind and relieving agitation.

Chuanxiong harmonizes the functional activities of Qi and facilitates the movement of liver-Qi. When suanzaoren and chuangxiong are teamed, sour astringency and acrid dispersal occur together. These two actions constrain yet enhance each other, resulting in the ability to generate blood and regulate the liver.

Raw gancao harmonizes the middle-jiao. It serves as envoy herb.

Through their interactions, the herbs in this formula generate blood and nourish the liver. Through these actions they calm the heart and the mind on the one hand and purge endogenous Heat to eliminate agitation on the other.

5 *Comments*

Both Tian Wang Bu Xin Dan and Suanzaoren Tang are representative of formulas that nourish and calm the mind. They are both used to treat restlessness, insomnia, palpitation and forgetfulness. They differ in that Tian Wang Bu Xin Dan emphasizes the augmentation of Yin and the generation of blood whereas Suanzaoren Tang emphasizes the nourishment of the heart, the harmonization of liver function and the elimination of agitation. Thus, Tian Wang Bu Xin Dan is indicated for Yin and blood deficiency in the Heart Meridian, with palpitation and insomnia; and Suanzaoren Tang is indicated for insufficiency of liver-blood, restlessness and insomnia.

6 *Clinical Study: Insomnia*

Thirty-one patients were treated with Suanzaoren Tang extract, 2.5 g 3 times daily for 4 weeks. Result: by the measures of falling asleep and sound sleep, there was marked improvement after 2 weeks of treatment. The overall effective rate was 90%.

(Source: *Journal of Chinese Medicine*, 1986, 1:185.)

Section 9 Formulas That Open Orifices (Resuscitate)

This group comprises all formulas that use an aromatic and resuscitative herb as chief herb. These formulas act to open orifices and restore consciousness. They are used for treating coma of the "closed" type (see Volume 2, Part II, Chapter 7, Section 15), which is due to strength of exogenous pathogenic evil. The clinical characteristics are unconsciousness or coma, heavy breathing, tight jaw, clenched fists, and a forceful pulse. Depending on the clinical symptoms, orifice-blockage illnesses can be categorized in two groups: Cold-blockage and Heat-blockage. Accordingly, formulas that resuscitate can be divided into the two categories of warm-resuscitation and cool-resuscitation.

In clinical practice, pay special attention to the following points. (1) Resuscitative formulas are contradicted in the "prostrate" type of coma (illnesses of orifice incompetence), which is characterized by loss of consciousness, flaccidity, profuse sweating, cold extremities, incontinence of feces and urine, and an indistinct pulse. (2) In general these formulas are not administered as decoctions. (3) They must used with utmost caution in pregnant women. (4) They should be discontinued as soon as the patient shows significant response.

Moreover, many illnesses of exogenous Heat in the visceral organs affect the level of consciousness. Careful differential diagnosis is necessary. For example, loss of consciousness due to exogenous Heat in the organs of the Yangming Meridian is treated by cooling and purging Heat from Yangming, and must not be erroneously treated with a resuscitative formula.

I An Gong Niuhuang Wan (Palace-Calming Gallstone Pill)

1 Source: Wen Bing Tiao Bian (Analysis of Febrile Illnesses)

2 Composition

Chief Herbs: niuhuang (*Bos taurus domesticus*) 30 g
shexiang* (*Moschus moschiferus*) 75 g

Deputy Herbs: shuiniujiao (*Bubalus bubalis*) 30 g
huanglian (*Coptis chinensis*) 30 g
huangqin (*Scutellaria baicalensis*) 30 g
zhizi (*Gardenia jasminoides*) 30 g
bingpian (*Dryobalanops aromatica*) 75 g
yujin (*Curcuma wenyujin, aromatica*) 30 g

Assistant Herbs: xionghuang (realgar) 30 g
husha (cinnabar) 30 g
henzhu (pearl) 15 g

Envoy Herbs: honey
gold leaf (as coating for the pills)

*Nowadays, natural shexiang is replaced by artificial shexiang.

Dosage of each herb in the formula is used only for making pills, but not for prescription of making decoction.

3 Application

Actions: purges Heat and opens the orifices; removes Phlegm and eliminates poison.

Indications: (1) Exogenous Heat trapped in the Pericardium Meridian. (2) Stroke-induced coma and infantile seizures due to Heat evil trapped internally.

Main Symptoms: high fever; irritability and agitation; impaired consciousness with delirium; a dry mouth and a dry crimson tongue; much thick sputum; and a rapid pulse.

4 Analysis of the Formula

An Gong Niuhuang Wan is designed primarily for Heat-induced "closed" coma caused by strong exogenous Heat penetrating into the Pericardium Meridian.

It has two chief herbs. Niuhuang purges Heat from the heart, eliminates poison, extinguishes Wind, calms anxiety, dissolves sputum and opens orifices. The formula also uses the acridity and warmth of shexiang to course through all 12 meridians, and especially to open orifices and restore consciousness. These two herbs assist each other to cool the heart and open orifices.

For deputies the formula uses six herbs. Shuiniujiao cools the heart and blood, and eliminates poison. Huangqin, huanglian and zhizi dispel Heat, purge Fire and eliminate poison. They assist niuhuang to cool Heat in the pericardium. Bingpian and yujin are aromatic; they can ward off pestilential evils, open orifices and remove blockage. They are included to enhance shexiang's ability to open orifices and restore consciousness.

For assistants the formula uses zhusha, zhenzhu and xionghuang. Zhusha and zhenzhu sedate the heart and calm the mind, thereby relieving agitation and restlessness. Xionghuang assists niuhuang to dislodge sputum and eliminate poison.

The formula is made into pills using honey, which settles the stomach and the middle-jiao. The gold leaf is used to coat the pills because it is also potent in calming the mind.

5 Comments

An Gong Niuhuang Wan is designed for treating orifice-blockage illnesses caused by Heat penetrating the Pericardium Meridian. It is a commonly prescribed herbal formula for purging Heat and opening orifices. The core of its construction is the teaming of herbs that clear Heat, cool blood and remove poison with aromatic herbs that open orifices. On this foundation, additional herbs are added, as dictated by the patient's illness, to calm the mind, dissolve sputum and to induce catharsis. This is a characteristic of the construction of cool-resuscitative herbal formulas.

6 Case Study: Acute Hepatic Coma in a 5-Year-Old Boy

Two days prior to coming to hospital the patient developed a yellow color in his face, with weakness of his limbs and weariness. He had mild chills and fever. He was treated elsewhere with Yinchenhao Tang and other formulas that clear Heat and eliminate Dampness as well as penicillin for 2 days. There was no response, and the patient drifted into coma. He was transferred to another hospital, but en route his jaw became clenched and he had tetany in his extremities. He was thought to be moribund and was brought to this hospital.

On examination, his entire body was yellow, his fingertips were purple in color, and his tongue and coating were both yellow and greasy. His countenance was expressionless. His body temperature was 38.5°C (101.3°F). His urine was reddish.

Diagnosis: Heat-type of orifice-blockage illness ("closed" coma).

Therapeutic Principle: Purge heat and open orifices.

Treatment: One pill of An Gong Niuhuang Wan was administered, in two divided portions. On re-examination the following day all his symptoms were alleviated. He was given another half of a pill of An Gong Niuhuang Wan and another Chinese herbal formula to clear Heat, eliminate Dampness and the icterus. He was also given an infusion of glucose solution. After 3 days, the child's mental status became normal and his condition was much improved.

(Source: *Jiangxi Journal of Chinese Medicine*, 1960, 12:31.)

II Suhexiang Wan (Storax Pill)

1 Source: Tai Ping Hui Min He Ji Ju Fang (Prescriptions from the Taiping Benevolent Pharmaceutical Bureau)

2 Composition

Chief Herbs: suhexiang (*Liquidambar orientalis*) 30 g
anxixiang (*Styrax tonkinensis*) 60 g
shexiang (*Moschus moschiferus*) 60 g
bingpian (*Dryobalanops aromatica*) 30 g

Deputy Herbs: muxiang (*Aucklandia lappa*) 60 g
chenxiang (*Aquilaria sinensis, agallocha*) 60 g
dingxiang (*Syzygium aromaticum*) 60 g
xiangfu (*Cyperus rotundus*) 60 g
ruxiang (*Boswellia carterii*) 30 g
tanxiang (*Santalum album*) 60 g

Assistant Herbs: biba (*Piper longum*) 60 g
hezi (*Terminalia chebula*) 60 g
baizhu (*Atractylodes macrocephala*) 60 g
zhusha (cinnabar) 60 g
shuiniujiao (*Bubalus bubalis*) 60 g

Dosage of each herb in the formula is used only for making pills. They are not for prescription of making decoction.

3 Application

Actions: aromatic opening of the orifices; facilitation of Qi movement; and warming of the interior.

Indications: (1) Cold type of orifice-blockage illnesses ("closed" coma). (2) Wind invasion (stroke).

Main Symptoms: sudden fainting with clenched jaw and loss of consciousness; in some cases, sudden pain in the abdomen and heart; in severe cases, coma. The tongue coating is white and the pulse slow.

4 Analysis of the Formula

Suhexiang Wan is designed primarily for the Cold type of orifice-blockage illnesses, so-called "closed" coma.

The four chief herbs are all aromatic orifice-opening herbs. They readily penetrate into the interior, transform turbidity, regulate Qi and dispel Cold.

They are supported by six deputy herbs that promote Qi circulation, relieve stagnation, dispel Cold, relieve pain, ward off pestilence, remove impurities, facilitate blood circulation and dissolve stasis.

Biba is acrid in flavor and hot in nature. It warms the middle-jiao and dispels Cold, and enhances the actions of the ten chief and deputy herbs to dispel Cold, stop pain and alleviate blockage. Baizhu augments Qi, strengthens the spleen, dries Dampness and dissolves impurities. Hezi astringes and restrains Qi. These last two herbs assist the aromatic herbs in augmenting Qi and in astringency, thereby preventing damage to genuine Qi by their excesses of acridity and aromaticity. The formula also includes shuiniujiao, which cools the heart and removes poison, and zhusha, which calms the mind. These five herbs serve as assistant herbs.

5 Comments

Suhexiang Wan is representative of warm-resuscitative formulas. It is particularly suitable for treating illnesses in which Cold–Dampness or Phlegm–Dampness impedes Qi circulation and blocks the orifices.

The strategy in the construction of this formula is to combine resuscitative herbs with Qi-activating and blockage-alleviating herbs. Consequently the formula is effective in simultaneously eliminating impurities and warming the middle-jiao.

Suhexiang Wan is absolutely contraindicated in orifice-blockage illnesses caused by Heat, or in illnesses of depletion of genuine Qi caused by the incompetence of the orifices ("prostrate" coma).

III Section Summary

An Gong Niuhuang Wan and **Suhexiang Wan** are both formulas that resuscitate by opening orifices. However, An Gong Niuhuang Wan is typical of cool-resuscitative formulas whereas Suhexiang Wan is typical of warm-resuscitative formulas. An Gong Niuhuang Wan is very effective for purging Heat, removing poison and dissolving sputum. It is most suitable for treating Heat lodged in the Pericardium Meridian causing loss of consciousness and delirium. Suhexiang Wan is very effective for opening orifices blocked by Cold. In addition to opening the orifices and removing impurities, it is also effective for facilitating Qi circulation, warming the middle-jiao and stopping pain. For pain in the heart and the abdomen due to impeded Qi and congealed Cold it produces excellent clinical response.

Section 10 Formulas That Regulate Qi

This group comprises all formulas that are constructed around herbs that regulate Qi. These formulas facilitate Qi movement or suppress abnormally rising Qi. They are used to treat illnesses in which Qi movement is impeded or obstructed or in which Qi rises abnormally.

Stagnation of Qi is mostly seen as stagnation of lung-Qi or of stomach-Qi. Abnormally rising Qi is mostly seen as the abnormal rising of lung-Qi or of stomach-Qi. When Qi is stagnant the treatment is to facilitate Qi movement. When Qi rises abnormally the treatment is to suppress it. Hence, Qi-regulating formulas fall in two large categories: formulas that facilitate Qi movement, and formulas that suppress Qi.

In the clinical application of Qi-regulating formulas, the first task is to differentiate between deficiency and strength. Strength of the pathogenic evil must not be mistaken for deficiency of body function, as that may result in the erroneous use of a restorative formula. If body deficiency is mistaken for strength of disease evil, a Qi-regulating formula may be erroneously used to suppress Qi, thereby causing further damage to Qi and leading to complications.

Furthermore, Qi-regulating formulas are mostly acrid, aromatic, drying and hot substances. In clinical application, their use should be stopped as soon the patient shows significant response. They must be used with the utmost caution in the aged, the debilitated, in those with blazing Fire in Yin deficiency, or in pregnant women.

I Yue Ju Wan (Stagnation-Releasing Pill)

1 Source: Dan Xi Xin Fa (Danxi's Experience in Medicine)

2 Composition

Chief Herb: xiangfu (*Cyperus rotundus*) 6 g

Deputy and Assistant Herbs: chuanxiong (*Ligusticum chuanxiong, wallichii*) 6 g
zhizi (*Gardenia jasminoides*) 6 g
cangzhu (*Atractylodes lancea*) 6 g
shenqu (medicated leaven) 6 g

3 Application

Actions: facilitates Qi movement and releases Qi stagnation.

Indications: illnesses of stagnation.

Main Symptoms: chest tightness with subcostal and abdominal pain; eructation, acid regurgitation; nausea and vomiting; and indigestion.

4 Analysis of the Formula

For chief herb Yue Ju Wan uses xiangfu to facilitate Qi movement and release stagnation.

The other four herbs all serve as deputy and assistant herbs. Chuanxiang is primarily an herb for the facilitation of blood circulation and the breaking up of blood stasis, but it also helps xiangfu to facilitate Qi movement and release stagnation. Zhizi clears Heat and purges Fire from the sanjiao. Cangzhu dries Dampness and strengthens the spleen to remove congealed Dampness. Shenqu promotes digestion and intestinal motility to cure food retention.

Gelling of Phlegm is mostly due to insufficiency of the spleen, but is also related to Qi, Fire and food. When Qi can move freely, all the various types of stagnation can be released, including gelling of Phlegm. This is the principle of "in treating an illness seek the root."

5 Comments

The construction of this formula illustrates the strategy for treating illnesses of stagnation. When clinically assessing the six types of stagnation illnesses, the physician must carefully identify cause and effect and the major and the minor. Herbs are then selected and teamed, or an established formula is modified, in accordance with the constellation of symptoms. Doing so will enhance the efficacy of the treatment.

If stagnation of Qi is predominant, xiangfu may be used as chief herb. It is then complemented with houpo (*Magnolia*), muxiang (*Aucklandia*), zhiqiao (*Poncirus trifoliata*) and others, to enhance the ability to facilitate Qi movement and remove stagnation.

If stagnation (accumulation and gelling) of Dampness is predominant, cangzhu (*Atractylodes*) may be used as chief herb. It is then complemented with fuling (*Poria*), zexie (*Alisma*) and huoxiang (*Agastache*), to enhance the ability to eliminate Dampness.

If stagnation (retention) of food is predominant, shenqu may be used as chief herb. It is then complemented with maiya (*Hordeum*), shanzha (*Crataegus*) and others, to enhance the ability to digest and remove the retained food.

If stagnation (accumulation and gelling) of Phlegm is predominant, processed banxia (*Pinellia*) may be used as chief herb. It is then complemented with bile-treated tiannanxing (*Arisaema consanguineum*, *erubescens*) and gualou (*Trichosanthes*), to enhance the ability to dissolve and eliminate Phlegm.

If stagnation (stasis) of blood is predominant, chuanxiong may be used as chief herb. It is then complemented with taoren (*Prunus persica*), honghua (*Carthamus*) and yujin (*Curcuma*), to enhance the ability to facilitate blood circulation and remove stasis.

If stagnation (accumulation and gelling) of Fire is predominant, zhizi (*Gardenia*) may be used as chief herb. It is then complemented with huanglian (*Coptis*), huangqin (*Scutellaria*) and qingdai (*Baphicacanthus cusia*), to enhance the ability to clear Heat and purge Fire.

6 Case Study: Chronic Cholecystitis in a 38-Year-Old Female

The patient had recurrent distention and pain in the right subcostal region for over 3 years. It became more severe during the past month. The pain was aggravated by pressure. It was accompanied by chest tightness, dyspepsia with intolerance of fats, reduced appetite and indigestion. She was weak and without energy. Her tongue was pale, with small sores along the edges, and the tongue coating was greasy. The pulse was taut. Liver function tests were normal. B-type ultrasound study indicated chronic cholecystitis.

Diagnosis: Chronic cholecystitis due to stagnation of liver-Qi and blood, with Dampness and Heat causing obstruction in the middle-jiao.

Therapeutic Principle: Mobilize stagnant liver-Qi, release the blockage, facilitate Qi and blood circulation, clear Heat and dry Dampness.

Treatment: Yue Ju Wan, with additions, was prescribed. The expanded composition was: xiangfu 15 g, cangzhu 15 g, zhizi 15 g, yujin (*Curcuma*) 15 g, zhiqiao

(*Poncirus trifoliata*) 15 g, shenqu (medicated leaven) 12 g, chuanxiong 12 g and chaihu (*Bupleurum*) 12 g. The herbs were decocted in water.

After three doses, the subcostal pain and distention were alleviated and appetite improved. The same formula, with minor modifications, was continued for 2 weeks, and all symptoms resolved. The patient had a relapse a year later. She was treated with the same herbal formula and again recovered.

(Source: *Sichuan Journal of Chinese Medicine*, 1990, 3:26.)

II Banxia Houpo Tang (Pinellia and Magnolia Decoction)

1 Source: Jin Gui Yao Lue (Essentials of the Golden Cabinet)

2 Composition

Chief Herb: processed banxia (*Pinellia ternata*) 12 g

Deputy Herb: houpo (*Magnolia officinalis*) 9 g

Assistant Herbs: fuling (*Poria cocos*) 12 g
shengjiang (*Zingiber officinale*) 9 g

Envoy Herb: zisu (*Perilla frutescens*) 6 g

3 Application

Actions: facilitates Qi movement, dissipates stagnation, suppresses abnormally rising Qi and dissipates Phlegm.

Indications: globus hystericus.

Main Symptoms: a sensation of a foreign body lodged in the throat that can neither be swallowed nor coughed up; chest tightness and distention; or, cough or vomiting. The tongue coating is white and moist or white and greasy. The pulse is taut and slow or taut and slippery.

4 Analysis of the Formula

Processed banxia is acrid–bitter in flavor and warm and dry in nature. It dissipates Phlegm, breaks up masses, suppresses abnormally rising Qi and settles the stomach. It serves as chief herb.

Houpo is acrid–bitter in flavor and warm in nature. It facilitates Qi movement, breaks up stagnation, directs Qi downward and relieves distention. It helps processed banxia to break up accumulations and suppress abnormally rising Qi, and serves as deputy herb.

Fuling is sweet and bland. It promotes the excretion of Dampness, strengthens the spleen, and aids banxia to dissipate Phlegm. Shengjiang is acrid and warm. It disperses and promotes movement, and helps banxia to settle the stomach and stop vomiting. These two herbs serve as assistant herbs.

Zisu is aromatic and is volatile in nature. It facilitates the flow of lung and liver Qi, and aids houpo to facilitate Qi movement and remove blockage. It serves as envoy herb.

These herbs acting in concert use their acridity to facilitate Qi movement and break up blockage, and their bitterness to dry Dampness and suppress abnormally rising Qi.

5 *Comments*

In general, globus hystericus results when the Seven Passions are pent up. That in turn leads to Qi flowing abnormally in the lung and the stomach, and therefore stagnation of Qi and accumulation of Phlegm. It is manifested by the sensation of having a lump in the throat causing obstruction, and the lump can be neither swallowed nor coughed up.

Banxia Houpo Tang facilitates the normal flow of Qi and relieves the blockage. Suppression of the abnormally rising Qi and dissipation of Phlegm will lead to resolution of all the symptoms.

However, the formula contains several herbs that are acrid–bitter in flavor and warm and dry in nature. They can easily harm Yin and the fluids. It is therefore appropriate to use only in illnesses of pent-up passions and congealed Phlegm. If there is significant damage to the body fluids or Yin deficiency, it must not be used.

6 *Case Study: Globus Hystericus in a 52-Year-Old Female*

For about half a year, the patient felt as though she had an object in the throat causing obstruction. It felt like a plum pit, or a piece of thread or a membrane. She was unable to cough it up or swallow it. Her abdomen became distended, and she felt upward pressure. She had constipation with discomfort that was relieved by the passing of gas. Her tongue coating was thin and greasy. Her pulse was deep and taut.

Diagnosis: Globus hystericus due to stagnation of Qi with congealed Phlegm blocking Qi movement.

Therapeutic Principle: Dissipate Phlegm and release stagnation to mobilize Qi.

Treatment: The patient was prescribed Banxia Houpo Tang with added zhishi (*Citrus aurantium*) 9 g, zhuru (*Phyllostachys nigra*) 9 g, laifuzi (*Raphanus*) 9 g, gualou (*Trichosanthes*) 12 g and raw gancao (*Glycyrrhiza*) 1.5 g. After two daily doses, the blockage in the throat disappeared, and her mental status improved.

(Source: *Experience in Clinical Practice.*)

7 *Case Study: Dizziness in a 46-Year-Old Male*

The patient suffered from dizziness, blurred vision, tinnitus, and vomiting for 2 days. When he fastened his vision on objects they seemed to rotate. Turning his head worsened the dizziness. He had no appetite, and eating led to vomiting. A western medical doctor diagnosed it as Meniere's Syndrome. The patient then consulted Chinese medical doctors. He was found to be mildly obese. He had the additional symptoms of photophobia and periodic nausea. His tongue was pale and plump, with a thin white coating. His pulse was taut and slippery.

Diagnosis: Qi stagnation and Phlegm accumulation in the stomach, with abnormal rise of Qi and Phlegm.

Therapeutic Principle: Suppress the abnormally rising Qi, dissipate Phlegm, settle the stomach, and extinguish liver-Wind.

Treatment: Banxia Houpo Tang was prescribed, with modifications as follows: processed banxia 10 g, houpo 10 g, fuling 10 g, zisu root (*Perilla frutescens*) 10 g, zhenzhumu (*Pteria magaritifera, martensii*) (decocted first) 15 g, Guangdong chenpi (*Citrus tangerina*) 5 g, stir-fried cangzhu (*Atractylodes*) 10 g, and zexie (*Alisma*) 10 g.

After three doses, the dizziness and blurred vision were subjectively improved, and the patient was able to eat. After five doses, he was able to function normally.

(Source: *Jiangsu Journal of Chinese Medicine*, 1980, 6:23.)

III Suzi Jiang Qi Tang (Perilla Qi-Suppressing Decoction)

1 *Source: Tai Ping Hui Min He Ji Ju Fang (Prescriptions from the Taiping Benevolent Pharmaceutical Bureau)*

2 *Composition*

Chief Herb: zisuzi (*Perilla frutescens*) 9 g

Deputy Herbs: processed banxia (*Pinellia ternata*) 9 g
qianhu (*Peucedanum praeruptorum*) 6 g
houpo (*Magnolia officinalis*) 6 g

Assistant Herbs: danggui (*Angelica sinensis*) 6 g
rougui (*Cinnamomum cassia*) 3 g
zisu leaf (*Perilla frutescens*) 5 pieces
shengjiang (*Zingiber officinale*) 2 pieces

Envoy Herbs: fried gancao (*Glycyrrhiza uralensis*) 6 g
dazao (*Ziziphus jujuba*) 1 piece

3 *Application*

Actions: suppresses abnormally rising Qi, relieves wheezing, eliminates Phlegm and stops cough.

Indications: asthma due to strength of pathogenic evil.

Main Symptoms: tightness and fullness in the chest, wheezing, dyspnea, cough with copious sputum; or, pain and weakness of the lower back and legs, sometimes edema of the extremities. A white and smooth or white and greasy tongue coating; and a taut and slippery pulse.

4 *Analysis of the Formula*

Zisuzi suppresses abnormally rising Qi, relieves wheezing, stops cough and dissipates Phlegm. It serves as chief herb.

Processed banxia suppresses abnormally rising Qi and dissipates Phlegm. Houpo suppresses abnormally rising Qi, stops wheezing, loosens the chest and eliminates distention. Qianhu unblocks the lung, suppresses abnormally rising Qi, dissipates Phlegm and stops cough. These three herbs help zisuzi suppress abnormally rising Qi, dissipate Phlegm and relieve wheezing. They serve together as deputy herbs.

Since kidney-Qi is deficient, acrid-warm rougui is used to warm and augment it, and to nourish the kidney, thereby stopping wheezing. Acrid–sweet and warm danggui can suppress abnormally rising Qi and stop cough, and also can generate blood and moisten Dryness. It acts with rougui to warm and augment kidney-Qi. These two form one group of assistant herbs. Small amounts of shengjiang and zisu leaf are used to facilitate the flow of lung-Qi and to dispel Cold. The herbs of both groups serve together as assistant herbs.

Dazao and fried gancao harmonize the middle-jiao and coordinate the actions of all the other herbs. They serve as envoy herbs.

The formula as a whole treats the symptoms in the upper body and the deficiencies in the lower body, and takes into account both cause and effect. It therefore suppresses abnormally rising Qi and dissipates Phlegm, so that wheezing also stops.

5 Comments

Suzi Jiang Qi Tang is designed to treat illnesses of strong exogenous evil in the upper body and deficiency in the lower. The upper strength refers to Phlegm causing blockage of the lung, so that Qi cannot move freely in the lung. The lower deficiency refers to deficiency of kidney-Yang, so that the kidney is unable to receive Qi or move fluids normally.

The formula is intended for the group of these illnesses in which the upper strength is primary and the lower deficiency is secondary. In illnesses of deficiency of both the lung and the kidney, with wheezing, it is not appropriate.

6 Case Study: Chronic and Acute Asthma in a 56-Year-Old Male

The patient suffered from asthma for about 10 years. In recent days his condition deteriorated, so that he had difficulty breathing and the wheezing and cough made it difficult for him to lie down. He had copious thin and white sputum. His pulse was taut, and his tongue moist and plump. He was thought to suffer from Cold and Phlegm lodging in the lung and impeding lung-Qi. He was initially treated with Ling Gan Wu Wei Jiang Xin Tang to warm the lung, dissipate Rheum, restrain the lung and stop wheezing, but the response was insignificant.

He was further examined. Careful palpation showed his pulse to be taut in the cun position but soft in the two chi positions. He now had polyuria, fatigue, and weakness in the lower back and legs.

Diagnosis: Asthma due to upper strength and lower deficiency (Cold–Phlegm lodged in the lung causing abnormal Qi movement), so that the kidney is unable to receive Qi normally.

Therapeutic Principle: Warm the kidney and the lung, dissipate Phlegm–Rheum and restrain the lung.

Treatment: The patient was treated with Suzi Jiang Qi Tang, with added chenxiang (*Aquilaria*), renshen (*Panax*) and dongchongxiacao (*Cordyceps*). With one dose the wheezing was much decreased and the patient was able to lie down. His mental status and body strength both also improved. Altogether nine daily doses were administered, and he recovered completely.

(Source: *Jiangsu Journal of Chinese Medicine*, 1980, 6:23.)

IV Ding Chuan Tang (Asthma-Relieving Decoction)

1 *Source: She Sheng Zhong Miao Fang (Effective Prescriptions for Health Conservation)*

2 *Composition*

Chief Herbs: baiguo (*Ginkgo biloba*) 9 g
mahuang (*Ephedra sinica*) 9 g

Deputy Herbs: kuandonghua (*Tussilago farfara*) 9 g
processed banxia (*Pinellia ternata*) 9 g
xingren (*Prunus armeniaca*) 9 g
zisuzi (*Perilla frutescens*) 6 g

Assistant Herbs: sangbaipi (*Morus alba*) 6 g
huangqin (*Scutellaria baicalensis*) 6 g

Envoy Herb: gancao (*Glycyrrhiza uralensis*) 3 g

3 *Application*

Actions: suppresses abnormally rising Qi, stops wheezing, dissipates Phlegm and stops cough.

Indications: asthma.

Main Symptoms: cough with copious yellow sputum and labored breathing; wind and cold aversion; a yellow greasy tongue coating; and a slippery and rapid pulse.

4 *Analysis of the Formula*

Ding Chuan Tang uses mahuang and baiguo for chief herbs. Mahuang is acrid and warm. It facilitates the flow of lung-Qi and stops wheezing. It also releases the exterior and dispels pathogenic evils. Baiguo is sweet and astringent. It dissipates Phlegm and stops cough. These two herbs, one dispersing and the other astringing, enhance each other's ability to stop wheezing. Baiguo also prevents damage to lung-Qi by mahuang's strong acridity and dispersion.

Kuandonghua, processed banxia, xingren and zisuzi all have the ability to suppress abnormally rising Qi, dissolve Phlegm and stop cough. They enhance the ability of the chief herbs to stop wheezing and dissipate Phlegm. They serve together as deputy herbs.

The formula further uses the sweet and cold sangbaipi and the bitter and cold huangqin to purge Heat from the lung and to stop cough and wheezing. They serve as assistant herbs. The deputy and assistant herbs act together to remove congealed Phlegm and Heat from the interior.

Gancao harmonizes the actions of the other herbs, and is the envoy.

Acting in concert these herbs suppress abnormally rising Qi, stop cough and wheezing, purge Heat and dissipate Phlegm.

5 Comments

The illness Ding Chuan Tang is designed to treat is wheezing caused by Cold and Wind binding the exterior and Phlegm and Heat smoldering in the interior. The key symptoms are wheezing, cough and dyspnea, copious yellow sputum, wind and cold aversion, a yellow and greasy tongue coating, and a slippery and rapid pulse.

Both Ding Chuan Tang and Xiao Qing Long Tang (Section 1) facilitate Qi movement, release the exterior, dissipate Phlegm and stop wheezing. They can both be used to treat wheezing caused by Wind and Cold in the interior and Phlegm in the interior. However, Xiao Qing Long Tang is most importantly used where there is Cold-induced fluids in the interior and more severe Cold in the exterior. Ding Chuan Tang emphasizes the treatment of Wind and Cold in the exterior and Heat and Phlegm in the interior. There are subtle differences between them.

V Xuanfu Daizhe Tang (Inula and Hematite Decoction)

1 Source: Shang Han Lun (Treatise on Cold-Attack)

2 Composition

Chief Herb: xuanfuhua (*Inula japonica, britannica*) 9 g

Deputy Herb: zheshi (hematite) 9 g

Assistant Herbs: shengjiang (*Zingiber officinale*) 10 g
processed banxia (*Pinellia ternata*) 9 g
renshen (*Panax ginseng*) 6 g
dazao (*Ziziphus jujuba*) 4 pieces

Envoy Herb: fried gancao (*Glycyrrhiza uralensis*) 9 g

3 Application

Actions: suppresses abnormally rising Qi, dissipates Phlegm, augments Qi and settles the stomach.

Indications: deficiency of stomach-Qi, with Phlegm and impurities causing blockage in the interior.

Main Symptoms: fullness and hardness in the epigastrium; persistent belching; or, vomiting and hiccup, and spitting up saliva; a pale tongue with white and slippery coating; and a string-taut but depletive pulse.

4 Analysis of the Formula

Xuanfuhua suppresses abnormally rising Qi, dissipates Phlegm and stops belching. It is the chief herb.

Zheshi is sweet in flavor, cold in nature and heavy. It also suppresses abnormally rising Qi, enhancing xuanfuhua in this action, and stops vomiting and belching. It is the deputy herb.

Processed banxia is acrid and warm. It dries Dampness, dissipates Phlegm, suppresses abnormally rising Qi and settles the stomach. Shengjiang is also acrid and warm. It dissipates Phlegm, breaks up accumulations, suppresses abnormally rising Qi and stops vomiting. These two together enhance the actions of the chief and deputy herbs to suppress abnormally rising Qi and to stop vomiting. Since stomach-Qi is deficient, renshen, dazao and fried gancao are included to augment Qi and tonify the middle-jiao in order to compensate for the deficiency of Stomach-Qi, and to prevent stomach injury by zheshi. These five serve as assistant herbs.

In its action of harmonizing the actions of the other herbs fried gancao serves as envoy herb as well.

5 Comments

The illnesses for which Xuanfu Daizhe Tang is designed fall into two groups. One is hiccup due to insufficiency of the stomach and blockage of Qi by Phlegm, preventing it from descending. The other is vomiting due to abnormally rising Qi. The key manifestations are epigastric distention, frequent belching, vomiting, a white and smooth tongue coating, and a taut and slippery pulse.

In clinical practice pay attention to the amount of zheshi used. If the insufficiency of the stomach is not marked, a larger amount may be used; but if the insufficiency of the stomach is marked, then smaller amounts must be used.

If the underlying problem is insufficiency of the stomach but there is concomitant hiccup or vomiting due to Heat in the stomach, then the proper approach is suppression of the abnormally rising Qi to stop the vomiting. The mainstay of treatment is **Jupi Zhuru Tang**, which has the following composition: jupi (*Citrus tangerina*) 12 g, zhuru (*Phyllostachys nigra*) 12 g, dazao 10 pieces, shengjiang 9 g, gancao 6 g and renshen 3 g. This formula is mainly used to treat hiccup or vomiting caused by Heat in an already insufficient stomach, with abnormally risen Qi not descending properly.

6 Case Study: Morning Sickness in a 24-Year-Old Female

The patient had been pregnant for 2 months when frequent nausea and vomiting began. Even merely touching food to her lips aggravated the vomiting. Her complexion was dull and sallow. She appeared fatigued. Her mouth had a slightly bitter taste. She was thirsty, but dared not drink as drinking was followed promptly by more vomiting. Her tongue was pale, with a thin white coating. Her pulse was slippery.

Diagnosis: Insufficiency of the spleen causing Qi to rise abnormally and the stomach to function improperly.

Therapeutic Principle: Strengthen the spleen to settle the stomach, facilitate normal Qi movement and suppress the abnormally risen Qi.

Treatment: Xuanfu Daizhe Tang with modifications was prescribed. The composition was: xuanfuhua 15 g, zheshi 20 g, banxia 12 g, hongshen (processed renshen) 8 g, wuzhuyu (*Evodia*) 6 g, huanglian (*Coptis*) 10 g, pipaye (*Eriobotrya japonica*) 12 g, gancao 3 g, shengjiang 3 slices, and dazao 3 pieces. The herbs were boiled in water. The patient was instructed to rub her throat with roasted ginger. When she felt some numbness she was to take several swallows of the decoction, wait half an hour, then take the remainder of the decoction. After two doses, the vomiting stopped, and she was able to eat small amounts. Her vivaciousness returned. Her prescription was then changed to the original Xuanfu Daizhe Tang, without wuzhuyu and huanglian. After two doses she recovered sufficiently to leave the hospital. She subsequently gave birth at full term.

(Source: *Heilongjiang Journal of Chinese Medicine*, 1985, 2:25.)

VI Section Summary

The five formulas selected for this section fall into the two categories of facilitation of Qi movement and suppression of abnormally rising Qi.

Yue Ju Wan and **Banxia Houpo Tang** are representative of those that facilitate Qi movement. Yue Ju Wan is particularly efficacious for facilitating Qi movement and releasing blockage. It is mainly used to treat the six types of stagnation. The main action of Banxia Houpo Tang is to release stagnation and to suppress abnormally risen Qi. It is mainly used to treat globus hystericus caused by emotional distress and gelling of Phlegm.

Suzi Jiang Qi Tang, **Ding Chuan Tang** and **Xuanfu Daizhe Tang** all vigorously suppress abnormally risen Qi, but they differ in emphasis. Suzi Jiang Qi Tang emphasizes the suppression of abnormally risen lung-Qi. It relieves wheezing and warms the kidney, enabling it to receive Qi. Ding Chuan Tang emphasizes releasing the exterior for removing Wind and Cold and clearing the interior for removing Heat and Phlegm. It is used in illnesses of wheezing caused by Wind and Cold attacking the exterior and Heat and Phlegm blocking the interior. Xuanfu Daizhe Tang emphasizes warming the stomach to stop vomiting and belching. It is most appropriate for illnesses of hiccup or vomiting caused by deficiency-Cold in the stomach and blocking of Qi by Phlem.

Section 11 Formulas That Regulate Blood

Herbal formulas that regulate blood comprise all those that are constructed around herbs that regulate blood. They have the ability to improve blood circulation and mobilize static blood, or the ability to stop bleeding.

Blood is an important nutritive substance. In normal circumstances it circulates in its channels throughout the body and nourishes all the limbs and organs. If blood does not circulate smoothly, blood stasis may occur, or blood may leave its channels and move about abnormally, or it may become depleted. In all these situations, illness may develop. Examples include hematoma, bleeding and blood deficiency. Therefore, the treatment of illnesses of blood includes the three aspects of mobilizing static blood, stopping bleeding and generating blood.

Though technically part of this group formulas that generate or nourish blood are not included in this section since they have been discussed in Section 6. The blood-regulating formulas discussed in this section fall in two main groups: those that stop bleeding and those that break up static blood.

In the clinical application of formulas that mobilize blood and break up stasis, be careful not to harm genuine Qi. Moreover, these formulas are mostly substances that break up the firm and gelled; hence great caution is necessary if they are to be used, if at all, in women who have excessive menstrual flow or who are pregnant.

In the clinical application of formulas that stop bleeding, the physician must determine the cause of the bleeding and take care to ascertain whether the illness is one of deficiency or strength, and whether it is one of Cold or Heat.

I Taohe Cheng Qi Tang (Peach Pit Qi-Activating Decoction)

1 Source: Shang Han Lun (Treatise on Cold-Attack)

2 Composition

Chief Herbs: dahuang (*Rheum palmatum*) 12 g
taoren (*Prunus persica*) 12 g

Deputy Herbs: mangxiao (*Mirabilite*) 6 g
guizhi (*Cinnamomum cassia*) 6 g

Assistant and Envoy Herb: fried gancao (*Glycyrrhiza uralensis*) 6 g

3 Application

Actions: breaks up static blood and drains Heat.

Indications: blood stasis in the lower-jiao.

Main Symptoms: acute lower abdominal pain and incontinence of urine. In severe cases: delirious speech or agitation or manic behavior; night fever; dysmenorrhea or amenorrhea; and a deep, replete yet impeded pulse.

4 Analysis of the Formula

Tao He Cheng Qi Tang is derived from Tiao Wei Cheng Qi Tang (see under Da Cheng Qi Tang, Section 2) by reducing the amount of mangxiao and adding taoren and guizhi.

It uses taoren and dahuang together as chief herbs. Taoren enhances blood circulation and breaks up static blood. Dahuang breaks up static blood and purges Heat. The two herbs together eliminate both blood stasis and Heat.

Guizhi and mangxiao serve as deputy herbs. Guizhi warms the meridians and promotes blood circulation, thereby strengthening the action of taoren to enhance blood flow and break up static blood. When teamed with herbs of cold nature its acrid flavor and warm nature also prevents the risk of the cold herbs congealing blood. Mangxiao dispels Heat and softens hard masses, thereby helping dahuang to dispel Heat and break up static blood.

Fried gancao, which serves as both assistant and envoy herb, protects the stomach and normalizes the middle-jiao by blunting the harshness of the other herbs.

These five herbs together have the ability to break up and eliminate blood stasis. Administration of the formula leads to mild diarrhea, which indicates the breaking up of static blood and accumulated Heat.

5 Comments

The illnesses Taohe Cheng Qi Tang is designed to treat are of blood stagnating in the lower-jiao. The key manifestations are cramps in the lower abdomen but normal urination. In severe cases, there may be delirium and agitation, even manic behavior.

Nowadays, the clinical use of Tao He Cheng Qi Tang has been extended. It is now prescribed also for traumatic bruises, and disturbances in menstruation or amenorrhea. However, it is a formula that breaks up blood stasis, and is therefore contraindicated in pregnancy.

6 Case Study: Ectopic Pregnancy in a 40-Year-Old Female

The patient was over 50 days past her last menses. For the last 20 days or more, she had irregular vaginal bleeding. She now had intermittent pain and pressure in the left lower abdomen, with a sensation of having to defecate. She had difficulty walking or bending over. She had slow but persistent vaginal bleeding, sometimes with small clots. There was no fever, and her urination and defecation were normal. She was admitted to hospital.

Her complexion was withered and yellow. She was emaciated and mentally fatigued, and groaned incessantly from pain. Her chest was tight, and she had little appetite. Her tongue was dull and gray, with a white coating. Her pulse was taut and threadlike but slippery.

On gynecological examination, the vagina contained a small amount of bloody fluid. The uterus was abnormal in position and in size, and the recto-uterine cavity was distended. Elevation of the cervix was markedly tender. In the left adnexal region there was an egg-sized mass. Culdocentesis produced bloody fluid without clots.

Diagnosis: Ectopic pregnancy, resulting from obstruction of Qi circulation and with blood stasis in the pelvic abdomen.

Therapeutic Principle: Unclog the liver and promote normal Qi circulation; induce catharsis and eliminate stasis.

Treatment: Modified Taohe Cheng Qi Tang was prescribed, with the following composition: taoren 6 g, dahuang 6 g, mangxiao 6 g, gancao 5 g, guizhi 5 g, qingpi (*Citrus tangerina*) 5 g, zhishi (*Citrus aurantium*) 10 g, danggui (*Angelica*) 12 g, baishaoyao (*Paeonia*) 10 g, sumu (*Caesalpinia sappan*) 10 g and chaihu (*Bupleurum*) 5 g.

Following three daily doses of this prescription, the patient began having diarrhea and concomitant reduction in the abdominal pain. Her vaginal bleeding increased, with dark clots, but the adnexal mass shrank in size. The prescription was continued without change. After three more doses, the abdominal pain and the vaginal bleeding both ceased. The adnexal mass was markedly reduced in size. Her mental state improved greatly, and she now could savor her foods. The same prescription was continued, but omitting mangxiao and reducing the amount of dahuang, for seven more doses. Her abdomen became soft and the mass disappeared. Treatment was continued with Ba Zhen Tang (section 6) with added yimucao (*Leonurus*) to consolidate the clinical response.

II Xue Fu Zhu Yu Tang (Decoction for Releasing Blood Stasis)

1 Source: Yi Lin Gai Cuo (Corrections of Medical Errors)

2 Composition

Chief Herbs: taoren (*Prunus persica*) 12 g
honghua (*Carthamus tinctorius*) 9 g

Deputy Herbs: danggui (*Angelica sinensis*) 9 g
chuanxiong (*Ligusticum chuanxiong*, *wallichii*) 5 g
chishaoyao (*Paeonia lactiflora*) 6 g
chaihu (*Bupleurum chinense*, *scorzonerifolium*) 3 g

Assistant Herbs: shengdihuang (*Rehmannia glutinosa*) 9 g
zhiqiao (*Poncirus trifoliata*) 5 g
jiegeng (*Platycodon grandiflorum*) 6 g
niuxi (*Achyranthes bidentata*) 9 g

Envoy Herb: gancao (*Glycyrrhiza uralensis*) 3 g

3 Application

Actions: facilitates blood circulation, eliminates blood stasis, promotes Qi movement and relieves pain.

Indications: blood stasis inside the thorax.

Main Symptoms: needle-jab-like chest pain and chronic persistent headache in a fixed location; or, incessant hiccup for many days; or, internal feverishness with irritability; or, palpitations of the heart with insomnia, impatience and irascibility.

In addition: high fever in the evening; dark lips or dimmed vision; a dark red tongue that may have spots of ecchymosis; and an impeded or taut and tight pulse.

4 Analysis of the Formula

Xue Fu Zhu Yu Tang is constructed by combining Tao Hong Si Wu Tang (see Si Wu Tang, Section 6) and Si Ni San and adding jiegeng and niuxi.

It uses danggui, chuanxiong, chishaoyao, taoren and honghua to stimulate blood circulation and eliminate blood stasis. Jiegeng facilitates lung-Qi and guides other herbs upward. When jiegeng and zhiqiao are teamed, one raises and one suppresses, so that Qi can move freely in the lung, and as Qi moves freely so does blood. Shengdihuang cools blood and clears Heat. When teamed with danggui it also augments Yin and moistens Dryness, so that the circulation of blood can be facilitated without consuming blood and blood stasis can be released as new blood is generated.

Acting in concert these herbs eliminate blood stasis and promote Qi circulation, so that all symptoms can resolve.

5 Comments

The physician Wang Qingren was especially skilled in the clinical use of herbs that facilitate blood circulation and remove blood stasis. He used them to create a series of well-known formulas for these purposes. In addition to Xue Fu Zhu Yu Tang there are **Tong Qiao Huo Xue Tang**, **Ge Xia Zhu Yu Tang**, **Shao Fu Zhu Yu Tang** and **Shen Tong Zhu Yu Tang.** These four are presented in the accompanying table.

6 Case Study: Refractory Insomnia in a 42-Year-Old Male

The patient suffered from insomnia for over 2 years. It was accompanied by dizziness, headache and numbness of the lower limbs. He was treated many times with various sedative formulas. In each case, there was initial response but prompt relapse. Chinese herbs used included those that strengthen the spleen, those that harmonize the heart and the kidney and those that warm the gallbladder. He was severely depressed, had a very dark complexion and a scaly skin. On his chest and back his skin showed lesions of tinea versicolor. His tongue was purplish, with a yellow and greasy coating. His pulse was taut and threadlike but forceful.

Diagnosis: Blood stasis in the chest.

Therapeutic Principle: Facilitate blood circulation and eliminate blood stasis in the chest.

Treatment: Xue Fu Zhu Yu Tang with added cishi (magnetite) was prescribed. After one dose, the patient became overly excited and was unable to sleep. Other symptoms showed some improvement after a second dose. Following seven daily doses, the dizziness and headache improved markedly. The prescription was then changed to unmodified Xue Fu Zhu Yu Tang. After 14 daily doses, the patient was able to sleep restfully every night, and the other symptoms also subsided. Treatment was continued with Tian Wang Bu Xin Dan (Section 8) to consolidate the clinical response (see Table 9.3).

(Source: *Journal of the New Medicine*, 1977, 11:32.)

7 Case Study: Persistent Hiccup in a 24-Year-Old Female

Four months previously the patient suddenly felt a sharp pain and tightness in the chest, followed the same day by persistent hiccup. She was treated by Chinese and Western physicians in her area, without benefit. Though the hiccup had lasted several months, her strength had not been affected. Her pulse was taut and forceful. Her urination and defecation were normal. Her only associated symptom was that whenever she hiccuped she felt a blockage in the chest with sharp pain in the ribs.

Diagnosis: Blood stasis and Qi stagnation.

Therapeutic Principle: Facilitate blood circulation and release blood stasis and Qi stagnation.

Treatment: Xue Fu Zhu Yu Tang with added xuanfuhua (*Inula britannica*) and daizheshi (hematite) was prescribed. After one dose her chest felt more comfortable, and she no longer had the sensation of blockage or the sharp pain. The hiccup was also reduced by 70–80%. After two doses, the hiccup stopped. After three doses, she recovered completely.

(Source: *Zhejiang Journal of Medicine*, 1963, 2:3.)

III Bu Yang Huan Wu Tang (Yang-Tonifying Balance-Restoring Decoction)

1 Source: Yi Lin Gai Cuo (Corrections of Medical Errors)

2 Composition

Chief Herb: huangqi (*Astragalus membranaceus*) 120 g

Deputy Herb: danggui (*Angelica sinensis*) 3 g

Table 9.3 Formulas derived from Xue Fu Zhu Yu Tang

Formula Name	Formula	Actions	Indications
Tong Qiao Huo Xue Tang (orifice-unblocking blood-mobilizing decoction)	Chishaoyao 9 g Chuanxiong 9 g Taoren 9 g Honghua 9 g Congbai 3 g Dazao 7 pieces Shengjiang 9 g Shexiang 0.15 g Wine	Mobilizes blood, relieves blood stasis; opens orifices	Aches, weakness in waist and knees; dizziness, vertigo; tinnitus, deafness; diabetes; recurrent deficiency fever; hotness in palms and soles; dry tongue, sore throat; residual urine post voiding; red tongue with scant coating; deep, threadlike and rapid pulse
Ge Xia Zhu Yu Tang (decoction for relieving stasis below the diaphragm)	Fried wulin gzhi 9 g Danggui 9 g Chuanxiong 6 g Taoren 9 g Mudanpi 6 g Chishaoyao 6 g Wuyao 6–12 g Yanhusuo 3–15 g Gancao 9 g Xiangfu 4.5 g Honghua 9 g Zhiqiao 4.5 g	Mobilizes blood, relieves blood stasis, warms menses; alleviates pain	Abdominal masses, abdominal pain in fixed location
Shao Fu Zhu Yu Tang (decoction for relieving stasis in the lower abdomen)	Fried ganj iang 6 g Yanhusuo 3–15 g Danggui 9–12 g Chuanxiong 3–10 g Moyao 3–10 g Chishaoyao 6–15 g Puhuang 9 g Wulingzhi 6–10 g Xiaohuixiang 6–10 g Rougui 3–5g	Mobilizes blood; alleviates pain	Lower abdominal masses, with or without pain, or abdominal pain without mass, or lower abdominal distention; purple menses, or painful metrorrhagia
Shen Tong Zhu Yu Tang (decoction for relieving stasis and pain)	Chishaoy ao 6 g Qinjiao 3 g Chuanxiong 6 g Taoren 9 g Honghua 9 g Qianghuo3 g Moyao 3 g Danggui 9 g Wulingzhi 6 g Xiangfu 3 g Niuxi 9 g Dilong 6 g Gancao 6 g	Mobilizes blood and Qi, relieves blood stasis, unblocks collaterals; unblocks painful obstruction, alleviates pain	Pain in the shoulder, arm, waist, legs or generalized pain due to blood stasis blocking channels

Assistant and Envoy Herbs: chuanxiong (*Ligusticum chuanxiong, wallichii*) 3 g
taoren (*Prunus persica*) 3 g
chishaoyao (*Paeonia lactiflora*) 5 g
honghua (*Carthamus tinctorius*) 3 g
dilong (*Pheretima aspergillum*) 3 g

3 Application

Actions: augments Qi, facilitates blood circulation and unblocks the channels.

Indications: Wind-induced stroke.

Main Symptoms: hemiplegia; facial paralysis; slurred speech, drooling; frequent urination or urinary incontinence; a gray tongue with white coating; and a slow pulse.

4 Analysis of the Formula

Bu Yang Huan Wu Tang uses huangqi in large amount for vigorous augmentation of spleen and stomach-Qi. Once Qi is ample blood will circulate briskly, stagnant blood will be mobilized and all channels will become unblocked. It serves as chief herb.

Danggui facilitates blood circulation and eliminates blood stasis without damaging blood. It serves as deputy herb.

There are five assistant herbs. Chuanxiong, chishaoyao, taoren and honghua assist danggui to facilitate blood circulation and remove stasis. Dilong unblocks meridians and channels.

The characteristic in the construction of this formula is to complement large amounts of herbs that augment Qi with small amounts of herbs that facilitate blood circulation. Helping Qi to flourish ensures that blood circulates freely without incurring any damage to genuine Qi. Together these two groups of herbs achieve the goals of augmenting Qi, facilitating blood circulation and unblocking channels.

5 Comments

Bu Yang Huan Wu Tang is designed for treating hemiplegia caused by Qi deficiency and blood stasis. The key clinical findings are hemiplegia, wry mouth and eyes, a white tongue coating, and a slow or a threadlike and feeble pulse. Since Qi deficiency is the characteristic of this condition Qi-augmenting herbs are used in large amounts. Blood stasis is a consequence of deficient Qi not being able to move blood. Therefore, even small amounts of stasis-removing herbs, used in concert with Qi-augmenting herbs, will be effective.

6 Clinical Study: Hemiplegia due to Wind-Induced Stroke

Thirty-eight patients with hemiplegia caused by Qi deficiency and blood stasis were treated with Bu Yang Huan Wu Tang with modifications. The composition was as follows: huangqi 30–60 g, danggui 10–15 g, taoren 10–15 g, chuanxiong 10–15 g, chishaoyao 10–15 g, dilong 15–20 g, juluo (*Citrus tangerina*) 5–10 g, danshen (*Salvia*) 15–30 g, and sangzhi (*Morus alba*) 15–30 g.

Of the 38 patients, six had cerebral hemorrhage, 29 had cerebral thrombosis and three had cerebral embolism.

Results: Fourteen patients showed complete recovery. Fourteen showed marked improvement. Eight showed some improvement. Two showed no response.

(Source: *Sichuan Journal of Chinese Medicine*, 1985, 11:15.)

IV Wen Jing Tang (Meridian-Warming Decoction)

1 Source: Jin Gui Yao Lue (Essentials of the Golden Cabinet)

2 Composition

Chief Herbs: wuzhuyu (*Evodia rutaecarpa*) 9 g
guizhi (*Cinnamomum cassia*) 6 g

Deputy Herbs: danggui (*Angelica sinensis*) 6 g
chuanxiong (*Ligusticum chuanxiong, wallichii*) 6 g
baishaoyao (*Paeonia lactiflora*) 6 g
mudanpi (*Paeonia suffruticosa*) 6 g

Assistant Herbs: ejiao (*Equus asinus*) 6 g
maimendong (*Ophiopogon japonicus*) 9 g
renshen (*Panax ginseng*) 6 g
shengjiang (*Zingiber officinale*) 6 g
processed banxia (*Pinellia ternata*) 6 g

Envoy Herb: gancao (*Glycyrrhiza uralensis*) 6 g

3 Application

Actions: warms the meridians, dispels Cold, eliminates blood stasis and generates blood.

Indications: (1) deficiency-Cold in the Chong and Ren Meridians, with blood stasis causing blockage. (2) Female infertility.

Main Symptoms: irregular menses (early or late, or twice in 1 month, or skipping a month) or amenorrhea; evening fever, hotness in the palms and soles; irritability; dry lips and mouth.

4 Analysis of the Formula

There are two chief herbs in Wen Jing Tang. Wuzhuyu, which is acrid–bitter and hot, dispels Cold and stops pain. Guizhi, which is acrid–sweet and warm, can warm the meridians and dispel Cold. The two herbs enhance each other's actions.

Of the four deputy herbs, danggui, chuanxiong and baishaoyao can penetrate the Liver Meridian. They facilitate blood circulation, remove blood stasis, generate blood and normalize menses. Mudanpi facilitates blood circulation, removes blood stasis, and eliminates deficiency Heat.

Ejiao nourishes liver-blood and augments kidney-Yin. It can thus generate blood and fluids, and stop bleeding. Maimendong is sweet–bitter and cool. It augments Yin and clears Heat. As a team these two herbs augment Yin, generate fluids and eliminate deficiency-Heat. They also restrain the tendency of wuzhuyu and guizhi to induce Dryness through their warmth. Renshen and gancao are sweet and have the ability to penetrate the spleen, augment Qi and tonify the middle-jiao, thereby supporting the sources of blood and Qi. Banxia is acrid and warm. It also penetrates the spleen and the stomach, and can suppress abnormally rising stomach-Qi and break up accumulations. The team of processed banxia, renshen and gancao strengthens the spleen and settles the stomach, in that way helping to remove stasis and normalize menses. Shengjiang is also acrid in flavor and warm in nature. It warms the interior and dispels Cold.

Together the herbs of the formula warm the meridians, remove blood stasis, generate blood and clear deficiency-Heat, and normalize menses.

5 Comments

Wen Jing Tang is the original herbal formula for warming meridians and normalizing menses. It combines warming-dispelling and augmenting-eliminating actions, though it emphasizes the warming of meridians and removal of stasis. Also characteristic is the complementation of many warming–augmenting herbs with a few cold or cool herbs. This permits the formula to be warming without drying.

6 Case Study: Metrorrhagia in a 24-Year-Old Female

The patient suffered from uterine bleeding for 3 months, and her vaginal discharge contained many clots. She had cramp-like pelvic pain, fever, cold-aversion and sometimes even syncope. Her appetite was reduced, and when she did eat she developed distention in her stomach. Her pulse at the cun position was large and forceful, but in the chi position it was threadlike and feeble.

Diagnosis: Blood stasis in the uterus.

Therapeutic Principle: Warm the meridians, dispel Cold, and stop the bleeding.

Treatment: She was prescribed Wen Jing Tang, with added zisu leaf (*Perilla frutescens*), xuanfuhua (*Inula britannica*) and charred puhuang (*Typha angustifolia*). After three doses, several large clots were discharged vaginally, following which the bleeding stopped and all other symptoms resolved. In follow-up her menses remained normal.

(Source: *Journal of the Hunan College of Chinese Medicine*.)

V Sheng Hua Tang (Generation and Transformation Decoction)

1 Source: Fu Qingzhu Nu Ke (Fu Qingzhu's Obstetrics and Gynecology)

2 Composition

Chief Herb: danggui (*Angelica sinensis*) 24 g

Deputy Herbs: chuanxiong (*Ligusticum chuanxiong*, *wallichii*) 9 g
taoren (*Prunus persica*) 9 g

Assistant Herbs: roast ganjiang (*Zingiber officinale*) 6 g
yellow wine and child's urine

Envoy Herb: fried gancao (*Glycyrrhiza uralensis*) 2 g

3 Application

Actions: removes stasis, generates blood, warms meridians and eliminates pain.

Indications: post-partum blood stasis.

Main Symptoms: cold pain in the pelvis and persistent lochia.

4 Analysis of the Formula

Sheng Hua Tang uses danggui in large amount to generate blood and facilitate blood circulation. It is the chief herb.

Chuanxiong facilitates blood and Qi circulation. Taoren facilitates blood circulation and removes stasis. They serve together as deputy herbs.

Quick-fried ganjiang warms the meridians and eliminates pain. Yellow wine warms and disperses, in that way enhancing the actions of the other herbs. Child's urine is added for its ability to augment Yin and dissolve static blood. It also has the ability to conduct static blood downward. These serve together as assistant herbs.

Fried gancao harmonizes the actions of the other herbs, and serves as envoy herb.

This formula has only five ingredients (not counting wine and urine), but they are well matched. Together they act to release stasis and generate new blood, warm the meridians and stop pain.

5 Comments

In many parts of southern China, post-partum women of an entire generation were required to take this formula. It had a broad range of applicability. However, judging from its composition and the relative amounts of the ingredients, it is most appropriate for postpartum women who have contracted exogenous Cold and who have blood stasis in the uterus.

If there is Heat in blood causing blood stasis, this formula is not appropriate. If there is little pain then remove taoren (*Prunus persica*). If pain is severe and blood stasis is marked then add puhuang (*Typha angustifolia*), wulingzhi (*Pleropus pselaphon*) and yanhusuo (*Corydalis*) to enhance the ability to remove stasis and stop pain. If Cold pain in the pelvic abdomen is prominent then add rougui (*Cinnamomum*) to warm the meridians and dispel Cold.

VI Xiaoji Yin Zi (Thistle Decoction)

1 Source: Ji Sheng Fang (Life-Saving Prescriptions)

2 Composition

Chief Herb: shengdihuang (*Rehmannia glutinosa*) 30 g

Deputy Herbs: xiaoji (*Cephalanoplos segetum*) 15 g
oujie (*Nelumbo nucifera*) 9 g
puhuang (*Typha angustifolia*) 9 g

Assistant Herbs: huashi (talcum) 15 g
danzhuye (*Lophatherum gracile*) 9 g
mutong (*Akebia quinata, trifoliata*) 6 g
zhizi (*Gardenia jasminoides*) 9 g
danggui (*Angelica sinensis*) 6 g

Envoy Herb: fried gancao (*Glycyrrhiza uralensis*) 6 g

3 Application

Actions: cools blood, stops bleeding, promotes diuresis and relieves urethritis.

Indications: urethritis with hematuria.

Main Symptoms: hematuria; frequent urination; urgency, burning and pain during urination. A red tongue with a thin, yellow coating; and a rapid, forceful pulse.

4 Analysis of the Formula

Xiaoji Yin Zi uses a large amount of shengdihuang to cool blood, stop bleeding, augment Yin and clear Heat. It is the chief herb.

Xiaoji cools blood and stops bleeding. Oujie and puhuang cool blood and stop bleeding, and can also dissolve static blood. They therefore ensure that stopping the bleeding will not lead to blood stasis. These three are together the deputy herbs.

Huashi, danzhuye and mutong clear Heat, promote diuresis and unclog the urethra. Zhizi purges Heat from the sanjiao and conducts Heat downward and out. Danggui generates and harmonizes blood, and conducts blood back into its channels. It also prevents undesirable effects from the excessively cold nature of the other herbs. These five are the assistant herbs.

Fried gancao settles the middle-jiao and harmonizes the actions of the other herbs. It is the envoy herb.

Together these herbs constitute a formula that cools blood, stops bleeding, promotes diuresis and cures urethritis. The characteristic of its construction is to combine dissolution of static blood with stopping of bleeding, and augmentation of Yin with promotion of diuresis.

5 Comments

Xiaoji Yin Zi is a commonly used herbal formula for treating urethritis with hematuria. However, the causes of urethritis with hematuria are many. The key indication for this formula is urethritis caused by blood stasis and Heat in the lower-jiao. Therefore, the primary action is to clear Heat from the lower-jiao, complemented by promotion of diuresis and stopping of bleeding. It is not appropriate for chronic urethritis due to deficiency of genuine Qi.

6 *Case Study: Acute Glomerulonephritis in a 13-Year-Old Male*

Following exposure to other ill persons, the patient developed fever and sore throat. Half a month later, he developed edema over the face and lower limbs. He had dizziness, difficulty with urination, scant yellow urine, thirst and restlessness. There were sores at the corners of the mouth. His throat was red and swollen. The tongue tip was red and had scant coating.

His pulse was floating and rapid. The blood pressure was 120/90 mmHg. Urinalysis showed 3+ protein and 1+ red blood cells and casts.

Diagnosis: Heat accumulation in the lower-jiao.

Therapeutic Principle: Purge Heat and stop bleeding.

Treatment: Xiaoji Yin Zi, with subtractions and additions, was prescribed. The composition was as follows: xiaoji 15 g, shengdihuang 10 g, oujie 15 g, puhuang 10 g, mutong 6 g, danzhuye 10 g, huashi 12 g, danggui 10 g, zhizi 10 g, gouteng (*Uncaria*) 20 g, and xiakucao (*Prunella*) 20 g. The herbs were decocted in water.

After six doses, the edema resolved, the urine volume increased and its color became lighter. The urine also cleared of protein, though it still had 0–3 white blood cells. The blood pressure was lowered to 90/60 mmHg. The same prescription was administered for three more doses, and all symptoms resolved.

(Source: *Journal of the New Chinese Medicine*, 1982, 9:46.)

VII Section Summary

The six herbal formulas chosen for this section are divided by function into two groups: those that facilitate blood circulation and release stasis (all except for Xiaoji Yin Zi), and those that stop bleeding (Xiaoji Yin Zi).

Tao He Cheng Qi Tang, Xue Fu Zhu Yu Tang, Bu Yang Huan Wu Tang, Wen Jing Tang and Sheng Hua Tang are representative of those that facilitate blood circulation and release stasis. Their main application is in illnesses of blood stasis.

The main action of **Taohe Cheng Qi Tang** is to break up blood stasis by purging Heat and stasis. It is mainly used for illnesses of blood and Heat gelling together causing blood stasis in the lower-jiao. **Xue Fu Zhu Yu Tang** is mainly indicated for illnesses with chest and subcostal pain caused by stasis of blood and impedance of Qi in the chest. **Bu Yang Huan Wu Tang** is designed to augment Qi and remove stasis. It is mainly used to treat hemiplegia caused by deficiency of Qi and stasis of blood, which lead to blockage of meridians and channels.

Wen Jing Tang and Sheng Hua Tang are both commonly used formulas in gynecological illnesses. **Wen Jing Tang** warms the meridians, dispels Cold, nourishes both Qi and blood, and releases stasis. Its primary indication is the disturbance of menses caused by deficiency-Cold in the Chong and Ren Meridians and blood stasis causing internal blockage. **Sheng Hua Tang** facilitates blood circulation, releases stasis, warms meridians and stops pain. Its main application is for the treatment of persistent postpartum lochia, pelvic pain and Cold in depleted blood, with emphasis on releasing stasis and generating new blood. Sheng Hua Tang is a commonly used formula following childbirth.

Xiaoji Yin Zi is a commonly used formula for stopping bleeding. Its main action is to stop bleeding, clear the bladder and promote diuresis. Its main application is for treating urinary track irritation or inflammation, e.g., urethritis with hematuria.

Section 12 Formulas That Eliminate Dampness

All herbal formulas that are designed to disperse fluids and dissolve Dampness, thereby promoting diuresis and removing impurities, are included in the category of Formulas that Eliminate Dampness. They are intended for treating illnesses of fluid excess and Dampness accumulation. Among the Eight Methods, they fall in the category of the Method of Dissipation.

As a cause of illness, the Dampness evil can be separated into external Dampness and internal Dampness. In its location of injury Dampness can be grouped in three opposing pairs: exterior versus interior, superficial versus deep, and upper versus lower body. In the progression of Dampness illnesses there are the two categories of Cold–Dampness and Heat–Dampness.

Thus, in clinical application there are accordingly many different approaches. In general, Dampness in the exterior can be treated by dispersal. Deep Dampness in the lower body can be dried and eliminated by aromatic and bitter herbs, or by sweet and bland herbs. Dampness that accumulates and causes blockage can be expelled by catharsis. Dampness transformed from Cold can be dispelled by warming Yang and drying Dampness. Dampness transformed from Heat can be dispelled by cooling Heat. Florid Dampness in a patient with a weak constitution is managed by combining the drying of Dampness with support for genuine Qi.

Dampness is a Yin-type of pathogenic evil. Its nature is heavy, impure and viscous. It easily blocks the activities and movement of Qi in the various organs. Impedance of Qi movement in turn impairs the dispersal of Dampness. Hence, formulas that eliminate Dampness generally contain herbs that regulate Qi in order to dissipate Dampness through facilitation of Qi movement.

Formulas that eliminate Dampness are mostly constructed from herbs that are aromatic, warm and dry, or herbs that are sweet and bland and that promote diuresis. These herbs can easily deplete Yin-fluids. It is important to exercise great caution in their use when treating patients who have chronic Yin or fluid deficiency, who are still weakened following illness, or women who are pregnant.

I Ping Wei San (Stomach-Settling Powder)

1 Source: Tai Ping Hui Min He Ji Ju Fang (Prescriptions from the Taiping Benevolent Pharmaceutical Bureau)

2 Composition

Chief Herb: cangzhu (*Atractylodes lancea*) 15 g

Deputy Herb: houpo (*Magnolia officinalis*) 9 g

Assistant Herb: chenpi (*Citrus tangerina*, *reticulata*) 9 g

Envoy Herbs: fried gancao (*Glycyrrhiza uralensis*) 6 g
shengjiang (*Zingiber officinale*) 3 pieces
dazao (*Ziziphus jujuba*) 2 pieces

3 Application

Actions: dries Dampness, stimulates the spleen, facilitates Qi movement and settles the stomach.

Indications: Dampness lodged in the spleen and the stomach.

Main Symptoms: epigastric and abdominal fullness or distention, with loss of appetite, nausea and vomiting, belching or acid regurgitation. A heavy sensation in the limbs; lassitude with a desire to lie down; loose feces or diarrhea; a white, greasy and thick tongue coating; and a slow pulse.

4 Analysis of the Formula

Pin Wei San uses cangzhu for chief herb. Cangzhu is particularly efficacious at drying Dampness and at strengthening the spleen, so that Dampness can be dissipated and the spleen can function with vigor.

Accumulation of Dampness impedes Qi movement, and impedance of Qi movement in turn aggravates Dampness accumulation. Houpo is included as deputy herb to facilitate Qi movement and dissipate accumulations. Its aromatic and drying nature and its bitter flavor enable it to eliminate Dampness as well.

The chief and deputy herbs are assisted by chenpi, which regulates Qi and settles the stomach. Its aromaticity enables it to strengthen the spleen and enhance the actions of cangzhu and houpo.

Fried gancao is sweet and gentle, and it regulates the middle-jiao. It is included to harmonize the actions of the other herbs. Shengjiang and dazao are added to enhance the harmonizing of the spleen and the stomach.

The herbs together are particularly effective in drying Dampness and enhancing the functions of the spleen. They also facilitate Qi movement and dissipate accumulations, so that Dampness and impurities can be eliminated, Qi can function properly, spleen-Qi can circulate without impedance, and the stomach settled. In this manner all symptoms can resolve.

5 Comments

Ping Wei San is the basic formula for treating spleen and stomach dysfunction caused by accumulated Dampness. The key symptoms are epigastric fullness or distention and a thick and greasy tongue coating. Since the formula is designed to dry Dampness, it is not appropriate to use in Yin deficiency, Qi stagnation and weak spleen and stomach.

II Huoxiang Zheng Qi San (Hyssop Qi-Regulating Powder)

1 Source: Tai Ping Hui Min He Ji Ju Fang (Prescriptions from the Taiping Benevolent Pharmaceutical Bureau)

2 Composition

Chief Herb: huoxiang (*Agastache rugosa*) 15 g

Deputy Herbs: zisu leaf (*Perilla frutescens*) 5 g
baizhi (*Angelica dahurica, anomala, taiwaniana*) 5 g
processed banxia (*Pinellia ternata*) 10 g
chenpi (*Citrus tangerina, reticulata*) 10 g
baizhu (*Atractylodes macrocephala*) 10 g
fuling (*Poria cocos*) 5 g

Assistant Herbs: houpo (*Magnolia officinalis*) 10 g
dafupi (*Areca catechu*) 5 g
jiegeng (*Platycodon grandiflorum*) 10 g

Envoy Herbs: shengjiang (*Zingiber officinale*) 1 slice
fried gancao (*Glycyrrhiza uralensis*) 12 g
dazao (*Ziziphus jujuba*) 3 pieces

3 Application

Actions: releases the exterior, dries Dampness, regulates Qi and harmonizes the middle-jiao.

Indications: invasion by exogenous Wind and Cold causing internal injury and accumulation of Dampness.

Main Symptoms: vomiting and diarrhea; chills and fever; headache; fullness and pain in the epigastrium and the abdomen; and a white and greasy tongue coating.

4 Analysis of the Formula

Huoxiang is used as chief herb for its ability to release the exterior of Wind–Cold and disperse Dampness. It can also ward off impurities and harmonize the middle-jiao, as well as raise the pure and suppress the impure.

There are three groups of deputy herbs. Zisu leaf and baizhi are acrid and aromatic. They aid huoxiang to vent Wind and Cold from the exterior. Their aromaticity also helps to disperse Dampness and eliminate impurities. Banxia leaven and chenpi dry Dampness and settle the stomach, suppress abnormally rising Qi and stop vomiting. Baizhu and fuling strengthen the spleen, mobilize accumulated Dampness, moderate the middle-jiao and stop diarrhea.

Houpo and dafupi facilitate Qi movement and disperse Dampness. Jiegeng facilitates lung-Qi and stimulates the diaphragm. It enhances the other herbs' ability to release the exterior and to dissolve Dampness. These three serve as assistant herbs.

Shengjiang, fried gancao and dazao all harmonize the Nutritive and the Defensive Levels, and coordinate the actions of the other herbs.

With these herbs working in concert, the formula is able to release both the exterior and the interior, disperse Dampness and eliminate impurities, regulate Qi and harmonize the middle-jiao. These actions bring about the venting of Wind and Cold and the dissipation of internal Dampness, so that Qi can circulate freely and the spleen and stomach function normally.

5 Comments

Although Huoxiang Zheng Qi San can expel Wind–Cold from the exterior, its main action is to eliminate Dampness and normalize the stomach. The key symptoms for its use are chills and fever, vomiting and diarrhea, and a white tongue coating. It is most suitable for treating illnesses of Cold and Dampness in summer, with dysfunction of the spleen and the stomach.

6 *Clinical Study: Acute Gastroenteritis*

In a comparative study of ordinary acute gastroenteritis without complication, 30 patients were treated with Huoxiang Zheng Qi San and 30 patients with Western formulas (sulfa formulas, calcium carbonate, belladonna formulas).

The patients had diarrhea 4–8 times a day. The diarrhea was often accompanied by borborygmus. Most of them also had mild abdominal distention, pri-umbilical pain and slight tenderness on pressure. There was no tenesmus. Seven hand mild fever up to 38°C (100.4°F). The feces were gruel-like or watery, light yellow in color and foamy, and mucoid without pus or blood.

Results: Using the number of days required for the symptoms to subside and for cure, Huoxiang Zheng Qi San was clearly more effective than the western formulas.

(Source: *Guangdong Journal of Chinese Medicine*, 1960, 9:442.)

III Ba Zheng San (Eight-Herb Rectification Powder)

1 *Source: Tai Ping Hui Min He Ji Ju Fang (Prescriptions from the Taiping Benevolent Pharmaceutical Bureau)*

2 *Composition*

Chief Herbs: qumai (*Dianthus superbus*) 9 g
bianxu (*Polygonum aviculare*) 9 g

Deputy Herbs: zhizi (*Gardenia jasminoides*) 9 g
dahuang (*Rheum palmatum*) 9 g
mutong (*Akebia quinata, trifoliata*) 9 g
Assistant Herbs: huashi (talcum) 9 g
cheqianzi (*Plantago asiatica*) 9 g

Envoy Herb: gancao (*Glycyrrhiza uralensis*) 9 g

3 *Application*

Actions: clears Heat, purges Fire, promotes diuresis and cures urethritis.

Indications: urethritis due to Dampness–Heat in the lower-jiao.

Main Symptoms: polyuria and urinary urgency; urethral dysuria; dribbling of urine; cloudy and red urine. In severe cases: inability to urinate with suprapubic abdominal distention. In addition: a dry mouth and throat, a yellow and greasy tongue coating; and a slippery and rapid pulse.

4 Analysis of the Formula

Ba Zheng San gathers together five herbs – mutong, huashi, cheqianzi, qumai, and bianxu – that promote diuresis, cure urethritis, clear Heat and dissipate Dampness. To complement them, zhizi, dahuang and gancao are included: zhizi purges Dampness–Heat from the sanjiao; dahuang drains Heat and suppresses Fire; and gancao harmonizes the actions of the other herbs and relieves urethral pain. A small amount of dengxincao (*Juncus effusus*) may be added to conduct Heat downward.

These herbs in concert have the ability to clear Heat, purge Fire, promote diuresis and cure urethritis.

5 Comments

The illnesses this formula is designed to treat are those in which Dampness and Heat attack the lower body. When Dampness and Heat lodge in the urinary bladder they impair the channels, so that urinary flow becomes impeded and urination painful, sometimes even completely blocked. Hence, the formula uses herbs that clear Heat and promote diuresis to expel the pathogenic evils downward in the urine. It also uses herbs that induce catharsis to expel the Heat evil in the feces. In this way, Dampness and Heat are eliminated in both the urine and the feces, and all symptoms can resolve.

6 Clinical Study: Pyelonephritis (Inflammation of the Kidney Pelvis)

Sixty-seven patients with acute pyelonephritis, caused by accumulated Dampness–Heat, were studied. The patients were treated with Ba Zheng San, with the addition of huanglian (*Coptis*), huangbai (*Phellodendron*) and other herbs as needed for additional symptoms.

Results: Fifty-four patients recovered completely, with resolution of all symptoms and abnormalities in urinalysis and two urine cultures. Five patients showed resolution of symptoms, but the urine culture still showed some bacterial growth. Eight patients showed no response.

(Source: *Liaoning Journal of Chinese Medicine*, 1986, 1:19.)

IV San Ren Tang (Three-Seeds Decoction)

1 Source: Wen Bing Tiao Bian (Analysis of Febrile Illnesses)

2 Composition

Chief Herbs: xingren (*Prunus armeniaca*) 12 g
doukou (*Amomum kravanh*) 6 g
yiyiren (*Coix lacrhyma-jobi*) 18 g

Deputy Herbs: huashi (talcum) 18 g
tongcao (*Tetrapanax papyriferus*) 6 g
danzhuye (*Lophaterum gracile*) 6 g

Assistant Herbs: processed banxia (*Pinellia ternata*) 10 g
houpo (*Magnolia officinalis*) 6 g

3 Application

Actions: promotes and facilitates Qi activities and dispels Dampness–Heat.

Indications: (1) Initial stages of Dampness–Heat illnesses. (2) Dampness complicating Summer Heat.

Main Symptoms: headache and chills; heaviness and pain in the body; a yellow complexion; tightness in the chest; loss of appetite; afternoon fever; absence of thirst; a white tongue coating; and a taut, threadlike and soft pulse.

4 Analysis of the Formula

Three herbs are used as chiefs. Xingren facilitates the activities of lung-Qi in the upper-jiao. As Qi moves, Dampness may be dispersed. Doukou is an aromatic herb that eliminates Dampness and promotes Qi circulation centrally. It normalizes spleen and stomach-Qi in the middle-jiao. Yiyiren, which is sweet-bland and cold, disperses Dampness, clears Heat and strengthens the spleen. It can open the channels in the lower-jiao, and makes possible the elimination of Dampness and Heat in the urine.

Three herbs are used as deputies. Huashi dissipates Dampness–Heat and relieves Summer Heat. Tongcao and danzhuye enhance the dispersal of Dampness and Heat.

The assistant herbs banxia and houpo are acrid–bitter and warm. They promote Qi circulation and disperse Dampness, so that accumulations can be dissipated. In addition, they prevent the herbs with cold nature from interfering with the elimination of Dampness.

These herbs acting in concert clear Dampness and Heat from the sanjiao. All symptoms then resolve.

5 Comments

In the initial stages of Dampness–Heat illnesses, the pathogenic evils are still at the Qi Level. The situation is one of Dampness being silent and Heat being hidden. If only acrid–bitter, warming and drying herbs are used to dissipate Dampness, then Heat can blaze. Or, if only bitter and cold herbs are used to clear Heat, then Dampness still remains. The most appropriate treatment is a formula that is aromatic and acrid–bitter and that promotes the circulation and activities of Qi. This unclogs the sanjiao and eliminates both Dampness and Heat. This approach is particularly suitable in conditions in which Dampness is more severe than Heat.

6 Case Study: Illness of Dampness–Heat in a 35-Year-Old Male

The patient suffered from fever, worst in the afternoon and often accompanied by sweating. He felt tired and weak, and had tightness in his chest. He was restless and slept very little. Though thirsty he did not desire to drink. His tongue was red, with a yellow and greasy coating; and his pulse was slippery and rapid.

Diagnosis: Intermixed Dampness and Heat causing loss of normal functions.

Therapeutic Principle: Dissipate Dampness with aromatic herbs and simultaneously clear Heat.

Treatment: San Ren Tang was prescribed with modifications as follows: xingren 12 g, doukou 10 g, yiyiren 15 g, huashi 30 g, processed banxia 12 g, danzhuye 15 g, xiangru (*Mosla chinensis*) 10 g, yinchaihu (*Stellaria dichotoma*) 12 g, lianqiao (*Forsythia*) 20 g, cheqiancao (*Plantago*) 20 g and chenpi (*Citrus tangerina*) 12 g. After six doses the patient recovered completely.

(Source: *Central China Journal of Medicine*, 1983, 5:23.)

V Zhen Wu Tang (True Warrior Decoction)

1 Source: Shang Han Lun (Treatise on Cold-Attack)

2 Composition

Chief Herb: processed fuzi (*Aconitum carmichaeli*) 9 g

Deputy Herbs: fuling (*Poria cocos*) 9 g
baizhu (*Atractylodes macrocephala*) 6 g

Assistant Herbs: shengjiang (*Zingiber officinale*) 9 g
baishaoyao (*Paeonia lactiflora*) 9 g

3 Application

Actions: warms Yang and promotes diuresis.

Indications: deficiency of spleen and kidney Yang, with internal stagnation of fluids.

Main Symptoms: difficulty with urination; heaviness and pain in the limbs; abdominal pain and diarrhea; or, edema of the limbs. A white tongue coating; absence of thirst; and a deep pulse.

4 Analysis of the Formula

For chief herb Zhen Wu Tang uses fuzi. Fuzi is very acrid and very hot, and it warms the kidney and supports its Yang, mobilizes Qi and fluids and promotes diuresis. It also warms the spleen (Earth Element) to eliminate Dampness (Water Element).

For deputy herbs, it uses fuling and baizhu to strengthen the spleen and to disperse Dampness. Doing so promotes diuresis and allows the excess water to leave as urine.

For assistant herb it uses shengjiang for its warmth and its ability to disperse. Shengjiang not only aids fuzi in supporting Yang and dispelling Cold, but also assists fuling and baizhu in dispersing Dampness. The formula also uses baishaoyao for assistant herb, on the one hand for its ability to mobilize fluids and facilitate urination and on the other for its ability to soften the liver and stop abdominal pain.

These five herbs act in concert to warm the spleen and the kidney, and mobilize water from Dampness, thereby supporting Yang and promoting diuresis.

5 Comments

The kidney is the organ of water. It governs the movement of Qi and facilitates diuresis. If kidney-Yang is deficient then Qi cannot move water. This leads to the formation of internal Dampness, which then infiltrates the entire body to cause illness. Such an illness is the consequence of deficiency-Cold attacking the lower-jiao. Zhen Wu Tang acts primarily to support kidney-Yang, but also to strengthen the spleen and promote water movement, so that Dampness can be dissipated and dispersed and all symptoms can resolve.

6 Case Study: Edema in a 59-Year-Old Male

The patient first noted pitting edema on his face and in the lower extremities, but only in the afternoon. The edema progressed, however, and became generalized, affecting the entire body except his chest, abdomen and palms. His urine became scant in volume. He had no appetite. Though thirsty he did not drink. He was somnolent and his body felt cold despite bundling up. His complexion was gray and lusterless. His tongue coating was black but smooth and moist, and his tongue was bright red. His pulse was large, floating but rootless.

Diagnosis: Deficiency of vital Yang, so that the Earth Element (spleen) is unable to restrain the Water Element (kidney).

Therapeutic Principle: Support Yang and disperse the water of Dampness.

Treatment: Modified Zhen Wu Tang was prescribed, with the following composition: processed fuzi 60 g, baizhu 24 g, fuling 24 g, dangshen (*Codonopsis*) 60 g, rougui (*Cinnamomum*) 6 g, fried gancao (*Glycyrrhiza*) 24 g, and shengjiang 30 g. The herbs were cooked 3 times. The decoction from the first cooking was taken promptly. The decoction from the second and third cooking was combined and taken in portions throughout the day but consumed on the same day.

Following three successive doses, the edema was reduced by 60–70%, the tongue coating was no longer black, and the pulse was no longer floating but deep. These changes indicated that deficiency-Fire was dying and vital Yang was reviving. The formula was further modified, by cutting the amounts of fuzi, dangshen, rougui and shengjiang in half. After four successive doses the patient recovered completely.

(Source: *Journal of Chinese Medicine*, 1965, 7: 39.)

Note: Precessed fuzi was prescribed with dosage of 60 g which is not the common dosage in clinical prescription.

VI Section Summary

Both Ping Wei San and Huo Xiang Zheng Qi San are representative of herbal formulas that dry Dampness and settle the stomach. However, **Ping Wei San** focuses on drying Dampness and mobilizing Qi. It is the principal formula for treating Dampness clogging the spleen and the stomach, with the key symptoms of distention of the epigastrium and abdomen and a thick and greasy tongue coating. **Huoxiang Zheng Qi San**, on the other hand, focuses on dispersing Wind and Cold from the exterior and dispersing Dampness from the interior. It is a commonly used formula for treating gastroenteritis, with the key symptoms of chills and fever, headache, distention of the epigastrium and abdomen, vomiting and diarrhea.

San Ren Tang is representative of herbal formulas that clear Heat and dissipate Dampness. Its Dampness-dissipating action is stronger than its Heat-clearing action. It is suitable in the early stages of illnesses of Dampness–Heat, when the pathogenic evils are still at the Qi Level. The key symptoms are cold-intolerance, headache, heaviness and pain in the body, chest tightness, anorexia, absence of thirst and a white tongue coating.

The primary application of **Ba Zheng San** is to clear Heat, promote water circulation and relieve urinary irritation or inflammation. It is primarily indicated for treating urethritis caused by Dampness and Heat in the lower-jiao.

Zhen Wu Tang is representative of formulas that support spleen and kidney Yang and mobilize the water of Dampness. Its main actions are to warm the spleen and the kidney and to help Yang move fluids. It is a commonly used formula for treating edema caused by Yang deficiency.

Section 13 Formulas That Dissipate Phlegm

Formulas for dissipating Phlegm are constructed around herbs that eliminate accumulated Phlegm, and are indicated for various Phlegm illnesses. The causes of Phlegm are manifold, and the strategies for treating Phlegm correspondingly vary with the nature of its cause. According to the actions, the Phlegm-eliminating formulas can be classified in five types: formulas for drying Dampness and eliminating Phlegm, formulas for clearing Heat and eliminating Phlegm, formulas for moistening Dryness and eliminating Phlegm, formulas for warming and eliminating Cold–Phlegm and formulas for dispelling Wind and eliminating Phlegm.

Phlegm results from the accumulation of Dampness, and the spleen is the organ that generates Phlegm. Herbs that strengthen the spleen and eliminate Dampness are usually used together in prescriptions for expelling Phlegm. Furthermore, because Phlegm can easily block Qi movement and Qi blockage in turn often causes the accumulation of Phlegm, formulas for expelling Phlegm generally also include herbs that can regulate Qi circulation. In illnesses in which Phlegm affects the channels and sinews, methods for softening masses and dispersing accumulations are generally used in combination with those that address the concomitant deficiency or strength and Cold or Heat.

In the clinical application of Phlegm-eliminating formulas, the physician must first identify the nature of the Phlegm, that is, whether it is associated with Cold or

Heat, Dryness or Dampness. At the same time, pay close attention to the illness to ascertain what is appearance and what is root, as well as the degree of urgency.

I Er Chen Tang (Two Aged-Herbs Decoction)

1 Source: Cheng Fang Qie Yong (Applications of Established Formulas)

2 Composition

Chief Herb: processed banxia (*Pinellia ternata*) 15 g

Deputy Herbs: chenpi (*Citrus tangerina, reticulata*) 15 g
fuling (*Poria cocos*) 9 g

Assistant Herbs: shengjiang (*Zingiber officinale*) 7 pieces
wumei (*Prunus mume*) 1 piece

Envoy Herb: fried gancao (*Glycyrrhiza uralensis*) 4.5 g

3 Application

Actions: dries Dampness, dissipates Phlegm, regulates Qi and harmonizes the middle-jiao.

Indications: cough due to accumulation of Dampness–Phlegm.

Main Symptoms: copious sputum that is clear and easily brought up; tightness in the chest and diaphragm; nausea and vomiting; fatigue with limb weakness, or dizziness and palpitation; a white and greasy or white and moist tongue coating; and a slow and slippery pulse.

4 Analysis of the Formula

Er Chen Tang uses processed aged banxia as chief herb in order to dry Dampness, eliminate Phlegm, regulate the stomach and suppress abnormally ascending Qi. It uses chenpi as deputy herb in order to regulate Qi, relieve the middle-jiao, dry Dampness and dissipate Phlegm. The choice of this combination is based on the approach of treating Phlegm by regulating Qi, since Phlegm will spontaneously dissipate when Qi circulates smoothly.

Since Phlegm comes from Dampness and Dampness from the spleen, the formula also uses fuling as deputy herb in order to invigorate the spleen and eliminate Dampness. When the spleen is strengthened and Dampness is eliminated, there will no longer be a source for Phlegm.

Of the assistant herbs, shengjiang reinforces the actions of aged banxia to control nausea and dispel Dampness, and wumei counterbalances the dispersing tendencies of banxia, thereby preventing the dissipation of lung-Qi.

Fried gancao serves as envoy herb to harmonize the effects of the other herbs and to strengthen the spleen.

5 Comments

Er Chen Tang is the principal formula for eliminating Phlegm. It is widely used in treating all types of illnesses involving Phlegm. In clinical application, however, modifications are frequently made with it as foundation.

For example, for illnesses of Wind–Phlegm add tiannanxing (*Arisaema consanguineum, erubescens*), baifuzi (*Typhonium giganteum*), zaojia (*Gleditsia sinensis*) and zhuli (*Phyllostachys nigra*) to expel Wind and dissolve Phlegm.

For Fire–Phlegm illnesses add shigao (gypsum) and qingdai (*Baphicacanthus cusia*) to eliminate Heat and Phlegm.

For Dampness–Phlegm add cangzhu (*Atractylodes lancea*) and baizhu (*Atractylodes macrocephala*) to dry Dampness and eliminate Phlegm.

For Dryness-Phlegm add gualou (*Trichosanthes*) and xingren (*Prunus armeniaca*) to moisten the lung and eliminate Phlegm.

For Phlegm-induced indigestion add shanzha (*Crataegus*), maiya (Hordeum) and shenqu (medicated leaven) to promote digestion and eliminate Phlegm.

6 Case Study: Teeth Grinding in a 25-Year-Old Male

Every night upon falling asleep the patient ground his teeth together. The grinding was so loud that it could be heard outside the room and it often woke his roommates. On examination, he was found to be obese, with a shiny and light complexion.

Diagnosis: Phlegm accumulation in the middle-jiao. (Note: the Stomach Meridian of Foot-Yangming passes through the teeth. Blockage of this meridian by Phlegm impedes Qi circulation and sometimes leads to unconscious teeth grinding.)

Therapeutic Principle: Eliminate Phlegm.

Treatment: Er Chen Tang was augmented with charred heye (*Nelumbo nucifera*) to dry Dampness and eliminate Phlegm. After five doses, the frequency and the loudness of the teeth grinding diminished. The patient was instructed to take several doses more in order to consolidate the therapeutic gains.

(Source: *Case Records of Dr. Yue Meizhong*.)

7 *Case Study: Night Cough in an Adult Male*

The patient suffered from cough with sputum and chest tightness for more than 3 months. The symptoms were mild during the day but severe during the night. His tongue coating was white and thin, and his pulse was taut and slippery.

Diagnosis: Dampness–Phlegm in the lung.

Treatment: The patient was treated with Er Chen Tang augmented with danggui (*Angelica*). The symptoms were much alleviated after five doses. The basic Er Chen Tang was continued for five more doses, resulting in complete cure.

(Source: *Zhejiang Journal of Chinese Medicine*, 1981, 1:36.)

II Wen Dan Tang (Gallbladder-Warming Decoction)

1 *Source: San Yin Ji Yi Bing Zheng Fang Lun (Treatise on the Three Categories of Pathogenic Factors of Illnesses)*

2 *Composition*

Chief Herb: processed banxia (*Pinellia ternata*) 6 g

Deputy Herb: zhuru (*Phyllostachys nigra*) 6 g

Assistant Herbs: zhishi (*Citrus aurantium*) 6 g
chenpi (*Citrus tangerina, reticulata*) 9 g
fuling (*Poria cocos*) 45 g

Envoy Herbs: shengjiang (*Zingiber officinale*) 5 pieces
dazao (*Ziziphus jujuba*) 1 pieces
fried gancao (*Glycyrrhiza uralensis*) 3 g

3 *Application*

Actions: regulates Qi, dissipates Phlegm, clears the gallbladder and harmonizes the stomach.

Indications: Phlegm–Heat disturbing the interior causing disharmony between the gallbladder and the stomach.

Main Symptoms: fearfulness; restlessness; insomnia with much dreaming; nausea and vomiting; hiccup; and epilepsy.

4 Analysis of the Formula

The main action of Wen Dan Tang is to purge Heat from the gallbladder and to regulate stomach-Qi. It is mainly used in disharmony of the gallbladder and stomach, with disturbance of the interior caused by Phlegm–Heat.

Processed banxia is selected to be chief herb to dry Dampness, eliminate Phlegm, suppress abnormally ascending Qi and harmonize the stomach. Zhuru is selected to be deputy herb to clear Heat from the gallbladder and stomach, and relieve vomiting and restlessness. Together these two herbs act to clear Heat from the gallbladder, settle the stomach and eliminate Phlegm.

Zhishi and chenpi are added to assist in Qi regulation. When Qi can course through the meridians freely, Phlegm dissipates spontaneously. Fuling is included as assistant herb to strengthen spleen function and cut off Phlegm at the source.

Shengjiang, dazao and gancao are added as envoy herbs to further strengthen the spleen and the stomach and to harmonize the actions of the other herbs.

The herbs acting in concert achieve the effect of purging Heat from the gallbladder, harmonizing the stomach, regulating Qi circulation and eliminating Phlegm. Doing so brings about spontaneous resolution of the restlessness and fearfulness, nausea and vomiting, hiccup, and insomnia.

5 Comments

Wen Dan Tang is basically Er Chen Tang with zhuru and zhishi added, and is therefore not merely a formula for drying Dampness and eliminating Phlegm. Zhuru is sweet and cold, and is efficacious in purging Heat, relieving restlessness and stopping vomiting. It is unsurpassed by other herbs in its ability to purge Heat from the gallbladder. Consequently, Wen Dan Tang is particularly useful for purging Heat from the gallbladder and the stomach and for eliminating Phlegm.

In clinical application, Wen Dan Tang is indicated in illnesses in which the following symptoms are prominent: a bitter taste in the mouth, a tongue coating that is greasy and yellow, and a pulse that is taut and slippery or rapid.

6 Case Study: Dizziness in a 56-Year-Old Male

For over a month the patient suffered from periodic dizziness, accompanied by nausea, vomiting, tinnitus, and vertigo with loss of balance. Symptoms were alleviated on lying down with the eyes closed. Another hospital diagnosed this as "Meniere's syndrome." He was treated in hospital for 20 days, without improvement.

On examination, his pulse was found to be taut and slippery. His tongue was pink and was covered by a greasy coating that was white in parts and yellow in parts.

Diagnosis: Phlegm–Rheum disturbing the orifices.

Therapeutic Principle: Dissipate Phlegm–Rheum and stop vomiting.

Treatment: Wen Dan Tang was prescribed, but with modification in amounts, as follows: banxia 12 g, chenpi 6 g, fuling 10 g, fried gancao 6 g, zhishi 10 g, zhuru 10 g, and shengjiang 3 slices. After one dose, the frequency of attacks was reduced to only once a day, lasting about 20 min. Following four doses, all symptoms resolved and his mental status improved. Three more doses were prescribed to consolidate the therapeutic gains.

III Banxia Baizhu Tianma Tang (Pinellia-Atractylodes-Gastrodia Decoction)

1 Source: Yi Xue Xin Wu (Insights from Medical Studies)

2 Composition

Chief Herb: processed banxia (*Pinellia ternata*) 9 g

Deputy Herbs: baizhu (*Atractylodes macrocephala*) 15 g
tianma (*Gastrodia elata*) 6 g

Assistant Herbs: fuling (*Poria cocos*) 6 g
juhong (*Citrus tangerina*, *reticulata*) 6 g

Envoy Herb: fried gancao (*Glycyrrhiza uralensis*) 3 g

3 Application

Actions: dries Dampness, dissipates Phlegm, pacifies the liver and extinguishes Wind.

Indications: illnesses of Wind–Phlegm causing upward disturbance.

Main Symptoms: vertigo; nausea and vomiting; headache; tightness in the chest; a white and greasy tongue coating; and a taut and slippery pulse.

4 Analysis of the Formula

Banxia Baizhu Tianma Tang uses processed banxia as chief herb. It dries Dampness, eliminates Phlegm, lowers abnormally rising stomach-Qi and stops vomiting.

It uses tianma and baizhu as deputy herbs. Tianma is particularly efficacious in normalizing the liver and extinguishing Wind, thereby relieving headaches. In combination with processed banxia it is an essential herb for treating illnesses caused by Wind–Phlegm. Used together, baizhu, banxia and tianma are even more active in eliminating Dampness and Phlegm, and in relieving dizziness.

When fuling, which strengthens the spleen and eliminates Dampness, is used with baizhu, they are highly efficacious for removing the source of Phlegm. Juhong regulates Qi circulation and dissipates Phlegm, helping Qi flow smoothly and clearing sputum.

For envoy herbs the formula uses three herbs. Shengjiang and dazao harmonize the spleen and the stomach and assist the chief herb in drying Dampness. Gancao is added for its ability to harmonize centrally and to coordinate the effects of the other herbs.

With these herbs acting in concert the formula is very effective in eliminating Phlegm and extinguishing Wind.

5 *Comments*

The aim of Banxia Baizhu Tianma Tang is to treat dizziness due to upward attack by Wind–Phlegm. Dizziness can result from many causes, such as accumulation of Dampness in the middle-jiao or lower-jiao. The dizziness under consideration is due principally to the internal stirring of liver-Wind in the presence of Phlegm and Dampness accumulation. Such dizziness is more marked, and is often accompanied by vomiting. It is important in clinical practice to differentiate these causes carefully.

This formula is derived from Er Chen Tang by the addition of baizhu and tianma. The method is to combine the actions of strengthening the spleen, dissipating Phlegm and extinguishing Wind. The combined method eliminates Phlegm–Dampness and induces the spleen, which belongs to the Earth element, to function smoothly. Achieving these results will extinguish liver-Wind and resolve headache.

In clinical application, the key symptoms calling for this formula are dizziness or heaviness of the head, headache, vomiting, and a white and greasy tongue coating.

6 *Case Study: Meniere's Syndrome in a 70-Year-Old Female*

Ten days prior to consultation, the patient was exposed to Cold in winter, which resulted in dizziness and headache with vertigo. She was diagnosed to have Meniere's syndrome and was treated with a western medication, without effect.

She had dizziness, with severe vomiting of salivary fluid, palpitation, and shortness of breath with tightness in the chest. Her appetite was poor. She had a sticky and greasy sensation in the mouth, and numbness in the tip of her tongue. She changed clothing frequently. Her scant feces were thin and soft. Her body was huge and fat. The tongue coating was white and greasy. Her pulses were soft and feeble in all six positions.

Diagnosis: Accumulated Wind–Phlegm attacking upward, with chronic deficiency of central Qi.

Therapeutic Principle: Dry Dampness and dissipate Phlegm.

Treatment: The prescription was Banxia Baizhu Tianma Tang with modifications as follows: banxia 10 g, tianma 10 g, chenbi 10 g, baizhu 12 g, fuling 15 g, dangshen (*Codonopsis*) 15 g, shanzha (*Crataegus*) 15 g, wuzhuyu (*Evodia*) 6 g, shengjiang 6 g, and fried gancao 3 g. After three doses all symptoms improved. After three more doses she recovered completely.

(Source: *Journal of the Anhui School of Chinese Medicine*, 1985, 1:17.)

IV Mengshi Gun Tan Wan (Chlorite Phlegm-Expelling Pill)

1 Source: Dan Xi Xin Fa Fu Yu (Supplement to Danxi's Methods of Treatment)

2 Composition

Chief Herb: mengshi (chlorite schist) 3 g

Deputy Herb: dahuang (*Rheum palmatum*) 15 g

Assistant Herbs: huangqin (*Scutellaria baicalensis*) 15 g
chenxiang (*Aquilaria sinensis*, *agallocha*) 2 g

3 Application

Actions: purges Fire and eliminates Phlegm.

Indications: illnesses of accumulation of Heat and thick Phlegm.

Main Symptoms: The principal symptoms are: (1) madness, anxiety, palpitation, and fright; or, coma; or (2) cough and dyspnea with thick sputum; or, tightness in the chest and diaphragm; or (3) dizziness or vertigo, with tinnitus. Additional symptoms include constipation, a yellow and greasy tongue coating, and a slippery, rapid and forceful pulse.

4 Analysis of the Formula

In Mengshi Gun Tan Wan mengshi serves as chief herb to eliminate chronically accumulated Phlegm.

For deputy herb dahuang is selected for its bitter flavor and cold nature and for its ability to purge Heat and open a downward path (catharsis) for expelling Phlegm–Heat.

Huangqin has bitter flavor and cold nature. As assistant herb it focuses on clearing Heat from the upper-jiao.

Chenxiang is included to guide the abnormally risen Qi downward. This is also based on the principle of regulating Qi circulation in order to eliminate Phlegm.

When these four herbs are used in concert their action in purging Fire and expelling Phlegm is especially strong. They are thus able to eliminate Phlegm and other accumulated matters downward through the intestines. This formula is most appropriate for treating patients who are ill from the accumulation and gelling of Phlegm–Fire but otherwise have a stout and vigorous body.

5 Comments

The action of Mengshi Gun Tan Wan is aimed at purging Fire and eliminating accumulated Phlegm, and is indicated for treating illnesses due to strong Heat and chronic Phlegm causing malfunction of the liver, the lung, the stomach and the kidney.

In clinical application, pay close attention to the four keys: namely, strength, Heat, Phlegm and fright. Treatment revolves around the elimination of Phlegm. The formula is generally applicable to illnesses of exogenous Phlegm–Heat as well as abnormal functions of the visceral organs and abnormal circulation of Qi caused by endogenous Phlegm–Fire due to excesses of the Seven Passions.

6 Case Study: Asthma with Cough in a 45-Year-Old Male

The patient suffered from asthma with cough for years. He was treated with both Chinese and western medications, without improvement. In mid-summer the dyspnea and cough abruptly worsened, with resulting difficulty in breathing.

He now had a purplish complexion and bright red neck. He was short of breath with a gurgling noise from sputum, and was not able to lie down on his back. His sputum was thick and yellow, which could be expectorated only with difficulty. He moved his bowels only once in several days, producing very dry feces followed by much mucus; it had a foul odor. He was thirsty for cold drinks and was restless. His tongue was red, with a thick, yellow, greasing but dry coating. His pulse was taut, slippery and rapid.

Diagnosis: Strong exogenous Heat with Phlegm–Fire.

Therapeutic Principle: Clear Fire and eliminate accumulated Phlegm.

Treatment: The initial treatment was 50 g of Mengshi Gun Tan Wan taken with water. An hour later, there were sounds of water movement from the intestines. The patient went to the toilet several times. One piece of dry feces was released, followed by mucoid feces with an unbearable malodor. Simultaneously, the dyspnea and the gurgling of sputum improved. An additional 50 g of Mengshi Gun Tan Wan was prescribed, divided into two portions. Three days later, the patient was able to return to the office by himself. He reported that his symptoms were all much alleviated. He was then prescribed formulas for purging Heat, eliminating Phlegm, strengthening the spleen and regulating Qi circulation, to ensure complete recovery.

(Source: *Jiangxi Journal of Chinese Medicine*, 1984, 2:33.)

V Section Summary

Of the four formulas in this section, **Er Chen Tang** is the principal formula for eliminating Phlegm. It has the actions of drying Dampness, dissolving Phlegm, regulating Qi and harmonizing centrally. It is mainly indicated for treating illnesses of Dampness and Phlegm accumulating in the interior, with cough and copious sputum. **Wen Dan Tang** has the ability to regulate Qi and dissipate Phlegm, clear the gallbladder and settle the stomach. It is indicated for illnesses of disharmony between the gallbladder and the stomach, with Phlegm and Heat causing disturbance in the interior and manifesting restlessness, insomnia, vomiting, hiccup and fearfulness. **Banxia Baizhu Tianma Tang** is a fine formula for extinguishing Wind and eliminating Phlegm. It acts mainly to dry Dampness and dissipate Phlegm, normalize the liver and extinguish Wind. It is very effective in treating the headache, dizziness and other symptoms produced when Wind and Phlegm rise and cause disturbance upward. **Mengshi Gun Tan Wan** is designed to purge Heat and dissipate tenacious Phlegm. It is mainly used to treat chronic illnesses of Heat and persistent Phlegm.

Section 14 Formulas That Dispel Wind

Formulas for dispelling Wind are constructed around acrid herbs that dispel exogenous Wind or extinguish endogenous Wind and stop spasms. They are used to treat illnesses due to attack by the exogenous Wind evil or due to movement of endogenous liver-Wind.

Illnesses of Wind are of two types. One type is caused by attack by the exogenous Wind evil, which enters the exterior of the body, the meridians or the joints. For attacks mainly in the exterior, treatment is principally based on formulas that release the exterior. For attacks that have reached the meridians or joints, treatment is principally based on formulas that dispel Wind. The other type is caused by Wind that arises endogenously out of dysfunction of the visceral organs. This type of illnesses tends to be sudden and acute, and highly changeable. The most important source of endogenous Wind is the liver, and the main types are the stirring of liver-Wind and the upward attack by liver-Wind. Endogenous Wind illnesses comprise abnormally vigorous and rising liver-Yang, Wind movement in Yin deficiency, Wind movement in blood deficiency, and others.

In treatment, exogenous Wind should primarily be dispelled, whereas endogenous Wind should primarily be extinguished. Therefore, in clinical practice it is necessary first to determine whether a Wind illness is caused by exogenous or endogenous Wind. In addition, pay attention to factors that may be associated with the pathogenic evil and the weaknesses or vigor of the bodily functions.

In selecting which formulas to apply, bear in mind that the acrid and dispelling herbs used in Wind-dispelling formulas act to warm and dry, and thus can easily injure body fluids and contribute to the rise of Fire. Wind-dispelling formulas should be avoided, or used with great care, when there is insufficiency of fluids or deficiency of Yin, or excessively active Yang producing endogenous Heat.

I Xiao Feng San (Wind-Extinguishing Powder)

1 Source: Wai Ke Zheng Zong (Orthodox Exogenous Illnesses)

2 Composition

Chief Herbs: jingjie (*Schizonepeta tenuifolia*) 6 g
fangfeng (*Saposhnikovia divaricata*) 6 g
niubangzi (*Arctium lappa*) 6 g
chantui (*Cryptotympana atrata, pustulata*) 6 g

Deputy Herbs: cangzhu (*Atractylodes lancea*) 6 g
kushen (*Sophora flavescens*) 6 g
mutong (*Akebia quinata, trifoliata*) 3 g

Assistant Herbs: zhimu (*Anemarrhena asphodeloides*) 6 g
shigao (gypsum) 6 g
danggui (*Angelica sinensis*) 6 g
shengdihuang (*Rehmannia glutinosa*) 6 g
heizhima (*Sesamum indicum*) 6 g

Envoy Herb: gancao (*Glycyrrhiza uralensis*) 3 g

3 Application

Actions: disperses Wind, nourishes blood, clears Heat and eliminates Dampness.

Indications: urticaria and eczema.

Main Symptoms: itchy skin, reddish rashes or weepy skin lesions over large parts of the body; a yellow or white tongue coating; and a forceful, floating and rapid pulse.

4 Analysis of the Formula

Xiao Feng San uses four chief herbs: jingjie, fangfeng, niubangzi and chantui. These herbs dispel exogenous Wind from the exterior and unblock the interstices and pores, thereby achieving the goal of relieving the itch.

Three deputies complement the chiefs. Cangzhu disperses Wind and Dampness, and strengthens the spleen. Kushen purges Heat, dries Dampness, and promotes diuresis. Mutong purges Heat and promotes diuresis.

The Wind–Dampness and Wind–Heat evils can attack blood and the meridians, and easily exhaust Yin-blood. The herbs for dispelling Wind and promoting diuresis also easily exhaust Yin-blood. In such conditions endogenous Fire and Dryness can arise. Dryness is also induced by blood deficiency and often exacerbates the itch. For these reasons, shigao and zhimu are included to purge Heat and drain Fire. Danggui, shengdihuang and heizhima are included to nourish Yin, generate blood and moisten Dryness. They replenish the injured Yin and blood, and restrict the ability of the Wind-dispelling and diuresis-promoting herbs from injuring Yin and blood. These serve as assistant herbs.

Raw gancao clears Heat, detoxifies poison and harmonizes the effects of the other herbs. It is the envoy herb.

The formula as a whole is designed to have several actions. It disperses Wind–Heat and Wind–Dampness from the exterior. It purges Heat, dries Dampness and promotes diuresis, which actions eliminate Dampness and Heat by draining them downward. It generates blood and stimulates its circulation, nourishes Yin and moistens Dryness. Acting in concert the herbs in the formula achieve the goal of releasing the exterior and purifying the interior.

5 Comments

Xiao Feng San is composed principally of herbs that dispel Wind. These are complemented by herbs that clear Heat, eliminate Dampness and generate blood. It is highly suitable for treating urticaria and eczema, which result from Wind–Dampness or Wind–Heat invading the meridians and injuring Yin and blood. The formula includes herbs that generate blood, promote its circulation, nourish Yin and moisten Dryness. These herbs not only replenish the injured Yin and blood, but also restrains the tendency of Wind-expelling and Dampness-drying herbs to induce Dryness and injure the fluids. It employs the principle of "when treating Wind first treat blood, so that as blood circulates well Wind dies spontaneously."

6 Clinical Study: Eczema

Forty-four patients with eczema were treated with Xiao Feng San with appropriate modifications. For the five patients with more severe cases, wet compresses with fresh machixian (*Portulaca oleracea*) were applied in addition. Patients were prescribed this herb at the dosage of one dose per day. During treatment, all other anti-allergy drugs were discontinued. The shortest duration of treatment was 5 days and the longest 23 days, with an average of 20 days.

Results: Thirty-eight patients showed complete resolution of the skin lesions. Six showed essential resolution (subjective recovery, with only slight skin damage remaining). Of the 38 who had complete resolution 27 were followed for about a year. Twenty-six had an uneventful course, and only one had recurrence. During the course of treatment, a light and bland diet was emphasized, with avoidance of spicy and rich foods.

(Source: *Journal of New Medicine*, 1976, 8:15.)

II Duhuo Jisheng Tang (Pubescens and Loranthus Decoction)

1 Source: Bei Ji Qian Jin Yao Fang (Essential Prescriptions for Emergency)

2 Composition

Chief Herb: duhuo (*Angelica pubescens*) 9 g

Deputy Herbs: fangfeng (*Saposhnikovia divaricata*) 6 g
qinjiao (*Gentiana macrophylla, crassicaulis*) 6 g
rougui (*Cinnamomum cassia*) 6 g
xixin (*Asarum heterotropoides, sieboldi*) 6 g

Assistant Herbs: sangjisheng (*Loranthus parasiticus*) 6 g
niuxi (*Achyranthes bidentata*) 6 g
duzhong (*Eucommia ulmoides*) 6 g
danggui (*Angelica sinensis*) 6 g
baishaoyao (*Paeonia lactiflora*) 6 g
shengdihuang (*Rehmannia glutinosa*) 6 g
chuanxiong (*Ligusticum chuanxiong, wallichii*) 6 g
renshen (*Panax ginseng*) 6 g
fuling (*Poria cocos*) 6 g

Envoy Herb: gancao (*Glycyrrhiza uralensis*) 6 g

3 Application

Actions: expels Wind and Dampness; relieves the pain of rheumatism; strengthens the liver and the kidney; augments Qi and blood.

Indications: chronic rheumatism caused by insufficiency of the liver and the kidney, and deficiency of Qi and blood.

Main Symptoms: cold pain in the lower back and the knees; hampered joint mobility; palpitations; shortness of breath; a pale tongue with a white coating; and a threadlike and weak pulse.

4 Analysis of the Formula

Duhuo is acrid–bitter in flavor and warm in nature. It specializes in dispelling Wind–Cold–Dampness from the lower-jiao, in so doing relieving rheumatism and its pain. It is the chief herb.

Fangfeng and qinjiao dispel Wind and eliminate Dampness. Rougui warms the interior, dispels Cold, and clears channels. Xixin uses its acridity and warmth to disperse gelled Cold and to relieve pain. These four herbs are the deputies.

There are nine assistant herbs. Sangjisheng, niuxi and duzhong nourish the liver and the kidney, and strengthen tendons and bones. Danggui, baishaoyao, shengdihuang and chuanxiong invigorate and generate blood. Renshen and fuling augment Qi, strengthen the spleen, and support genuine Qi.

In addition to its ability to harmonize the actions of the other herbs, gancao also augments Qi and strengthens the spleen. It serves as both assistant and envoy herb.

5 Comments

Rheumatism usually manifests as aching pain in the muscles, tendons and bones, with heaviness, numbness and reduced joint mobility. It is caused by simultaneous attack by the intermingled Wind, Cold and Dampness evils, and their accumulation in the meridians, tendons and bones.

Duhuo Jisheng Tang is designed to treat illnesses in which long-standing Wind, Cold and Dampness in the tendons and bones have caused insufficiency of the liver and the kidney, and deficiency of Qi and blood. For that purpose, the composition of this formula emphasizes herbs that nourish the liver and the kidney, and augment Qi and blood. As complement it uses herbs that dispel Wind, eliminate Cold and dry Dampness. The two groups together can make Qi and blood full, so that Wind–Cold–Dampness can be eliminated and the spleen and the kidney invigorated. Doing so relieves the rheumatism and pain.

6 Case Study: Rheumatism in a 31-Year-Old Female

The patient suffered from kidney inflammation for 5 years. She insisted on treatment with a combination of Chinese and Western formulas. Though her symptoms diminished somewhat, she had persistent albumin in the urine, fluctuating between 2+ and 3+. She also continued to have weakness and aches in her waist and knees and mild intermittent edema in the face and limbs. Not long prior to consultation she was caught in the rain. This led to coldness and pain in her waist and knees, which hampered their mobility. She developed cold-aversion with preference for warmth, dizziness and general weakness.

Her face had edema and a lusterless complexion. She was emaciated and both lower limbs had mild pitting edema. Her tongue was pale, with a thin, white and greasy coating. Her pulse was threadlike and feeble. Urinalysis showed 3+ albumin.

Diagnosis: Rheumatism brought about by pathogenic evils attacking a weakened body.

Therapeutic Principle: Dispel Wind and Dampness, stop the rheumatic pain, strengthen the liver and the kidney, augment Qi and generate blood.

Treatment: Modified Duhuo Jisheng Tang was prescribed. The composition was: duhuo 10 g, duzhong 10 g, niuxi 10 g, qinjiao 10 g, fangfeng 10 g, baishaoyao 10 g, shengdihuang 10 g, xixin 3 g, rougui 3 g, chuanxiong 6 g, gancao 6 g, dangshen (*Codonopsis*) 10 g, fuling 10 g, and danggui 10 g.

One dose was administered each day. After ten doses the pain and the edema were relieved. She felt more vigorous and the other symptoms also diminished. Urinalysis now showed only 1+ albumin. The same formula was prescribed for 1 month. All the symptoms resolved. Repeated urinalysis thereafter showed normal findings. Another evaluation of kidney function showed completely normal results.

(Source: *Sichuan Chinese Medicine*, 1988, 4.)

III Lingjiao Gouteng Tang (Horn and Uncaria Decoction)

1 Source: Tong Su Shang Han Lun (Popular Treatise on Exogenous Febrile Illnesses)

2 Composition

Chief Herbs: lingyangjiao (*Saiga tatarica*) 45 g
gouteng (*Uncaria rhynchophylla*) 9 g

Deputy Herbs: sangye (*Morus alba*) 6 g
juhua (*Chrysanthemum morifolium*) 9 g

Assistant Herbs: shengdihuang (*Rehmannia glutinosa*) 15 g
baishaoyao (*Paeonia lactiflora*) 9 g
raw gancao (*Glycyrrhiza uralensis*) 3 g
Sichuan beimu (*Fritillaria cirrhosa*, *verticillata*) 12 g
zhuru (*Phyllostachys nigra*) 15 g
fushen (*Poria cocos*) 9 g

Envoy Herbs: gancao (*Glycyrrhiza uralensis*) 3 g

3 Application

Actions: cools the liver, extinguishes Wind, increases fluid and relaxes the sinews.

Indications: Heat in the Liver Meridian giving rise to endogenous Wind.

Main Symptoms: persistent high fever; restlessness; spasms of the extremities, sometimes developing into convulsions; in severe cases, loss of consciousness. A tongue that is red and dry, or dark and hairy; and a pulse that is taut and rapid.

4 Analysis of the Formula

Lingyangjiao (usually replaced by shuiniujiao, *Bubalus bubalis*) cools the liver and extinguishes Wind. Gouteng purges Heat and normalizes the liver, extinguishes Wind and stops convulsion. They are the chief herbs.

Two herbs complement the chief herbs: sangye and juhua. Acrid and cool together these two are dispersing herbs that clear Heat, normalize the liver and suppress Wind. They enhance the actions of the chief herbs to cool the liver and to suppress Wind. They are the deputy herbs.

When Heat is extreme, endogenous Wind is engendered. When Wind and Fire stimulate each other, Yin and fluids are especially easily damaged. So shengdihuang, baishaoyao and raw gancao are included to nourish Yin, generate fluids, soften the liver and soothe the sinews. When these herbs are used in concert with lingyangjiao, gouteng and other herbs that clear Heat, cool the liver and suppress Wind, both cause and effect are attended to and the ability to extinguish Wind and relieve spasms is enhanced. When the Heat evil flourishes, the body fluids become overheated and form Phlegm. So Sichuan beimu and fresh zhuru are included to clear Heat and dissipate Phlegm. Heat can disturb the heart and the mind. So fushen is included to calm the heart and the mind. These six herbs are assistants.

Gancao harmonizes the actions of the other herbs. It is the envoy herb.

The characteristic of this formula is to use herbs that cool liver and suppress Wind as the core and to complement them with herbs that augment Yin, dissipate Phlegm and calm the spirit. This is what makes it the representative formula for cooling the liver and extinguishing Wind.

5 *Comments*

Lingjiao Gouteng Tang is designed for illnesses brought about when exogenous Wind and Heat enter the Liver Meridian, where blazing Fire can develop and engender endogenous liver-Wind. These are illnesses of Heat and of strength of exogenous disease evil. For this reason the formula relies on herbs that cool the liver, extinguish Wind and relieve convulsions. Also, because blazing Fire gives rise to Wind and injures Yin and fluids, herbs that are sour–sweet, augment Yin and generate fluids are used to complement the other herbs. Doing so ensures that Yin and Yang are properly balanced.

If there is loss of consciousness brought on by Heat lodging in the Heart Meridian, then Zi Xue Dan (Purple-Snow Pill) is used at the same time to open orifices and to resuscitate by its acrid-coolness. Zi Xue Dan has the following composition: shigao (gypsum), hanshuishi (sodium sulfate), huashi (talcum), cishi (magnetite), xijiao powder (rhinoceros horn), lingyangjiao powder (*Saiga tartarica* horn), qingmuxiang (*Aristolochia debilis, contorta*), chenxiang (*Aquilaria*), xuanshen (*Scrophularia*), shengma (*Cimicifuga*), gancao (*Glycyrrhiza*), dingxiang (*Syzygium*), shexiang (*Moschus*), zhusha (cinnabar), and huangjin (gold foil). Note: nowadays, water shuiniujiao (buffalo horn) is used in place of xijiao and lingyangjiao.

6 *Case Study: Psychosis in a 24-Year-Old Male*

The patient had a history of psychosis. Recently, because of overwork on a summer day and because of dejection, he had a relapse. For about a week he had insomnia through the entire night, fearfulness and anxiety, limb spasms and loss of self-control. He drooled saliva, refused to speak, and had occasional incontinence of urine and feces. He did not eat unless urged by others. His tongue was red, with a thin and yellow tongue coating; and his pulse was taut and slippery.

Diagnosis: Recurrent psychosis caused by abnormally rising liver-Yang with movement of endogenous Wind.

Therapeutic Principle: Extinguish Wind, stop the spasms, clear Heat and dissipate Phlegm.

Treatment: Modified Lingjiao Gouteng Tang was prescribed, with the following composition: lingyangjiao 2 g, gouteng 12 g, fuling 12 g, jiangcan (*Bombyx mori*) 12 g, tianzhuhuang (*Bambusa textilis*) 12 g, shengdihuang 30 g, shijueming (*Haliotis*) 20 g, baishaoyao 20 g, beimu 10 g, zhuru 10 g, dilong (*Pheretima*) 6 g, sangye 6 g and wugong (*Scolopendra*) 2 pieces. In addition acupuncture was employed. Altogether over 20 doses were administered. The patient recovered and was able to leave the hospital.

(Source: *Zhejiang Journal of Chinese Medicine*, 1982, 9:413.)

IV Zhen Gan Xi Feng Tang (Liver-Sedating and Wind-Extinguishing Decoction)

1 Source: Yi Xue Zhong Zhong Can Xi Lu (Discourse on Integrated Chinese and Western Medicine)

2 Composition

Chief Herb: niuxi (*Achyranthes bidentata*) 30 g

Deputy Herbs: longgu (fossil bone) 15 g
muli (*Ostrea gigas*, *rivularis*) 15 g
guiban (*Chinemys reevesii*) 15 g
baishaoyao (*Paeonia lactiflora*) 15 g
zheshi (hematite) 30 g

Assistant Herbs: xuanshen (*Scrophularia ningpoensis*) 15 g
tiandong (*Asparagus chochinchinensis*) 15 g
yinchenhao (*Artemisia capillaris*) 6 g
maiya (*Hordeum vulgare*) 6 g
chuanlianzi (*Melia toosendan*) 6 g

Envoy Herb: gancao (*Glycyrrhiza uralensis*) 5 g

3 Application

Actions: sedates the liver, extinguishes Wind, nourishes Yin, and submerges Yang.

Indications: apoplexy.

Main Symptoms: dizziness with blurred vision, pressure in the eyes, tinnitus, feverish sensation and pain in the head; restlessness; flushed face; or, frequent eructation; or, progressive loss of motor function, with wry mouth; or, sudden faint; or, loss of consciousness with loss of motor function upon awakening. The pulse is taut, long and forceful.

4 Analysis of the Formula

Zhen Gan Xi Feng Tang uses a large amount of niuxi to conduct blood downward (from the head) and to nourish the liver and the kidney. It serves as chief herb.

Daizhushi is included to regulate the liver and suppress the abnormally rising Qi. Longgu, muli, guiban and baishaoyao are included to augment Yin, suppress excessive Yang, regulate the liver and extinguish Wind. They serve as deputy herbs.

Xuanshen and tiandong augment Yin and cool Heat (stimulate the Water Element and control the Wood Element). Since it is the nature of the liver to prefer smooth functioning and to abhor impedance, using only herbs that suppress it may hamper its functions. For this reason, yinchenhao, chuanlianzi and raw maiya are included to purge Heat from the liver and to facilitate and regulate liver-Qi, so that excessive liver-Yang can be more easily normalized. These five serve as assistant herbs.

Gancao harmonizes the actions of the other herbs. Teamed with raw maiya it also settles the stomach and regulates Qi in the middle-jiao, counteracting the adverse effects on the stomach of mineral herbs. It serves as envoy herb.

The characteristic feature in the construction of this formula is the use of herbs that suppress excessive Yang and complementing them with herbs that augment Yin. The Yang suppression aims at the appearance and the Yin augmentation at the root. Thus, both cause and effect are attended to, though the treatment of the effects is primary. These herbs acting in concert have the ability to calm the liver and extinguish Wind.

5 Comments

Zhen Gan Xi Feng Tang is a commonly used formula in treating apoplexy. If an illness is ascertained to be one of Yin deficiency with Yang excess, so that liver Wind stirs internally, it may be used, whether before or after the development of the stroke. The key symptoms are dizziness, blurred vision, sensation of fullness and pain in the head, flushed face, restlessness, and a taut, long and forceful pulse.

The purpose of emphasizing herbs that suppress and regulate is to design a formula that normalizes the liver, conducts blood downward from the head, augments Yin and restrains excess Yang.

In clinical application, if there is much Phlegm as well, zhuli (*Phyllostachys nigra*) and bile-treated tiannanxing (*Arisaema consanguineum*, *erubescens*) may be added to clear Heat and flush Phlegm. If the pulse is weak at the chi position in both wrists, then add shudihuang (*Rehmannia*) and shanzhuru (*Cornus*) to strengthen the spleen and restrain the liver.

6 Clinical Study: Headache

Zhen Gan Xi Feng Tang was used to treat 70 patients with vascular headache. If the headache was sudden, gouteng (Uncaria) and baizhi (Angelica dahurica) were added. If the headache was persistent, danshen (Salvia) and chuanxiong (Ligusticum) were added. Each course of treatment was 15 days, one dose daily.

Results: Twenty-three patients responded promptly, and 41 responded by the end of the treatment course. Six patients did not respond. The overall effective rate was 91%.

(Source: *Journal of Integrated Chinese and Western Medicine*, 1989, 9:563.)

V Tianma Gouteng Yin (Gastrodia and Uncaria Drink)

1 Source: Za Bing Zheng Zhi Xin Yi (New Concepts for the Diagnosis and Treatment of Miscellaneous Illnesses)

2 Composition

Chief Herbs: tianma (*Gastrodia elata*) 9 g
gouteng (*Uncaria rhynchophylla*) 12 g

Deputy Herbs: shijueming (*Haliotis diversicolor*) 18 g
Sichuan niuxi (*Achyranthes bidentata*) 12 g

Assistant Herbs: zhizi (*Gardenia jasminoides*) 9 g
huangqin (*Scutellaria baicalensis*) 9 g
yimucao (*Leonurus heterophyllus*, *japonicus*) 9 g
duzhong (*Eucommia ulmoides*) 9 g
sangjisheng (*Loranthus parasiticus*) 9 g
yejiaoteng (*Polygonum multiflorum*) 9 g
fushen (*Poria cocos*) 9 g

3 Application

Actions: normalizes the liver, extinguishes endogenous Wind, and strengthens the liver and the kidney.

Indications: excessive liver-Yang, with upward disturbance by liver-Wind.

Main Symptoms: headache; vertigo; insomnia; a red tongue with a yellow coating; and a taut pulse.

4 Analysis of the Formula

Tianma and gouteng have the ability to normalize the liver and extinguish endogenous Wind. They are the chief herbs.

Shijueming normalizes the liver, suppresses Yang, clears Heat and improves vision. It enhances the ability of tianma and gouteng to normalize the liver and extinguish Wind. Niuxi conducts blood downward. These two are the deputy herbs.

There are seven assistant herbs. Zhizi and huangqin clear Heat and purge Fire, thereby preventing the upward attack by the Heat from the Liver Meridian. Yimucao invigorates blood and promotes diuresis. Duzhong and sangjisheng nourish the liver and the kidney, especially their Yin. Yejiaoteng and fushen calm the spirit and bolster decisiveness.

Acting in concert, the herbs together constitute a formula that normalizes the liver, extinguishes endogenous Wind, clears Heat, invigorates blood, and nourishes the liver and the kidney.

5 Comments

The prominent characteristic in the construction of this formula is the emphasis on herbs that normalize the liver and extinguish endogenous Wind and the complementation with herbs that clear Heat, conduct blood downward, nourish the liver and the kidney, calm the spirit and bolster decisiveness. The key symptoms at which the formula aims are headache, vertigo and insomnia.

Since the liver is the reservoir for blood, and excessive liver-Yang tends to rise, such illnesses often develop deficiency of liver-Yin. It is important to include herbs that augment Yin and generate blood, so that both root and appearance can be treated.

6 Case Study: Meniere's Syndrome in a 39-Year-Old Female

Initially the patient suffered from dizziness, which was diagnosed as Meniere's syndrome. Treatment with western formulas proved to be ineffective. At consultation, her main symptoms were dizziness, vertigo, tinnitus, headaches in the temples; blurred vision, sensation of rotation of objects viewed obliquely; unsteady gait requiring much care when turning corners; palpitation of the heart; insomnia, and much dreaming when able to sleep; intermittent thirst; and yellow urine. Her menses were normal, as was her blood pressure. Her body was plump. Her tongue was red, with a thin and yellow coating. Her pulse was taut and rapid.

Diagnosis: Meniere's syndrome, caused by deficiency of liver and kidney Yin, so that the Water Element (kidney) is unable to nourish the Wood Element (liver), permitting excessively active liver-Yang.

Therapeutic Principle: Augment the Water Element, enabling it to nourish the Wood Element, normalize the liver and extinguish endogenous Wind.

Treatment: Tianma Gouteng Yin, with added shudihuang (*Rehmannia*) 20 g and gouqizi (*Lycium*) 20 g, was prescribed. Altogether 15 doses were administered, after which all her symptoms, including vertigo, palpitations of the heart, insomnia and frequent dreams, resolved. She recovered fully and was able to return to work.

(Source: *Journal of Countryside Medicine*, 1985, 12:18.)

VI Da Ding Feng Zhu (Major Wind-Extinguishing Pearls)

1 Source: Wen Bing Tiao Bian (Analysis of Febrile Illnesses)

2 Composition

Chief Herbs: jizihuang (egg yolk) 2 pieces
ejiao (*Equus asinus*) 9 g

Deputy Herbs: baishaoyao (*Paeonia lactiflora*) 18 g
shengdihuang (*Rehmannia glutinosa*) 18 g
maimendong (*Ophiopogon japonicus*) 18 g
guiban (*Chinemys reevesii*) 18 g
biejia (*Amyda sinensis*) 18 g

Assistant Herbs: huomaren (*Cannabis sativa*) 6 g
muli (*Ostrea gigas, rivularis*) 12 g
wuweizi (*Schisandra chinensis*) 6 g

Envoy Herb: fried gancao (*Glycyrrhiza uralensis*) 12 g

3 Application

Actions: augments Yin and extinguishes Wind.

Indications: (1) Heat injuring Yin, and Yin deficiency giving rise to movement of endogenous Wind. (2) Depleted Yin on the verge of collapse.

Main Symptoms: symptoms of late stage Heat illnesses; convulsion, fatigue; a crimson tongue with little coating; and a depletive and feeble pulse.

4 *Analysis of the Formula*

For chief herbs Da Ding Feng Zhu uses jizihuang and ejiao. They nourish Yin and fluids, and extinguish endogenous Wind.

The formula further uses large amounts of baishaoyao, shengdihuang and maimendong to nourish Yin and soften the liver, thereby strengthening the Water Element and nourishing the Wood Element. Guiban and biejia augment Yin and suppress excess Yang. These five are the deputy herbs.

Huomaren is moist and high in fat. It augments Yin and moistens Dryness. Muli is salty and cold. It normalizes the liver and suppresses excess Yang. Wuweizi is sour in flavor, and is an astringent. Used with herbs that augment Yin it prevents vital Yin from dissipating. Used with fried gancao the sour and sweet flavors can induce the generation of Yin. These three are the assistant herbs.

Gancao harmonizes the actions of the other herbs, and is the envoy.

5 *Comments*

Da Ding Feng Zhu is designed to treat illnesses in which the Heat evil has injured Yin-fluids and endogenous Wind is moving. At this stage Yin and fluids are depleted and Yin is on the verge of collapse, whereas only residual amounts of the pathogenic evil still remain. Hence the formula emphasizes the rescue of Yin and fluids and the extinction of endogenous Wind. If the pathogenic evil is still vigorous then this formula is not appropriate to use, even if Yin and fluids are both depleted.

In clinical application, the key symptoms are fatigue, convulsion, an indistinct and feeble pulse and a red tongue with scant coating.

6 *Case Study: Post-radiation Tongue Atrophy in a 50-Year-Old Female*

The patient received radiation therapy for naso-pharyngeal cancer. Following radiation her cancer stabilized, but her tongue became atrophied and stiff. It deviated to the left and lost all sensation. Her speech became indistinct, and swallowing became difficult so that she could not eat or drink. Her pulse was taut and threadlike, and is forceless on pressure. Her tongue was atrophied and red, with scant coating.

Diagnosis: Tongue atrophy due to strong Heat injuring Yin, so that the body fluids were consumed and the body of the tongue lost its nourishment.

Therapeutic Principle: Nourish Yin and extinguish Wind.

Treatment: Da Ding Feng Zhu was administered at the dosage of one pearl a day. After 5 days her tongue became softer, her speech clearer, and she was able to eat thin rice gruel. After 17 uninterrupted doses, her speech became essentially normal and she was able to eat soft rice.

(Source: *Zhejiang Journal of Chinese Medicine*, 1985, 6:275.)

7 *Case Study: High Blood Pressure in a 65-Year-Old Male*

The patient was a chronic alcoholic, and had a hot temper. Because of overwork, 5 days prior to consultation he suddenly developed dizziness and fainting. Examination showed a ruddy complexion with flushed cheeks, dry lips and mouth, a red tongue with thin and yellow coating, and a threadlike and rapid pulse. His blood pressure was 180/90 mmHg.

Diagnosis: Deficiency of liver and kidney Yin, with loss of restraint over the Fire caused by the Passions.

Therapeutic Principle: Nourish Yin and Yang.

Treatment: Da Ding Feng Zhu, with modifications, was prescribed. The composition was: ejiao 10 g, jizihuang 2 pieces, baishaoyao 15 g, dihuang 15 g, huomaren 5 g, fresh muli 30 g, maimendong 10 g, fried gancao 5 g, guiban 15 g, wumei (*Prunus mume*) 10 g, and zhezhi (juice of the sugarcane, *Saccharum sinensis*) 100 mL (the last added to the decoction after cooking the rest). After four successive doses, the dizziness improved and the blood pressure lowered to 160/80 mmHg. After 12 additional doses, all symptoms resolved. In follow-up, there was no relapse for 1 year.

(Source: *Journal of Chinese Medicine*, 1983, 6:33.)

VII Section Summary

Of these five formulas, **Xiao Feng San** is particularly effective in dispelling Wind, generating blood, clearing Heat and eliminating Dampness. It is a commonly used treatment for urticaria and eczema.

The main actions of **Duhuo Jisheng Tang** are to dispel Wind and Dampness, relieve the pain of rheumatism, strengthen the liver and kidney, and augment Qi and blood. It is indicated for chronic rheumatism, deficiency of liver and kidney Qi and blood, and aches and weakness in the waist and knees.

Lingjiao Gouteng Tang, Tianma Gouteng Yin and Da Ding Feng Zhu are all efficacious for extinguishing endogenous Wind. However, **Ling Jiao Gouteng Tang** is stronger at purging Heat. It is most appropriate in illnesses of strong Heat in the Liver Meridian and endogenous Wind induced by extreme Heat. **Tianma Gouteng Yin** is capable of clearing Heat, invigorating blood circulation and calming the mind. It is suitable for treating excessive liver-Yang and upward attack by liver-Wind, causing headache, dizziness and insomnia. **Da Ding Feng Zhu** is a typical formula for augmenting Yin and extinguishing Wind. It is suitable for treating depletion of Yin caused by burning Heat, in late stages of Heat illnesses, and the stirring of endogenous Wind arising in Yin depletion.

Section 15 Formulas That Relieve Dryness

Dryness-relieving formulas contain mainly herbs that gently moisten Dryness or enrich Yin. They are applicable to illnesses of Dryness in either the exterior or the interior.

Dryness in the exterior is caused by exogenous Dryness, whereas Dryness in the interior is due to endogenous Dryness arising when Yin fluids in the visceral organs are exhausted. Dryness in the exterior and Dryness in the interior have different causes and manifest different clinical symptoms; so different treatments are required. Gentle moistening is used for exterior Dryness, whereas methods of augmenting Yin and generating fluids are used for interior Dryness. For illnesses involving interior and exterior Dryness concurrently, these treatments should be applied accordingly.

Dryness-relieving formulas generally contain nourishing and greasy herbs. These have a tendency to promote the formation of Dampness and to disrupt Qi movement. Therefore, caution should be exercised in a patient with a Dampness constitution, or with spleen deficiency, loose feces, stagnation of Qi and much Phlegm. Acrid and aromatic herbs that impair Yin should not be used in Dryness illnesses.

I Xing Su San (Apricot and Perilla Powder)

1 Source: Wen Bing Tiao Bian (Analysis of Febrile Illnesses)

2 Composition

Chief Herbs: zisu (*Perilla frutescens*) 9 g
xingren (*Prunus armeniaca*) 9 g

Deputy Herbs: qianhu (*Peucedanum praeruptorum*) 9 g
jiegeng (*Platycodon grandiflorum*) 6 g
zhiqiao (*Poncirus trifoliata*) 6 g

Assistant Herbs: processed banxia (*Pinellia ternata*) 9 g
chenpi (*Citrus tangerina, reticulata*) 6 g
fuling (*Poria cocos*) 9 g
gancao (*Glycyrrhiza uralensis*) 3 g

Envoy Herbs: shengjiang (*Zingiber officinale*) 3 pieces
dazao (*Ziziphus jujuba*) 3 pieces

3 Application

Actions: mildly disperses Cold-Dryness, regulates lung-Qi and dissipates Phlegm.

Indications: illnesses of exogenous Cold-Dryness.

Main Symptoms: headache; chills, absence of sweating; cough with watery sputum; nasal congestion; dry throat; a white tongue coating; and a taut pulse.

4 Analysis of the Formula

Of the chief herbs, zisu, which is acrid, warm and not dry, disperses Cold-Dryness from the exterior and muscles. It also facilitates the movement of lung-Qi. Xingren is bitter, warm and lubricating. It releases stagnant lung-Qi, suppresses cough and dissipates Phlegm.

One deputy herb, qianhu, disperses Wind, suppresses abnormally rising lung-Qi and dissipates Phlegm. It helps the chief herbs dispel exogenous pathogenic factors from the exterior and eliminate Phlegm. The other deputies, jiegeng, which is ascending in nature, and zhiqiao, which is descending, together enhance the ability of xingren to release stagnant lung-Qi.

The assistant herbs, banxia, chenpi and fuling, regulate Qi circulation and dissipate Phlegm. Gancao, on the other hand, works with jiegeng to release stagnant lung-Qi and to eliminate Phlegm.

Shengjiang and dazao harmonize Nutritive and Defensive Qi, thereby promoting the circulation of bodily fluids. They function as envoy herbs.

In combination, the herbs disperse Cold-Dryness from the exterior, eliminate Phlegm and regulate the movement of lung-Qi.

5 Comments

Xing Su San is designed for illnesses caused by exogenous Cold-Dryness, leading to dysfunction of the lung by impeding the movement of ascending and descending Qi and internal obstruction by Dampness and Phlegm. The key symptoms calling for it include cold-aversion, absence of sweating, a cough that produces watery sputum, a dry throat, a white coating on the tongue and a taut pulse. It is applicable to influenza, chronic bronchitis, emphysema, and related illnesses.

6 Clinical Study: Cough

Xing Su San was studied as treatment for cough due to Wind–Cold. Eighty-seven patients were treated, with satisfactory results.

Method: Replace qianhu with baiqian (*Cynanchum*) in Xing Su San. The herbs were decocted in boiling water. The formula was administered at the dosage of one dose daily, taken in two portions.

For more severe Wind–Cold symptoms add mahuang (*Ephedra*). For severe cough and dyspnea due to abnormally risen lung-Qi add xuanfuhua (*Inula britannica*). For Cold deficiency of lung-Qi add dangshen (*Codonopsis*). For chest tightness add houpo (*Magnolia*) and cangzhu (*Atractylodes*). For fever with cold-aversion, thirst, sore throat, a white tongue coating and a floating and taut pulse, add huangqin (*Scutellaria*) and lianqiao (*Forsythia*).

Results: Of the 87 patients 73 recovered completely and 12 had relief of symptoms. Two patients did not respond.

(Source: *Guangxi Journal of Chinese Medicine*, 1985, 6:37.)

II Qing Zao Jiu Fei Tang (Dryness-Moistening Lung-Rescuing Decoction)

1 Source: Yi Men Fa Lu (Principles and Regulations for the Medical Profession)

2 Composition

Chief Herb: sangye (*Morus alba*) 9 g

Deputy Herbs: shigao (gypsum) 8 g
maimendong (*Ophiopogon japonicus*) 4 g

Assistant Herbs: renshen (*Panax ginseng*) 2 g
huomaren (*Cannabis sativa*) 3 g
ejiao (*Equus asinus*) 3 g
xingren (*Prunus armeniaca*) 2 g
pipaye (*Eriobotrya japonica*) 3 g

Envoy Herb: gancao (*Glycyrrhiza uralensis*) 3 g

3 Application

Actions: clears warm Dryness and moistens the lung.

Indications: illnesses of Warm-Dryness attacking the lung.

Main Symptoms: fever; headache; a dry cough with scanty sputum; wheezing and dyspnea; dry throat; thirst; dry nasal passages; chest fullness; a dry tongue with little coating; a depletive, large and rapid pulse.

4 Analysis of the Formula

Qing Zao Jiu Fei Tang is designed for illnesses of Warm-Dryness attacking the lung. In this formula, sangye is used in large amount to eliminate and clear warm Dryness and Heat in the lung. It serves as chief herb.

For the treatment of Warm-Dryness in the lung, Heat should be cleared with cooling therapy while Dryness should be treated with moistening methods. Therefore, shigao, which is acrid–sweet and cold, is included to clear Heat from the lung, and maimendong, which is sweet and cold, is included to nourish Yin and moisten the lung. These two serve as deputy herbs.

The stomach belongs to the Earth Element, and the lung to the Metal Element. Earth gives birth to Metal. Thus gancao is used to strengthen the stomach (Earth) so as to invigorate the lung (Metal). Renshen promotes the production of fluid in the stomach and invigorates lung-Qi. Huomaren and ejiao nourish Yin and moisten the lung. Xingren and pipaye suppress abnormally rising lung-Qi. These six serve as assistant herbs.

Gancao serves as envoy herb to harmonize the effects of the other herbs.

Used in concert these herbs simultaneously free the lung from Dryness and Heat and suppress abnormally risen Qi, so that all the corresponding symptoms are relieved simultaneously. The dual action is the reason for the name of this formula.

5 Comments

In treating a Dryness illness, it is important at the beginning to differentiate between cold Dryness and Warm-Dryness. Qing Zao Jiu Fei Tang is designed for illnesses due to lung injury by warm Dryness during autumn when rain is rare.

When the lung is injured by Heat and Dryness, it loses its property of clearing, moistening and descending. Symptoms such as cough, dyspnea, dry throat, thirst, and a dry tongue with little coating appear. At this stage, acrid and aromatic herbs should be avoided; otherwise, Qi may become depleted. Herbs that are cold in nature or that purge Fire should also be avoided, as they too may damage Qi. Therefore, herbs that are gentle in nature are used in this formula to dispel Dryness and to moisten the lung.

Qing Zao Jiu Fei Tang is indicated when there are general Heat in the body, a cough with scanty sputum, wheezing, dyspnea, a reddish tongue with little coating, and a depletive, large and rapid pulse.

6 Case Study: Autumn Dryness in a 41-Year-Old Female

The patient had this illness for 5 days. She began with fever, cold-aversion, headache, cough, and dry throat. She had not defecated for 4 days and her urine was scanty and dark yellow. On the day of consultation, she suddenly developed severe vomiting, followed by aphasia and hemiplegia of the right limbs.

On examination, she was conscious but had difficulty opening her eyes. Her temperature was 38°C (100.4°F) her blood pressure 140/90 mmHg, and her heart rate 115 beats per min. Her complexion was pale red. Her tongue was pink; it was denuded centrally and the rest covered with a dry, thin and yellowish coating. She had a slow knee jerk reflex, and absence of reflexes in the right abdominal wall. She had no pain sensation on the right side of the body. The rest of the examination and her blood tests showed no abnormality.

She was initially treated with acupuncture in conjunction with western medicine, as well as Tianma Gouteng Yin, without apparent effect. The following day, she was further examined. She now had headache, fever and chills, a dry cough and a dry throat.

Diagnosis: Exogenous Dryness affecting the lung.

Therapeutic Principle: Clear warm Dryness and moisten the lung.

Treatment: Modified Qing Zao Jiu Fei Tang was prescribed, with the following composition: sangye 9 g, maimendong 9 g, heizhima (*Sesamum indicum*) 9 g, gualou seed (*Trichosanthes*) 9 g, pipaye 9 g, shigao 12 g, xiyangshen (*Panax quinquefolium*) 3 g, xingren 6 g, biemu (*Fritillaria*) 6 g, gancao 4.5 g, shengdihuang (*Rehmannia*) 15 g, zhuli (*Phyllostachys nigra*) 15 g. The formula was administered at one dose per day for 3 days. All symptoms were relieved.

(Source: *Fujian Journal of Chinese Medicine*, 1966, 1:45.)

III Yang Yin Qing Fei Tang (Yin-Nourishing Lung-Clearing Decoction)

1 Source: Chong Lou Yu Yao (Jade Key to the Private Chamber)

2 Composition

Chief Herb: shengdihuang (*Rehmannia glutinosa*) 12 g

Deputy Herbs: xuanshen (*Scrophularia ningpoensis*) 9 g
maimendong (*Ophiopogon japonicus*) 9 g

Assistant Herbs: mudanpi (*Paeonia suffruticosa*) 5 g
stir-fried baishaoyao (*Paeonia lactiflora*) 5 g
Sichuan beimu (*Fritillaria cirrhosa, verticillata*) 5 g
bohe (*Mentha haplocalyx*) 5 g

Envoy Herbs: gancao (*Glycyrrhiza uralensis*) 3 g

3 Application

Actions: nourishes Yin, clears the lung, relieves toxicity and soothes the throat.

Indications: "white throat" (diphtheria).

Main Symptoms: a white curd-like coating in the throat that is difficult to scrape off; a swollen and sore throat; dry nasal passages and parched lips; and a rapid pulse.

4 Analysis of the Formula

Yang Yin Qing Fei Tang is designed for "white throat" (diphtheria). In the formula, shengdihuang, which is sweet and cold, is used in large amount to nourish Yin and to clear Heat. It serves as chief herb.

Xuanshen nourishes Yin, promotes the production of fluid, clears Heat and removes toxins. Maimendong nourishes Yin and clears Heat from the lung. Together they function as deputy herbs.

Mudanpi purges Heat, cools blood and reduces swelling. Fried baishaoyao nourishes Yin and blood. Beimu moistens the lung and dissipates Phlegm, purges Heat and disperses stagnation. In small amounts bohe is acrid and cool and has the ability to disperse accumulations. It clears the exterior and eases the throat. These herbs assist the chief and deputies.

Raw gancao purges Fire, releases toxins and harmonizes the actions of the other herbs. It is used as envoy herb.

These herbs acting in concert have the actions of nourishing Yin, clearing Heat from the lung, releasing toxins and easing the throat.

5 *Comments*

This is a typical prescription for treating "white throat." This illness is always due to constitutional Yin deficiency and Heat accumulation in the upper-jiao, with consequent contraction of an epidemic toxin. In this light, treatment should focus on nourishing Yin and clearing Heat from the lung. At an early stage of the illness, clearing and dispersing herbs are added. For patients with severe Heat, herbs that purge Heat and release toxins may be applied in large amounts. Clinical indications for Yang Yin Qing Fei Tang include a white coating of the pharynx that cannot be scraped off, pain and swelling in the throat, dry nose and lips, and a rapid and large pulse.

6 *Case Study: Severe Sore Throat in a Female*

The patient suffered from sore throat with pain and swelling and inability to drink fluids or to take medicines. She also had swelling in the eyes and face, dyspnea with much sputum, and a sensation of suffocation. She was in critical condition.

Diagnosis: Severe Heat and accumulated toxins in the throat.

Therapeutic Principle: Purge Heat and remove toxins.

Treatment: Since there was danger that an attempt to swallow a medicine might precipitate obstruction, Lei Shi Liu Sheng Wan was first placed on the tongue, after moistening with warm water. The next day, the patient was able to drink fluids. Yang Yin Qing Fei Tang was then prescribed as the basic prescription, but with the amount of bohe halved and the amount of shengdihuang doubled. Seven days later, all symptoms disappeared.

(Source: *Case Records of Dr. Ran Xuefeng*.)

IV Section Summary

In this section three Dryness-relieving formulas are discussed. **Xing Su San** is often used for eliminating cold Dryness that attacks the lung. It is indicated for such symptoms as cold-aversion, cough with watery sputum, absence of sweating, headache and stuffy nose. **Qing Zao Jiu Fei Tang** is used for eliminating warm Dryness in addition to nourishing Yin. It is indicated for severe cases of warm Dryness attacking the lung, with the main symptoms of fever, thirst, dyspnea, a sensation of pain and fullness in the chest. **Yang Yin Qing Fei Tang** is applicable for illnesses due to Dryness in the lung as a result of Yin deficiency. The main symptoms include thirst, hotness in the five centers (soles, palms and precordium) and a dry cough.

Section 16 Formulas That Relieve Accumulations

Formulas for relieving accumulations are composed of herbs that promote digestion, relieve stagnation, eliminate a feeling of abdominal pressure, as well as dissolve abdominal masses. Among the Eight Methods, they fall within the category of the Method of Dissipation.

Food retention illness is closely linked to the normal functions of the stomach and the spleen. Dysfunction of the stomach and the spleen, obstruction or retrograde ascent of stomach-Qi, or unbalanced diet may all lead to food retention. The formation of abdominal masses is generally due to abnormal interaction of Heat, Phlegm, food and blood with Qi over a long period of time.

In application, formulas for relieving accumulations can be divided into two categories: those for relieving dyspepsia and food retention and those for eliminating fullness and masses. In constructing the formulas, herbs that regulate Qi circulation are usually added to eliminate stagnation. For patients with prolonged Qi deficiency or prolonged stagnation leading to deficiency of stomach and spleen Qi, it is important to use the combined approach of invigorating the vital force and eliminating stagnation and dyspepsia. Applying only the elimination of stagnation may permit the recurrence of stagnation because of Qi deficiency.

Formulas for dispersing stagnation are not recommended for prolonged administration since they may injure the spleen and the liver. Excessive administration of such formulas may injure genuine Qi, resulting in failure to eliminate the abnormal stagnation.

I Bao He Wan (Harmony-Preserving Pill)

1 Source: Dan Xi Xin Fa (Danxi's Experience in Medicine)

2 Composition

Chief Herbs: shanzha (*Crataegus pinnatifida*) 18 g

Deputy Herbs: shenqu (medicated leaven) 6 g
laifuzi (*Raphanus sativus*) 6 g

Assistant Herbs: processed banxia (*Pinellia ternata*) 9 g
chenpi (*Citrus tangerina, reticulata*) 6 g
fuling (*Poria cocos*) 9 g
lianqiao (*Forsythia suspensa*) 6 g

3 Application

Actions: digests retained food and settles the stomach.

Indications: illnesses of food retention.

Main Symptoms: fullness in the epigastrium and abdomen; rotten-smelling belching; acid regurgitation; aversion to food with reduced appetite; diarrhea; a thick and greasy tongue coating; and a slippery pulse.

4 Analysis of the Formula

In large amounts shanzha has the ability to relieve all types of food retention, especially that of meats and fatty foods. For that reason it is used as chief herb.

Shenqu is useful for eliminating stagnation and for strengthening the spleen, especially when the illness results from excess alcohol and food. Laifuzi suppresses abnormally risen Qi and eliminates food accumulation, and is particularly efficacious in removing accumulated Phlegm. These two are together used as deputy herbs. The chief herb and the deputy herbs interact synergistically to digest all kinds of retained food.

Since stagnated food obstructs Qi circulation and can lead to illnesses of stomach-Qi, processed banxia and chenpi are included to promote Qi movement, eliminate stagnation, settle the stomach and inhibit vomiting. Stagnated food may give rise to Heat and Dampness. Hence, fuling is included to disperse Dampness, strengthen the spleen, settle the stomach and relieve diarrhea; and lianqiao is included to purge Heat and remove stagnation. These four serve as assistant herbs.

Through the complementary actions of all the ingredients, this formula is effective in relieving stagnation, regulating stomach-Qi, purging Heat, and eliminating Dampness. It resolves all resulting symptoms simultaneously. Because all the herbs in this formula are gentle in action and nature, the formula is named "harmony-preserving."

5 Comments

Illnesses of food retention result from overindulgence in food or drinks of all types, leading to stagnation in the middle-jiao. For food retention in the upper-jiao, with symptoms of abnormally rising Qi, emesis therapy should be adopted. For food retention in the lower-jiao, with symptoms of solid masses forming, therapy to drain (catharsis) should be implemented. For food retention in the middle-jiao, which indicates that the accumulation has not been prolonged, neither vomiting nor draining therapy is appropriate. Only therapy that aims at dissolving and relieving stagnation is effective.

For choosing to apply this formula the key clinical indications are fullness in the stomach and epigastrium, rotten-smelling belching, a thick and greasy tongue coating, and a slippery pulse.

6 *Case Study: Indigestion in a 35-Year-Old Female*

The patient suffered spasmodic pain in the upper abdomen following overeating of greasy food. Her symptoms were chills and fever, vomiting, and a complexion indicative of acute pain. She had a slight distention of the abdomen, spasms of the abdominal muscles, abdominal tenderness, a bitter taste in the mouth, a reddish tongue with a yellowish, greasy and smooth coating, and a taut but soft pulse.

Diagnosis: Accumulation of Heat–Dampness in the gallbladder, with impairment of transformation and transportation in the middle-jiao.

Therapeutic Principle: Facilitate transportation, invigorate Qi circulation, relieve stagnation, mobilize liver-Qi and strengthen the gallbladder.

Treatment: Bao He Wan was used as the basic formula, with the addition of yanhusuo (*Corydalis*) 10 g, zhiqiao (*Poncirus trifoliata*) 10 g, and yinhua (*Lonicera*) 20 g. One dose was administered each day. Abdominal pain and nausea were relieved after three doses, but dyspepsia and anorexia did not resolve. For further treatment, yinhua, zhiqiao and yanhusuo were removed from the formula, and yujin (*Curcuma*) 10 g was added. After five doses of the new modified prescription, there was complete recovery.

II Zhishi Dao Zhi Wan (Orange Stagnation-Relieving Pill)

1 *Source: Nei Wai Shang Bian Huo Lun (Guide for the Perplexities of Internal and External Injuries)*

2 *Composition*

Chief Herb: dahuang (*Rheum palmatum*) 9 g

Deputy Herbs: zhishi (*Citrus aurantium*) 9 g
shenqu (medicated leaven) 9 g

Assistant Herbs: huangqin (*Scutellaria baicalensis*) 6 g
huanglian (*Coptis chinensis*) 6 g
fuling (*Poria cocos*) 6 g
zexie (*Alisma plantago-aquatica, orientale*) 6 g
baizhu (*Atractylodes macrocephala*) 6 g

3 Application

Actions: digests retained food, clears Heat and eliminates Dampness.

Indications: food retention with Dampness–Heat.

Main Symptoms: fullness or distention in the epigastrium and abdomen; dysentery, diarrhea or constipation; scanty and dark urine; a yellow and greasy tongue coating; and a deep and forceful pulse.

4 Analysis of the Formula

Zhishi Dao Zhi Wan depends heavily on dahuang for its purgative, bitter and cold nature. As chief herb it can relieve food retention and drain Heat downward to eliminate Heat–Dampness through defecation.

Zhishi promotes Qi movement to relieve food retention, remove accumulations and eliminate fullness. Shenqu eliminates food retention and settles the stomach. These two herbs help dahuang relieve food retention, and are together the deputy herbs.

Huangqin and huanglian, which are bitter and cold, remove Heat and Dampness to stop dysentery. Fuling and zexie remove Dampness and promote diuresis to stop diarrhea. Baizhu dries Dampness and strengthens the spleen, and facilitates the attack on accumulations without damaging genuine Qi. These five serve as assistant herbs.

The herbs in this formula complement one another and together act to promote food digestion, clear Heat and eliminate Dampness, thereby eliminating food retention, dispersing Dampness and Heat, and resolving all the symptoms.

5 Comments

Dampness–Heat and food retention blocking the intestines and the stomach will lead to diarrhea or dysentery. At the initial stage, reducing food retention, clearing Heat and eliminating Dampness are the main goals of therapy. If Dampness, Heat and food retention are not resolved, the abdominal pain cannot be relieved. Diarrhea or dysentery will resolve only if Dampness, Heat and food retention are cleared. This is the method of treating diarrhea by purgation.

6 Clinical Application: Impaired Intestinal Motility

Zhishi Dao Zhi Wan, especially with modified amounts, is quite effective in treating impaired motility of the intestines. The expanded formula has the following composition: dahuang 25 g, zhishi 10 g, shenqu 15 g, huangqin 15 g, huanglian 15 g, baizhu 10 g, fuling 10 g, and zexie 10 g.

If there is Heat accumulation with severe dysentery, add yinhua (*Lonicera*) 30 g and baitouweng (*Pulsatilla*) 40 g. If there is Heat accumulation in the middle-jiao, add mangxiao (*Mirabilite*) 20 g. If there is much vomiting, add zhuru (*Phyllostachys nigra*) 15 g and daizheshi (Hematite) 30 g.

Decoct in boiling water. Administer—one to two doses each day. Each dose should be taken on an empty stomach in three or four portions.

(Source: *Jilin Journal of Chinese Medicine*, 1983, 3:34.)

III Jian Pi Wan (Spleen-Invigorating Pill)

1 Source: Zheng Zhi Zhun Sheng (Standards of Diagnosis and Treatment)

2 Composition: The Herbs in This Formula Are Not Classified

baizhu (*Atractylodes macrocephala*) 15 g
muxiang (*Aucklandia lappa*) 6 g
huanglian (*Coptis chinensis*) 6 g
gancao (*Glycyrrhiza uralensis*) 6 g
fuling (*Poria cocos*) 10 g
renshen (*Panax ginseng*) 9 g
shenqu (medicated leaven) 6 g
chenpi (*Citrus tangerina, reticulata*) 6 g
sharen (*Amomum villosum*) 6 g
maiya (*Hordeum vulgare*) 6 g
shanzha (*Crataegus pinnatifida*) 6 g
shanyao (*Dioscorea opposita*) 6 g
roudoukou (*Myristica fragrans*) 6 g

3 *Application*

Actions: strengthens the spleen, harmonizes the stomach, relieves food retention and stops diarrhea.

Indications: insufficiency of the spleen with food retention.

Main Symptoms: fullness and distress in the epigastrium and abdomen; reduced appetite with difficulty in digestion; loose feces; a greasy and slightly yellow tongue coating; and an empty and weak pulse.

4 *Analysis of the Formula*

The 13 herbs in this formula are not grouped by the standard categorization.

Renshen, baizhu, fuling and gancao augment Qi and strengthen the spleen. Among these four, baizhu and fuling are used in relatively large amounts so as to stop diarrhea and promote diuresis by strengthening the spleen. Shanzha, shenqu and maiya are used to relieve food retention by promoting digestion. Shanyao and roudoukou assist in strengthening the spleen and relieving diarrhea. Muxiang, sharen and chenpi are used to regulate Qi movement, harmonize the stomach, augment transportation and eliminate masses. Huanglian eliminates Dampness–Heat by purging Heat and drying Dampness.

Acting in concert, these herbs form a formula that combines the actions of elimination and strengthening, thereby restoring spleen function, removing stagnation, dispelling Dampness and purging Heat.

Jian Pi Wan mainly uses herbs that strengthen the spleen. At the same time, as stagnation is relieved spleen function is further enhanced. For this reason it is named "spleen-strengthening."

5 *Comments*

The formula is indicated for illnesses due to stomach and spleen insufficiency accompanying Dampness and Heat, or weak spleen and food retention resulting from excessive eating and drinking. The stomach governs food digestion and the spleen controls the transformation and movement of food. Stomach dysfunction causes inability to digest food, whereas spleen dysfunction causes inability to push Qi upward and to fail in the transformation and movement of food.

Treatment should focus on both strengthening the spleen and eliminating the stagnation. The key clinical indications for using this prescription include distention and fullness in the epigastrium and abdomen, loss of appetite, indigestion, loose stools, a slightly yellow and greasy tongue coating and a weak pulse.

IV Section Summary

Bao He Wan, Zhishi Dao Ji Wan and Jian Pi Wan are typical formulas for relieving food retention. **Bao He Wan** is designed specifically for relieving food retention and settling the stomach, and is commonly used in various kinds of dyspepsia. **Zhishi Dao Ji Wan** is applicable for mild food retention and masses in association with Dampness. **Jian Pi Wan** is effective in strengthening the spleen and the stomach, promoting digestion, transforming Dampness and relieving diarrhea. It is indicated for illnesses involving spleen insufficiency, anorexia and diarrhea with loose stool.

Section 17 Formulas That Expel Worms

Formulas that expel worms comprise all those that suppress, expel or kill parasites that lodge in the human intestines. Only one such formula is described in this section.

Worm-expelling formulas should be taken on an empty stomach, so that they can reach the affected area directly and exert maximal effect.

I Wumei Wan (Mume Pill)

1 Source: Shang Han Lun (Treatise on Cold-Attack)

2 Composition

Chief Herb: wumei (*Prunus mume*) 30 g

Deputy Herbs: huajiao (*Zanthoxylum bungeanum*) 5 g
xixin (*Asarum heterotropoides, sieboldi*) 3 g

Assistant Herbs: huanglian (*Coptis chinensis*) 6 g
huangbai (*Phellodendron chinense, amurense*) 6 g
processed fuzi (*Aconitum carmichaeli*) 6 g
guizhi (*Cinnamomum cassia*) 6 g
ganjiang (*Zingiber officinale*) 9 g
danggui (*Angelica sinensis*) 6 g
renshen (*Panax ginseng*) 6 g

Envoy Herb: honey

3 Application

Actions: warms the *zang* organs and suppresses roundworms.

Indications: (1) Roundworm infestation. (2) Persistent diarrhea or dysentery.

Main Symptoms: intermittent abdominal pain; intermittent nausea and vomiting; vomiting of roundworms; cold hands and feet.

4 Analysis of the Formula

Wumei Wan uses a large amount of wumei for its sour flavor, which enables it to suppress roundworms and stop pain. It is the chief herb.

The roundworms move because the stomach is hot and the intestines cold. Huajiao and xixin are acrid and warm. Their acridity enables them to suppress the roundworms, their warmth to warm the *zang* organs and dispel Cold. These two serve as the deputy herbs.

Huanglian and huangbai are bitter and cold. Their bitter flavor enables them to expel the roundworms and their cold nature to clear stomach-Heat. Fuzi, guizhi and ganjiang are all acrid and hot. They aid the deputy herbs in warming the organs and dispelling Cold and their acridity also suppresses the roundworms. Danggui and renshen augment Qi and generate blood. They support genuine Qi. Together with guizhi they open the channels, regulate Yin–Yang and warm the cold limbs. These seven herbs all serve as assistant herbs.

Honey is sweet and harmonizes the middle-jiao. It is the envoy herb.

The formula uses both warm and cold and attends to both evil Qi and genuine Qi. Together the herbs warms the middle-jiao, clears Heat, suppresses the roundworms and augments what is deficient.

5 Comments

This formula uses wumei to astringe the intestines and stop diarrhea. Huanglian and huangbai are bitter and cold; they can clear Heat, dry Dampness and stop dysentery. Fuzi, guizhi, ganjiang, huajiao and xixin are all warming herbs; they warm the kidney and the spleen and help to enhance the transportation and transformation functions of the middle-jiao. Renshen and danggui augment Qi, nourish blood and support genuine Qi.

Used in concert these herbs have the effect of warming the middle-jiao, augmenting the deficient, clearing Heat, drying Dampness and stopping dysentery. Thus, the formula is also effective for treating chronic diarrhea or dysentery due to intermixed Heat and Cold with deficiency of genuine Qi.

6 *Case Study: Roundworm Infestation in a 22-Year-Old Female*

The patient had sharp pain of sudden onset in the right epigastrium. The pain was intermittent, but when it came it was sharp like stabs with a knife. She had associated nausea and vomiting of bitter fluids. She sweated profusely and her body was cold, especially the four limbs. She had chills and fever. The sclera of her eyes was slightly yellow. After 4 days she came to the clinic. The abdomen was not tense and there was no rebound tenderness. Intestinal sounds were loud. She was diagnosed to have roundworms in the bile ducts, and was treated over 3 days with formulas to relieve spasm, stop pain, or facilitate the gallbladder, as well as fluid infusion and antibiotics. None of these treatments had effect.

On examination, the patient had a taut and prominent pulse. Her tongue tip was red and the tongue coating yellow and smooth.

Diagnosis: Roundworm infestation.

Treatment: Wumei Wan was prepared as a decoction, with the amounts modified as follows: wumei 15 g, huanglian 9 g, huangbai 12 g, huajiao 9 g (stir-fried first for an hour) and danggui 9 g. Also, nanshashen (*Adenophora tetraphylla*) 12 g is added.

After two doses, all the symptoms resolved. Unmodified Wumei Wan was then used at the dosage of 3 g twice a day. After 5 days, the patient regained her body strength and normal activities.

(Source: *Chongqing Medicine*, 1980, 1:22.)

Guidance for Study

I Aim of Study

This chapter introduces the main groups of the complex herbal formulas that are commonly used in CM. It describes in detail a number of selected formulas within each section and lets students to know how they are constructed and how they are applied in therapeutics.

II Objectives of Study

Upon completion of this chapter, the learner will

1. Be familiar with the composition, actions, and indications of each commonly used formula;
2. Master the modification, characteristics and properties of each formula;
3. Understand the clinical usage of each formula.

III Exercises for Review

1. List all 17 sections in the classification of formulas. For each group, briefly describe its definition, characteristics, applications and any items of particular attention.
2. Within each section of formulas, illustrate the characteristics of each formula. Briefly describe how each formula is used clinically. In what way are the formulas used differently?
3. Within each section of formulas, list the main indications of each formula. List the key clinical symptoms for which the formula is indicated.
4. Describe the differences between Mahuang Tang and Guizhi Tang with respect to composition, actions, and indications. How are they used differently in clinical practice?
5. Is there any difference between Sang Ju Yin and Yin Qiao San? If so, illustrate the differences.
6. Explain the composition and indications of Da Cheng Qi Tang. Describe how to modify the formula based on the different syndromes.
7. What is the principle of construction of formulas that warm Yang and drain accumulation downward? Explain and provide examples.
8. What are the characteristics of the composition of Maziren Wan? How is this formula used clinically?
9. Compare the actions and usages of Xiao Chaihu Tang and Hao Qin Qing Dan Tang.
10. How should one construct a formula to regulate and harmonize the liver and the spleen? What are the clinical indications of such a formula? Give examples.
11. What are the characteristics of the composition of Banxia Xie Xin Tang? How is it modified based on clinical symptoms?
12. Describe the composition, indications, and modifications of Qing Wen Bai Du Yin.
13. Describe the characteristics and clinical usage of Longdan Xie Gan Tang, Qing Wei San, and Qinghao Biejia Tang.
14. Compare the compositional characteristics of formulas that clear Heat and open the orifices with those that warm and open the orifices.
15. Describe the uses and modifications of Si Ni Tang.
16. Compare the composition, indications, and actions of Zhishi Dao Zhi Wan and Bao He Wan.
17. Describe the principles of constructing formulas that regulate Qi and regulate blood. How should formulas that augment Yin and Yang be constructed? Give examples.
18. Explain the differences between Si Shen Wan and Zhen Ren Yang Zang Tang. What are the differences in their clinical usage?
19. Illustrate the differences in composition and usage of formulas that redirect abnormally rising lung-Qi, stomach-Qi and liver-Qi.
20. Explain how to combine herbs that regulate Qi and herbs that promote blood circulation in formulas. Give examples.

21. Why it is important to use herbs that tonify blood in formulas that promote blood circulation and remove blood stasis? Give examples.
22. Explain how to modify Xue Fu Zhu Yu Tang based on clinical symptoms.
23. Describe the clinical applications of Lingjiao Gouteng Tang and Tianma Gouteng Yin.
24. Discuss the composition and indications of formulas that clear Dampness–Heat. Give examples.
25. How are Qing Zao Jiu Fei Tang and Xing Su San applied clinically?
26. Explain how to integrate herbs that regulate Qi into formulas for treating Phlegm. Give examples.
27. Explain how to treat Phlegm. Give examples.

Index

MIX
Papier aus verantwortungsvollen Quellen
Paper from responsible sources
FSC® C105338

If you have any concerns about our products,
you can contact us on
ProductSafety@springernature.com

In case Publisher is established outside the EU,
the EU authorized representative is:
Springer Nature Customer Service Center GmbH
Europaplatz 3, 69115 Heidelberg, Germany

Printed by Libri Plureos GmbH
in Hamburg, Germany